Dietary Intake and Behavior in Children

Special Issue Editor
Sibylle Kranz

MDPI • Basel • Beijing • Wuhan • Barcelona • Belgrade

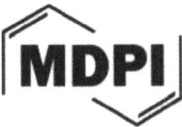

MDPI

Special Issue Editor
Sibylle Kranz
University of Virginia
USA

Editorial Office
MDPI
St. Alban-Anlage 66
Basel, Switzerland

This edition is a reprint of the Special Issue published online in the open access journal *Nutrients* (ISSN 2072-6643) from 2013–2014 (available at: http://www.mdpi.com/journal/nutrients/special_issues/behavior_children).

For citation purposes, cite each article independently as indicated on the article page online and as indicated below:

Lastname, F.M.; Lastname, F.M. Article title. *Journal Name* **Year**, *Article number*, page range.

First Edition 2018

ISBN 978-3-03842-893-0 (Pbk)
ISBN 978-3-03842-894-7 (PDF)

Table of Contents

About the Special Issue Editor

Sibylle Kranz is Associate Professor in the Department of Kinesiology in the Curry School of Education and Adjunct Associate Professor in the Department of Public Health Sciences in the School of Medicine at the University of Virginia, Charlottesville, VA. She is a Registered Dietitian Nutritionist and holds a PhD in Nutrition Epidemiology from the University of Carolina at Chapel Hill. She has held faculty positions at Pennsylvania State University, East Carolina University, Purdue University, and the University of Bristol. Her research interests include ways to improve children's diet quality as well as the relationships between food intake and children's learning and behavior. She studies these relationships through observational studies and in clinical trials in children of different ages and from a variety of socio-economic backgrounds. Dr. Kranz is a Fellow of the Obesity Society and member of the American Society for Nutrition and the Society of the Study for Ingestive Behavior.

Preface to "Dietary Intake and Behavior in Children"

Children's diet and nutrition has been an area of interest for researchers and practitioners from many different fields. For many years, the focus in child nutrition was on infant feeding and the safety of infant formulas. With the dawn of the childhood obesity epidemic, the need to understand how toddlers and young children develop food preferences and establish their intake patterns emerged and many studies indicate that the food intake patterns of early childhood remain part of the individual's lifestyle. Overall health, cognitive development and abilities, behavioral patterns and tracking of intake patterns are only some of the issues related to child nutrition research today. One of the important questions that remains open to date is the reciprocity of the relationship between diet and behavior. Observational data would indicate that some foods or food groups are more desired by children than others, however, the underlying mechanism for this relationship is not known. Furthermore, there is a potential relationship between the foods children are used to consuming and their behavior—much like a negative feedback loop, where children who are not used to eating vegetables will likely develop behaviors that allow them to continue eating small amounts or no vegetables at all.

At the time this book came together, the U.S. standards set forth in 2012 for the School Breakfast Program and the School Lunch Program had just been relaxed. While the overall goal of the U.S. school feeding program remained to provide access to balanced and nutritious food to children, the foci appeared to change. This recent modification was not unusual, since the American federal guidelines for school meals have undergone a number of changes in the past, based on information about disease prevention, cost, or food procurement, and production resources, to name a few reasons. Since children consume approximately 33%–50% of their daily food intake at school, the changes to the school meal guidelines affect large numbers of children and disproportionally higher amounts of children from low income families. Some school feeding programs worldwide reach similar proportions of the child population and face similar challenges and opportunities. The long-term consequences of average daily dietary intake on learning ability, career opportunities and lifestyle are not well understood at this time.

Conceptually, child nutrition can be divided into behavior that leads to specific intake choices and, conversely, intake choices that affect children's behavior. Current research endeavors to focus on the clarification of these relationships, possible interactions and confounding factors, and the development of guidelines that can be implemented as "best practices" to best support better diet quality in children. This book consists of a collection of research papers on the issue of child nutrition and child behavior that were selected for a Special Issue in Nutrients, which was highly successful. The research reports included epidemiologic and clinical studies and ramifications for predictors of intake (8), school feeding programs (3), school performance (5), picky eating and neophobia (2), and home food environment (2). Fruits and vegetables, which despite their high nutritional value appear to remain the food group that most children struggle with, were specifically addressed in several instances.

Sibylle Kranz
Special Issue Editor

nutrients

MDPI

Article

Which Diet-Related Behaviors in Childhood Influence a Healthier Dietary Pattern? From the Ewha Birth and Growth Cohort

Hye Ah Lee [1,*], Hyo Jeong Hwang [2], Se Young Oh [3], Eun Ae Park [4], Su Jin Cho [4], Hae Soon Kim [4] and Hyesook Park [1,*]

[1] Department of Preventive Medicine, School of Medicine, Ewha Womans University, Seoul 07985, Korea
[2] Biomaterials Research Institute, Sahmyook University, Seoul 01795, Korea; fullmoon0118@naver.com
[3] Department of Food & Nutrition, Research Center for Human Ecology, College of Human Ecology, Kyung Hee University, Seoul 02447, Korea; seyoung@khu.ac.kr
[4] Department of Pediatrics, School of Medicine, Ewha Womans University, Seoul 07985, Korea; pea8639@ewha.ac.kr (E.A.P.); sujin-cho@ewha.ac.kr (S.J.C.); hyesk@ewha.ac.kr (H.S.K.)
* Correspondence: khyeah@naver.com (H.A.L.); hpark@ewha.ac.kr (H.P.);
  Tel.: +82-2-2650-5753 (H.A.L.); +82-2-2650-5756 (H.P.); Fax: +82-2-2652-8325 (H.A.L. & H.P.)

Received: 19 September 2016; Accepted: 15 December 2016; Published: 23 December 2016

Abstract: This study was performed to examine how childhood dietary patterns change over the short term and which changes in diet-related behaviors influence later changes in individual dietary patterns. Using food frequency questionnaire data obtained from children at 7 and 9 years of age from the Ewha Birth and Growth Cohort, we examined dietary patterns by principal component analysis. We calculated the individual changes in dietary pattern scores. Changes in dietary habits such as eating a variety of food over two years were defined as "increased", "stable", or "decreased". The dietary patterns, termed "healthy intake", "animal food intake", and "snack intake", were similar at 7 and 9 years of age. These patterns explained 32.3% and 39.1% of total variation at the ages of 7 and 9 years, respectively. The tracking coefficient of snack intake had the highest coefficient ($\gamma = 0.53$) and that of animal food intake had the lowest ($\gamma = 0.21$). Intra-individual stability in dietary habits ranged from 0.23 to 0.47, based on the sex-adjusted weighted kappa values. Of the various behavioral factors, eating breakfast every day was most common in the "stable" group (83.1%), whereas consuming milk or dairy products every day was the least common (49.0%). Moreover, changes in behavior that improved the consumption of milk or dairy products or encouraged the consumption of vegetables with every meal had favorable effects on changes in healthy dietary pattern scores over two years. However, those with worsened habits, such as less food variety and more than two portions of fried or stir-fried food every week, had unfavorable effects on changes in healthy dietary pattern scores. Our results suggest that diet-related behaviors can change, even over a short period, and these changes can affect changes in dietary pattern.

Keywords: children; dietary pattern; diet-related behavior; longitudinal study

---

1. Introduction

To improve diet, understanding how dietary patterns develop is important in epidemiological studies related to chronic diseases and public health planning [1]. The critical period for the development of certain dietary patterns, during which time the development should be tracked, remains a major issue in nutritional epidemiology. Several studies have suggested that dietary patterns are determined in childhood [2–4]. One large prospective cohort study, the Avon Longitudinal Study of Pregnancy and Childhood (ALSPAC), indicated that the dietary pattern at 7 years old was a determinant of later dietary patterns based on the results of tracking coefficients from diverse statistical approaches [4]. However, previous studies focusing on the stability of dietary patterns yielded mixed results with only moderate [5,6] or slight tracking [1,7].

With regard to the critical period, children learn what, when, and how to eat through direct experience observing others [8]. Thus, it is important to identify critical intervention factors to suggest appropriate strategies for improving dietary behaviors. However, the effectiveness of interventions to modify dietary behaviors remains unclear [9,10]. One recent observational study from the NEXT Generation Health Study among American teens indicated within-individual correlations of 41%–51% in food group intake and meal practices over four years. It was also reported that time-varied frequencies of intake of fruit/vegetables or snacks were associated with time-varied meal practices, such as the frequency of fast food intake [6]. However, this study focused on intakes of specific food groups or eating behaviors.

Childhood dietary patterns could be reflected in underlying food preferences, diet-related behaviors, as well as environmental factors, such as household income and parental education level [8]. Studying dietary patterns is a reasonable approach because the net effect of a single food or nutrient cannot be separated from the total. Several methodologies have been introduced to explore dietary patterns [11,12]. Of these, principal component analysis (PCA) is a multidimensional reduction analysis method to examine the correlations of food intakes, and is commonly used in nutritional epidemiology [13]. Several studies using PCA reported several dietary patterns in children and adolescents as "healthy", "traditional", "Western", and "junk or processed food intakes", among others [5,14,15]. However, Hu suggested that much more research is necessary in diverse populations due to sociocultural differences [12]. In addition, many previous studies did not take into consideration changes in dietary pattern or related behaviors. A better understanding of changes in diet-related behaviors and dietary patterns may provide an opportunity to explore appropriate intervention strategies.

Using data from a Korean cohort study, we evaluated how childhood dietary patterns change in the short term, and which changes in diet-related behavior influence later changes in individual dietary patterns.

2. Methods

2.1. Study Subjects

This study was part of an ongoing Ewha Birth and Growth Cohort study by the Ewha Woman's University Mokdong Hospital, Seoul, Korea. It was established to longitudinally evaluate the growth and health of children, and it commenced in the early life of the subjects. Briefly, mothers (n = 940) were enrolled in the study between 2001 and 2006 during prenatal care visits when they were 24–28 weeks pregnant, and a follow-up was done with their children 3, 5, and 7 years later. About 30% of all possible subjects agreed to participate in the study [16]. A detailed description of the cohort composition, including methodology, has been published elsewhere [17]. Through follow-up at 7 or 9 years of age, a diet-related questionnaire survey was performed using a food frequency questionnaire (FFQ) and questions related to dietary habits. Follow-up at 7 years of age began in 2009, but data were collected using FFQs from 2010. A total of 364 and 380 children participated in follow-up at 7 years (follow-up years from 2009 to 2014) and 9 years of age (follow-up years from 2011 to 2015), respectively. Of these, completed FFQs were obtained for 279 and 360 children, respectively. FFQ data for both follow-up times were obtained for 154 children. Approximately 41.9% of cohort subjects were lost to follow-up (they changed their telephone numbers or withdrew) at the time of the 7-year follow-up, and an additional 3.4% were lost to follow-up at 9 years. Written informed consent for participation in the study was obtained from the parents or guardians of all study participants at the time of follow-up. The study protocol was approved by the Institutional Review Board of the Ewha Womans University Hospital.

2.2. Dietary Data and Dietary Pattern Analysis

Individual dietary data for the past year were collected by the parents or guardians and validated by trained interviewers using the FFQ (90 food items). Both the reproducibility (*r* value = 0.5–0.8) and validity (*r* value = 0.3–0.6) of the instrument were acceptable, as reported elsewhere [18,19]. We used the same questionnaire at both follow-ups. These food items were placed into nine non-overlapping categories according to the frequency of consumption, ranging from "rarely eaten" to "more than three times per day" during the preceding year, and portion size, namely, small, average, or large. In this study, we used food intake frequencies to construct dietary patterns [20]. Weekly intake from the FFQ was calculated by multiplying the consumption frequency of each food by the following values for each frequency option: never = 0; once a month = 0.23; two-to-three times a month = 0.58; one-to-two times a week = 1.5; three-to-four times a week = 3.5; five-to-six times a week = 5.5; once a day = 7; twice a day = 14; and three times a day = 21. Of the 90 food items, similar items were grouped to form 22 food groups (Table S1). Prior to PCA, data were standardized using means and standard deviations, and the dietary patterns at each time point were analyzed via PCA with varimax rotation. The first three components were appropriate, based on the screen plots and eigenvalues ≥1. The factor-loading values by dietary pattern are shown in Table 1. Factors with loading >0.3 were considered the principal contributors to a dietary pattern [5]. Factor scores were used as outcomes, which were defined as dietary pattern scores. To assess changes in the same dietary patterns over time, we calculated the z scores of food group intake from children aged 9 years using the means and standard deviations obtained when they were 7 years of age. These were multiplied by factor-loading values for each dietary pattern (it was obtained using the data for 7 years old), and then summed. This approach has been used in previous studies [5,21].

Table 1. Factor loading scores for the first three components derived from principal component analysis.

	Healthy Intake		Animal Food Intake		Snack Intake	
	7 Years	9 Years	7 Years	9 Years	7 Years	9 Years
Variance	13.83%	15.12%	10.23%	16.20%	8.21%	7.77%
Yellow vegetables	0.840	0.820	0.070	0.108	−0.020	0.050
Green vegetables	0.800	0.795	0.149	0.105	0.045	0.074
White vegetables	0.475	0.417	0.268	0.014	−0.040	0.057
Mushrooms	0.802	0.677	−0.066	0.081	−0.037	0.126
Beans	0.476	0.522	0.181	0.089	0.198	0.091
Potatoes	0.280	0.468	0.071	0.056	0.227	0.277
Fruit	0.271	0.341	0.160	0.038	0.151	0.148
Nuts	0.222	0.418	0.200	0.090	0.044	0.150
Shellfish	0.106	0.019	0.798	0.948	0.073	0.047
White fish	0.092	0.009	0.714	0.938	0.152	0.022
Blue fish	0.144	0.200	0.598	0.909	0.257	0.063
Meat	0.444	0.081	0.587	0.853	0.125	0.239
Eggs	0.276	0.136	0.120	0.400	0.268	−0.007
Rice	0.066	0.089	0.224	−0.037	0.063	0.072
Bread	0.108	0.078	−0.023	0.033	0.712	0.399
Jam	−0.006	0.192	0.023	0.005	0.617	0.396
Soda	0.047	0.226	0.094	0.024	0.394	0.559
Milk	0.235	0.388	0.028	0.065	0.346	0.459
Candy	−0.047	0.048	0.109	0.011	0.339	0.509
Pizza	−0.030	0.042	0.240	0.059	0.322	0.424
Noodles	0.054	0.070	0.175	0.075	0.251	0.433
Seaweed	0.089	0.529	0.138	0.083	0.234	0.127

2.3. Dietary Habits

We collected data regarding dietary habits using the following questions:

DH1. Do you eat more than two servings of milk or dairy products every day?

DH2. Do you eat meat, fish, egg, beans, or tofu with every meal?

DH3. Do you eat vegetables other than kimchi with every meal?

DH4. Do you eat one serving size of fruit or drink one portion of fruit juice every day?

DH5. Do you eat more than two servings of fried or stir-fried food every week?

DH6. Do you eat more than two servings of fatty meat (e.g., bacon, ribs, eel) every week?

DH7. Do you generally add table salt or soy sauce to food?

DH8. Do you eat three regular meals per day?

DH9. Do you eat ice cream, cake, snacks, and soda (e.g., cola, cider) as snacks more than twice a week?

DH10. Do you eat a variety of food every day?

The possible responses were "always", "generally", and "seldom". Questions DH1–4, DH8, and DH10 evaluated healthy dietary habits, and questions DH5–7 and DH9 evaluated unhealthy dietary habits. This mini-dietary assessment tool has been validated in previous studies [22,23]. In addition, the subjects were also asked "Do you eating breakfast every day?" to which they responded either "yes" or "no". Changes in individual behaviors were classified as "increased", "stable", or "decreased". If one subject at 7 years old replied "seldom" to the question "Do you eat over two servings of milk or dairy products every day?" and answered "always" or "generally" to the same question at 9 years old, the behavior was defined as "increased", while the opposite was classified as "decreased". Finally, those who gave the same answer at both follow-ups were defined as "stable".

2.4. Other Variables

We also evaluated data on household income, parental education, parental obesity, time spent watching television (TV), and child body mass index (BMI); previous studies have shown that these were potentially important factors [2,6,15,21]. Monthly household income was grouped as "low" (<3 million South Korean Won (KRW)), "middle" (3.0–4.9 million KRW), or "high" (>5 million KRW). Parental education level was classified into two levels (graduated from high school; some college or higher). Parental obesity was defined as BMI ≥ 25 kg/m^2, calculated by dividing weight by height squared. These data were collected by a self-reported questionnaire at follow-up. The daily amount of time spent watching TV was categorized as <1 h, 1–2 h, and >2 h. Child BMI was calculated by measuring height and weight at both follow-ups.

2.5. Statistical Analysis

The associations between dietary pattern scores and socioeconomic factors, parental factors, and dietary habits were analyzed using the *t* test or analysis of variance (ANOVA). Based on the findings from the univariate analyses, we selected potentially significant factors ($p < 0.2$) for inclusion in the multiple regression analyses. A factor was considered relevant if it was potentially related to any dietary pattern. However, paternal education was not considered, being strongly associated with household income (an indicator of socioeconomic status). In multiple regression analysis, responses to dietary habits were treated as continuous variables (e.g., "always" = 2, "generally" = 1 and "seldom" = 0 for questions related to healthy dietary habits and applied in reverse for questions about unhealthy dietary habits) by considering multicollinearity. Multicollinearity in multiple regression was assessed based on variance inflation factors and it had a value <2 across our results. Correlations between dietary pattern scores at the two time points were estimated using Spearman's correlation, and the changes in dietary pattern scores within an individual were assessed using the paired *t* test. To determine the changes in dietary habits, we used weighted kappa and proportion of dietary habit changes stratified according to sex. The independent effects of changes in individual behaviors were expressed as "increased", "stable", or "decreased" over time in terms of changes in dietary patterns after taking sex, household income, and other parameters, into consideration. The change in watching TV was excluded due to data on this variable being missing for a large proportion of the subjects (13.6%). In all analyses, $p < 0.05$ (two-tailed test) was taken to indicate statistical significance. All statistical analyses were conducted using SAS 9.3 (SAS Institute, Cary, NC, USA).

3. Results

With regard to the characteristics of the study subjects, about half were boys (49.46%) with an average BMI of 15.95 kg/m^2 (95% confidence interval: 15.71–16.20 kg/m^2). Most of the children ate breakfast daily (84.84%). Of all of the children, 41.73% watched television for more than 2 h per day. In terms of household income (an indicator of socioeconomic status), 20.59%, 41.54%, and 37.87% of children were in the low, middle, and high groups, respectively. Table 1 shows dietary patterns derived from PCA at each time point. The first three components accounted for 32.27% (PC1: 13.83%, PC2: 10.23%, and PC3: 8.21% at 7 years old) and 39.10% (PC1: 15.12%, PC2: 16.20%, and PC3: 7.77% at 9 years old) of total variation. The three components were referred to as "healthy intake", "animal food intake", and "snack intake". Healthy intake was positively associated with vegetable and bean items. Animal food intake showed weighted loading factors in meat and fish items. Finally, snack intake showed positive loading factors in candy, soda, and bread items. The patterns were similar at the older age, but some food types had more weighted loading factors. Healthy intake at 9 years of age showed more weighted loading factors in fruit, milk, nut, and seaweed food groups than at the younger age.

The results of univariate association are presented in Table S2. Higher household income status tended to show higher mean health intake pattern scores at 7 years of age. In addition, healthy intake was significantly associated with eating breakfast every day and all of the related healthy dietary habits. Animal food intake was associated with sex, eating fatty meat, and generally adding table salt or soy sauce to food. Subjects that spent a longer time watching TV had higher mean snack pattern scores. Snack intake also showed a significant association with eating milk or dairy products; eating fruit or drinking fruit juice every day; eating fried or stir-fried food; generally adding table salt or soy sauce to food; and eating ice cream, cake, snacks, and soda (e.g., cola, cider) as snacks.

In multiple regression analysis, eating breakfast every day and eating a variety of food every day showed independent effects on the healthy pattern with positive coefficients ($\beta = 0.24$, $\beta = 0.19$, respectively). With regard to animal food intake, female gender showed higher pattern scores, while unusual behaviors with regard to fatty meat and generally adding table salt or soy sauce to food showed lower pattern scores. Pattern scores in snack intake were also positively associated with watching TV ($\beta = 0.15$) and negatively associated with eating vegetables other than kimchi ($\beta = -0.23$). Moreover, several factors showed independent effects at both follow-up times. Eating a variety of food was consistently associated with healthy intake at both follow-up times. Eating vegetables other than kimchi with every meal was also negatively associated with snack intake. Otherwise, there were no significant associations with animal food intake (Table 2).

Table 3 shows the results regarding changes in dietary pattern scores and tracking coefficients of dietary patterns. The tracking coefficient of snack intake showed the highest coefficient (0.53, $p < 0.0001$) and animal food intake showed the lowest coefficient (0.21, $p < 0.01$). The mean dietary pattern scores from the earlier time point showed increasing tendencies across dietary patterns, and this score was highest for animal food intake ($\Delta = 0.20$, $p < 0.001$).

Figure 1 shows the intra-individual stability of dietary habits over two years by sex. The weighted kappa values of eating breakfast every day, watching TV, eating three regular meals a day, and eating ice cream, cake, snacks, and soda were markedly higher in girls than in boys, while those of eating a variety of food every day and eating meat, fish, egg, beans, or tofu with every meal were higher in boys than in girls. Sex-adjusted weighted kappa values ranged from 0.23 to 0.47. Of the behavior factors, eating breakfast every day showed the highest proportion for "stable" (83.1%), while eating milk or dairy products every day showed the lowest proportion (49.0%) (Table 4).

Table 2. Multiple regression analysis of the effects of potential factors on dietary pattern at two observation times.

Potential Factor at 7 Years	Dietary Pattern Scores at 7 Years Old						Dietary Pattern Scores at 9 Years Old					
	Healthy Intake		Animal Food Intake		Snack Intake		Healthy Intake		Animal Food Intake		Snack Intake	
	β	S.E.	β	S.E.	β	S.E.	β	S.E.	β	S.E.	β	S.E.
Sex	−0.010	0.06	0.183 [a]	0.06	−0.078	0.10	−0.027	0.10	0.056	0.13	0.127	0.18
Monthly household income	0.023	0.04	0.003	0.04	0.014	0.07	0.037	0.07	0.068	0.09	0.186	0.13
Body mass index (BMI)	−0.007	0.02	−0.0002	0.02	−0.016	0.03	−0.011	0.03	−0.021	0.04	0.005	0.05
Maternal obesity	0.007	0.08	−0.002	0.08	−0.222	0.14	−0.051	0.14	0.022	0.18	0.007	0.24
Watching television (TV)	−0.043	0.04	0.057	0.04	0.152 [a]	0.07	−0.004	0.07	−0.052	0.09	0.015	0.13
Eating breakfast every day	0.242 [a]	0.10	−0.071	0.10	−0.071	0.17	0.091	0.16	0.206	0.20	−0.296	0.28
Healthy dietary habits												
DH1	0.071	0.05	0.036	0.05	0.129	0.08	0.026	0.07	−0.0004	0.09	0.152	0.13
DH2	−0.002	0.05	0.071	0.05	0.016	0.09	−0.048	0.09	0.007	0.11	−0.114	0.16
DH3	0.068	0.05	0.026	0.05	−0.226 [a]	0.08	−0.153	0.08	−0.067	0.10	−0.435 [a]	0.14
DH4	0.048	0.05	−0.043	0.05	0.117	0.09	0.154	0.08	−0.120	0.10	0.028	0.14
DH8	0.075	0.06	0.069	0.06	−0.069	0.11	−0.083	0.10	0.069	0.13	0.063	0.18
DH10	0.190 [a]	0.05	0.047	0.05	0.114	0.08	0.166 [a]	0.07	−0.021	0.09	0.123	0.13
Unhealthy dietary habits												
DH5	0.064	0.05	0.021	0.05	−0.047	0.08	−0.129	0.07	−0.035	0.09	−0.245	0.13
DH6	−0.038	0.05	−0.154 [a]	0.05	−0.105	0.08	−0.047	0.08	−0.048	0.11	0.250	0.15
DH7	−0.005	0.06	−0.127 [a]	0.06	−0.152	0.10	−0.027	0.10	−0.052	0.12	−0.358 [a]	0.17
DH9	0.010	0.04	−0.007	0.04	−0.113	0.07	0.006	0.07	0.024	0.08	−0.160	0.12

[a] $p < 0.05$. S.E. = standard error. DH1: Eating more than two portions of milk or dairy products every day. DH2: Eating meat, fish, eggs, beans, or tofu with every meal. DH3: Eating vegetables other than kimchi with every meal. DH4: Eating one portion of fruit or drinking one portion of fruit juice every day. DH5: Eating more than two portions of fried or stir-fried food every week. DH6: Eating more than two portions of fatty meat (e.g., bacon, ribs, eel) every week. DH7: Generally adding table salt or soy sauce to food. DH8: Eating three regular meals a day. DH9: Eating ice cream, cake, snacks, and soda (e.g., cola, cider) as snacks more than twice a week. DH10: Eating a variety of food every day. The possible responses to dietary habits (DHs) were "always", "generally", or "seldom". The daily TV-watching time was categorized as <1 h, 1–2 h, and >2 h. Eating breakfast everyday was grouped as yes or no.

Table 3. Changes in dietary pattern scores between the two observational times.

Dietary Pattern Scores	Tracking Coefficient [†]	At 7 Years		At 9 Years [‡]		Differences of Dietary Pattern Scores [‡]		Paired *t* Test *p*
		Mean	S.D.	Mean	S.D.	Mean	S.D.	
Healthy intake	0.369 [a]	−0.106	0.498	0.062	0.613	0.176	0.624	<0.001
Animal food intake	0.215 [b]	−0.091	0.479	0.123	0.691	0.204	0.717	<0.001
Snack intake	0.526 [a]	−0.003	0.861	0.213	0.969	0.161	0.864	0.02

[†] The tracking coefficients between the dietary pattern scores at the two time points were estimated by deriving Spearman's correlations. [‡] Results are presented for those who participated in both follow-ups (*n* = 154). [a] *p* < 0.0001, [b] *p* < 0.01. S.D. = standard deviation.

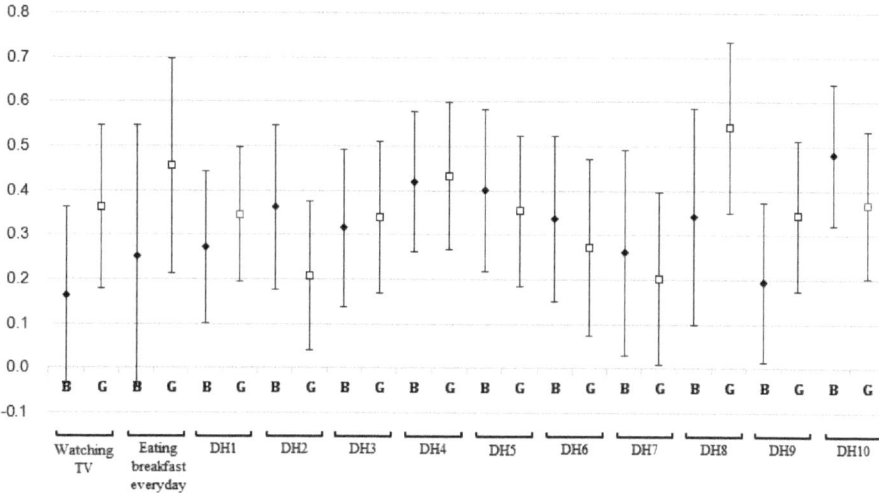

Figure 1. Weighted κ of two repeated measures for behaviors by sex. B: boys (black diamonds), G: girls (white squares), line indicates 95% confidence interval. DH1: Eating more than two portions of milk or dairy products every day. DH2: Eating meat, fish, egg, beans, or tofu with every meal. DH3: Eating vegetables other than kimchi with every meal. DH4: Eating one portion of fruit or drinking one portion of fruit juice every day. DH5: Eating more than two portions of fried or stir-fried food every week. DH6: Eating more than two portions of fatty meat (e.g., bacon, ribs, eel) every week. DH7: Generally adding table salt or soy sauce to food. DH8: Eating three regular meals per day. DH9: Eating ice cream, cake, snacks, and soda (e.g., cola, cider) as snacks more than twice a week. DH10: Eating a variety of food every day. The possible responses to dietary habits (DHs) were "always", "generally", or "seldom". The daily TV-watching time was categorized as <1 h, 1–2 h and >2 h. Eating breakfast everyday was grouped as yes or no.

Table 5 shows the effects of behavioral changes on changes in dietary patterns. Those with improved dietary habits (who ate vegetables other than kimchi with every meal and consumed more than two portions of milk or dairy products every day) exhibited improved healthy intake pattern scores over two years, whereas those with worsening habits (less food variety and more than two portions of fried or stir-fried food every week) exhibited decreased scores. In addition, worsening with regard to eating ice cream, cake, snacks, and soda as snacks increased in the animal food intake patterns. However, other dietary habit changes were not significantly related to dietary pattern changes.

Table 4. Changes in individual's behaviors over two years.

	Sex-Adjusted Weighted Kappa	Stable		Increased		Decreased	
		n	%	*n*	%	*n*	%
Watching TV	0.271	75	56.39	27	20.30	31	23.31
Eating breakfast	0.373	128	83.12	9	5.84	17	11.04
Healthy dietary habits							
DH1	0.314	75	49.02	30	19.61	48	31.37
DH2	0.277	82	53.95	34	22.37	36	23.68
DH3	0.328	83	54.25	39	25.49	31	20.26
DH4	0.427	90	59.21	25	16.45	37	24.34
DH8	0.466	115	75.66	18	11.84	19	12.5
DH10	0.427	88	57.52	42	27.45	23	15.03
Unhealthy dietary habits							
DH5	0.376	90	59.21	27	17.76	35	23.03
DH6	0.307	97	63.4	27	17.65	29	18.95
DH7	0.227	101	66.01	25	16.34	27	17.65
DH9	0.273	74	48.68	41	26.97	37	24.34

DH1: Eating more than two portions of milk or dairy products every day. DH2: Eating meat, fish, egg, beans, or tofu with every meal. DH3: Eating vegetables other than kimchi with every meal. DH4: Eating one portion of fruit or drinking one portion of fruit juice every day. DH5: Eating more than two portions of fried or stir-fried food every week. DH6: Eating more than two portions of fatty meat (e.g., bacon, ribs, eel) every week. DH7: Generally adding table salt or soy sauce to food. DH8: Eating three regular meals per day. DH9: Eating ice cream, cake, snacks, and soda (e.g., cola, cider) as snacks more than twice a week. DH10: Eating a variety of food every day. The possible responses to dietary habits (DHs) were "always", "generally", or "seldom". The daily TV-watching time was categorized as <1 h, 1–2 h, and >2 h. Eating breakfast everyday was grouped as yes or no.

Table 5. Effects of behavioral changes over two years within dietary patterns.

		Difference in Dietary Pattern 1 Score		Difference in Dietary Pattern 2 Score		Difference in Dietary Pattern 3 Score	
		β	S.E.	β	S.E.	β	S.E.
Eating breakfast	increased	−0.057	0.23	−0.483	0.29	0.251	0.35
	decreased	−0.175	0.17	−0.375	0.23	−0.013	0.27
Healthy dietary habits							
DH1	increased	0.374 [a]	0.15	0.122	0.20	0.240	0.23
	decreased	0.143	0.13	0.255	0.17	0.130	0.20
DH2	increased	−0.089	0.14	0.152	0.18	0.060	0.21
	decreased	−0.215	0.14	−0.233	0.17	−0.134	0.21
DH3	increased	0.272 [a]	0.13	−0.136	0.17	0.278	0.20
	decreased	0.167	0.15	0.078	0.19	0.263	0.23
DH4	increased	−0.073	0.15	0.128	0.20	0.021	0.24
	decreased	−0.196	0.13	−0.042	0.17	−0.174	0.20
DH8	increased	−0.108	0.17	0.141	0.23	−0.140	0.26
	decreased	0.037	0.17	0.235	0.22	−0.073	0.25
DH10	increased	0.117	0.13	0.099	0.17	0.090	0.20
	decreased	−0.301 [a]	0.15	0.021	0.20	−0.285	0.23
Unhealthy dietary habits							
DH5	increased	0.153	0.14	0.046	0.19	0.219	0.22
	decreased	−0.310 [a]	0.14	−0.199	0.18	−0.261	0.22
DH6	increased	0.095	0.15	−0.090	0.19	−0.176	0.22
	decreased	−0.070	0.14	0.166	0.19	−0.033	0.22
DH7	increased	−0.137	0.16	−0.287	0.20	−0.081	0.23
	decreased	−0.051	0.14	0.009	0.18	0.047	0.22
DH9	increased	−0.010	0.13	−0.227	0.17	0.019	0.20
	decreased	0.239	0.14	0.390 [a]	0.18	0.348	0.21

[a] $p < 0.05$. DH1: Eating more than two portions of milk or dairy products every day. DH2: Eating meat, fish, egg, beans, or tofu with every meal. DH3: Eating vegetables other than kimchi with every meal. DH4: Eating one portion of fruit or drinking one portion of fruit juice every day. DH5: Eating more than two portions of fried or stir-fried food every week. DH6: Eating more than two portions of fatty meat (e.g., bacon, ribs, eel) every week. DH7: Generally adding table salt or soy sauce to food. DH8: Eating three regular meals per day. DH9: Eating ice cream, cake, snacks, and soda (e.g., cola, cider) as snacks more than twice a week. DH10: Eating a variety of food every day. The possible responses to dietary habits (DHs) were "always", "generally", or "seldom". The daily TV-watching time was categorized as <1 h, 1–2 h, and >2 h. Eating breakfast everyday was grouped as yes or no. All of the results were obtained by multiple regression analyses after adjusting for sex, maternal obesity, body mass index at 7 years of age, and household income.

4. Discussion

We explored the childhood dietary patterns at 7 and 9 years of age and assessed the changes in individual dietary patterns. There were three dietary patterns, namely, "healthy intake", "animal food intake", and "snack intake", the contributions of which differed at each time point. The tracking coefficients ranged from 0.21 for animal food intake to 0.53 for snack intake. Overall, the mean dietary pattern scores tended to increase over time. Moreover, changes in behaviors that improved the consumption of milk and dairy products or vegetables with every meal exhibited improved healthy intake pattern scores over two years, whereas those with worsened habits, such as less food variety and more than two portions of fried or stir-fried food every week, exhibited decreased scores.

Individual dietary patterns change over time, even in childhood [5,21]. As individual diet-related behaviors can also change, the above findings appear reasonable. Supporting evidence from intervention studies is required to improve the dietary habits of children. Repeated measures in cohort design could also be used to assess the effects of natural changes in dietary behaviors. In this study, we examined the effects of changes in diet-related behaviors on changes in pattern scores. The results indicated that improved individual dietary behaviors related to eating vegetables with every meal independently attributed to increased healthier dietary patterns over time. The advantages of eating vegetables have been demonstrated by several systematic review studies with regard to diverse health effects, as well, they reflect the nutritional quality of meals [24–26]. However, interventions involving increasing the vegetable intake among children were unsuccessful [10]. One large study conducted in American teens estimated that within-person correlations for eating behaviors were >0.41 for the intake frequencies of fruit and vegetables, whole grains, soda, and snacks using four sets of repeated-measure data, and time-varying intake frequency of fruit and vegetables was positively associated with time-varying breakfast and family meals and negatively associated with fast food intake using a generalized estimating equations model. However, this previous study did not discuss the intake of various food [6]. In addition, eating a variety of food reflects adequate intake of essential nutrients, and is recommended in most dietary guidelines, including those in South Korea [27]. In addition, milk and dairy products are major sources of calcium for growing children. A national study found that more than half of all Korean children have inadequate calcium intake [28]. Although it is difficult to compare previous findings with ours because different assessment methods were used, we also found that it was beneficial to eat a variety of foods including milk and dairy products. In contrast, fried or stir-fried food was associated with high fat intake. We found that increased consumption of fried or stir-fried food unfavorably influenced a healthy dietary pattern. Thus, our results are meaningful in terms of epidemiological approaches. The unexpected results regarding the association between changes in eating ice cream, cake, snacks, and soda (e.g., cola, cider) as snacks seemed to be influenced by increased food frequency. Unlike other dietary habits, overall intake frequencies were higher for subjects with worsening behaviors regarding eating ice cream, cake, snacks, and soda as snacks compared with those with stable and increased behaviors. Indeed, all dietary pattern scores increased with a decrease of that behavior, as shown in Table 5.

As presented in Table 1, there were some changes in the composition of the three types of dietary patterns over two years. This was not surprising based on the results of previous studies [5,7]. Generally, the traditional diet in South Korea includes high levels of various vegetables and is low in fat [29,30]. These features were similar in our study. A previous study among South Korean adults also showed similar patterns to those in the present study [30], but little evidence was available regarding dietary patterns in South Korean children. For variation during two years, the intakes of most food items increased at 9 years old compared to those at 7 years old, with the exceptions of yellow vegetables, mushrooms, fruit, milk, and seaweed laver. Soda, potatoes, bread, and pizza showed relatively large increases (data not shown). Increased soda intake with increasing age was also observed in a previous growth and health study from the National Heart, Lung, and Blood Institute [31] and the Bogalusa Heart Study [32]. The environmental influences on food choice, preference, and accessibility vary over the lifespan. The opportunity to choose food oneself would increase with increasing age. Consistent with our study, the results regarding dietary pattern derived from the ALSPAC study showed that notable loading factors differed among food groups at 9 years old compared with those at 7 years old [4]. Another two studies using reduced rank regression and cluster analysis of the same cohort data indicated that dietary patterns at 7 years of age was a strong determinant of later dietary patterns [4,21]. Children starting school and participating in various activities are placed in a new environment, which may influence food choice. Therefore, further studies on changes in dietary habits and patterns over longer periods are required.

Several factors potentially related to dietary patterns have been reported, including low maternal education level [14,15,21]; socioeconomic status [15]; passive smoking and watching TV [14]; childhood obesity or maternal obesity [2]; diet-related factors, such as being vegetarian [33]; and TV meals, family meals, and breakfast [6]. However, most of these studies reported effects at a critical time on dietary patterns rather than changes in potential factors as mentioned above. Parental education level and birth- or infancy-related features were considered as time-independent factors. In this study, associations between household income and dietary patterns were more notable than parental education level. These observations may be explained by more highly educated parents having a better understanding of nutritional information and being more likely to restrict their children's intake of unhealthy food [34]. These observations may also be explained by the dependence of the ability to pay for food or groceries on household income, because a nutrient-dense diet is more expensive than an energy-dense diet [35]. However, any independent effects of household income were not significant as determined by multiple regression analyses. Moreover, we found no association with maternal obesity and child BMI.

Several points must be taken into consideration when interpreting the results of our study. Our results were derived from a smaller sample than previous studies. Bias due to follow-up loss would probably have an impact on the results. However, there were no differences in the distribution of demographic factors or dietary habits between subjects who successfully followed up or were lost to follow-up, except in eating a variety of food ($p_{chi} = 0.02$). Therefore, this did not seem to affect our results. To allow comparison, loading factors were applied to the calculated dietary pattern scores at the older age. This approach also has limitations in that it did not reflect the changes in characteristics of dietary patterns. Healthy intake pattern showed a positive loading factor for eating vegetables at the two time points, but eating fruit showed a higher weighting for a healthy diet at 9 years old. Thus, scores of a change within dietary patterns do not reflect the above-mentioned change. We used the same validated questionnaires at both follow-ups, and all of the data were collected by trained dieticians. Thus, any bias imparted by this procedure would be small. Moreover, there could be residual confounding effects of several factors that were not considered in this study.

This cohort study had several strengths. In this cohort study, we observed behavioral changes within individuals and were able to assess the associated effects, although the observational period was short. This work is the first step towards observationally determining whether behavioral changes in early life can modify dietary patterns, thereby improving health later in life. In addition, our results yield important data from a non-Western country. Future studies are needed to determine if the effects that we observed will persist in the long term.

5. Conclusions

Our results suggest that single measurements of food frequency intake and dietary habits during childhood may be insufficient to determine individual dietary patterns. In addition, diet-related behaviors can change, even in a short period, and such changes can affect dietary patterns.

Supplementary Materials: The following are available online at http://www.mdpi.com/2072-6643/9/1/4/s1, Table S1: Composition of food groups; Table S2: Univariate associations between potential factors and dietary pattern scores at 7 years of age.

Acknowledgments: This study was supported by National Research Foundation of Korea Grant funded by the Korean Government (NRF-2014R1A1A1007207). It had no role in the design, analysis or writing of this article.

Author Contributions: H.A.L. wrote the paper and performed the statistical analyses; S.Y.O., H.J.H., E.A.P., S.J.C. and H.S.K. provided advice about writing the paper, and H.P. provided advice about interpreting the data.

Conflicts of Interest: The authors declare no conflict of interest.

References

1. Patterson, E.; Wärnberg, J.; Kearney, J.; Sjöström, M. The tracking of dietary intakes of children and adolescents in Sweden over six years: The European Youth Heart Study. *Int. J. Behav. Nutr. Phys. Act.* **2009**, *6*, 91. [CrossRef] [PubMed]
2. Burke, V.; Beilin, L.J.; Dunbar, D. Family lifestyle and parental body mass index as predictors of body mass index in Australian children: A longitudinal study. *Int. J. Obes. Relat. Metab. Disord.* **2001**, *25*, 147–157. [CrossRef] [PubMed]
3. Wang, Y.; Bentley, M.E.; Zhai, F.; Popkin, B.M. Tracking of dietary intake patterns of Chinese from childhood to adolescence over a six-year follow-up period. *J. Nutr.* **2002**, *132*, 430–438. [PubMed]
4. Emmett, P.M.; Jones, L.R.; Northstone, K. Dietary patterns in the Avon longitudinal study of parents and children. *Nutr. Rev.* **2015**, *73*, 207–230. [CrossRef] [PubMed]
5. Northstone, K.; Emmett, P.M. Are dietary patterns stable throughout early and mid-childhood? A birth cohort study. *Br. J. Nutr.* **2008**, *100*, 1069–1076. [CrossRef] [PubMed]
6. Lipsky, L.M.; Haynie, D.L.; Liu, D.; Chaurasia, A.; Gee, B.; Li, K.; Iannotti, R.J.; Simons-Morton, B. Trajectories of eating behaviors in a nationally representative cohort of U.S. adolescents during the transition to young adulthood. *Int. J. Behav. Nutr. Phys. Act.* **2015**, *12*, 138. [CrossRef] [PubMed]
7. Mikkilä, V.; Räsänen, L.; Raitakari, O.T.; Pietinen, P.; Viikari, J. Consistent dietary patterns identified from childhood to adulthood: The cardiovascular risk in young Finns study. *Br. J. Nutr.* **2005**, *93*, 923–931. [CrossRef] [PubMed]
8. Birch, L.; Savage, J.S.; Ventura, A. Influences on the development of children's eating behaviours: From infancy to adolescence. *Can. J. Diet. Pract. Res.* **2007**, *68*, s1–s56. [PubMed]
9. Racey, M.; O'Brien, C.; Douglas, S.; Marquez, O.; Hendrie, G.; Newton, G. Systematic review of school-based interventions to modify dietary behavior: Does intervention intensity impact effectiveness? *J. Sch. Health* **2016**, *86*, 452–463. [CrossRef] [PubMed]
10. Evans, C.E.; Christian, M.S.; Cleghorn, C.L.; Greenwood, D.C.; Cade, J.E. Systematic review and meta-analysis of school-based interventions to improve daily fruit and vegetable intake in children aged 5 to 12 years. *Am. J. Clin. Nutr.* **2012**, *96*, 889–901. [CrossRef] [PubMed]
11. Hoffmann, K.; Schulze, M.B.; Schienkiewitz, A.; Nöthlings, U.; Boeing, H. Application of a new statistical method to derive dietary patterns in nutritional epidemiology. *Am. J. Epidemiol.* **2004**, *159*, 935–944. [CrossRef] [PubMed]
12. Hu, F.B. Dietary pattern analysis: A new direction in nutritional epidemiology. *Curr. Opin. Lipidol.* **2002**, *13*, 3–9. [CrossRef] [PubMed]
13. Borges, C.A.; Rinaldi, A.E.; Conde, W.L.; Mainardi, G.M.; Behar, D.; Slater, B. Dietary patterns: A literature review of the methodological characteristics of the main step of the multivariate analyzes. *Rev. Bras. Epidemiol.* **2015**, *18*, 837–857. [CrossRef] [PubMed]
14. Leventakou, V.; Sarri, K.; Georgiou, V.; Chatzea, V.; Frouzi, E.; Kastelianou, A.; Gatzou, A.; Kogevinas, M.; Chatzi, L. Early life determinants of dietary patterns in preschool children: Rhea mother-child cohort, Crete, Greece. *Eur. J. Clin. Nutr.* **2016**, *70*, 60–65. [CrossRef] [PubMed]
15. Pisa, P.T.; Pedro, T.M.; Kahn, K.; Tollman, S.M.; Pettifor, J.M.; Norris, S.A. Nutrient patterns and their association with socio-demographic, lifestyle factors and obesity risk in rural South African adolescents. *Nutrients* **2015**, *7*, 3464–3482. [CrossRef] [PubMed]
16. Lee, H.A.; Park, E.A.; Cho, S.J.; Kim, H.S.; Kim, Y.J.; Lee, H.; Gwak, H.S.; Kim, K.N.; Chang, N.; Ha, E.H.; et al. Mendelian randomization analysis of the effect of maternal homocysteine during pregnancy, as represented by maternal MTHFR C677T genotype, on birth weight. *J. Epidemiol.* **2013**, *23*, 371–375. [CrossRef] [PubMed]
17. Lee, H.A.; Kim, Y.J.; Lee, H.; Gwak, H.S.; Hong, Y.S.; Kim, H.S.; Park, E.A.; Cho, S.J.; Ha, E.H.; Park, H. The preventive effect of breast-feeding for longer than 6 months on early pubertal development among children aged 7–9 years in Korea. *Public Health Nutr.* **2015**, *18*, 3300–3307. [CrossRef] [PubMed]

18. Oh, S.Y.; Chung, J.; Kim, M.; Kwon, S.O.; Cho, B. Antioxidant nutrient intakes and corresponding biomarkers associated with the risk of atopic dermatitis in young children. *Eur. J. Clin. Nutr.* **2010**, *64*, 245–252. [CrossRef] [PubMed]

19. Chung, J.; Kwon, S.O.; Ahn, H.; Hwang, H.; Hong, J.S.; Oh, S.Y. Association between dietary patterns and atopic dermatitis in relation to *GSTM1* and *GSTT1* polymorphisms in young children nutrients. *Nutrients* **2015**, *7*, 9440–9452. [CrossRef] [PubMed]

20. Shin, K.O.; Oh, S.Y.; Park, H.S. Empirically derived major dietary patterns and their associations with overweight in Korean preschool children. *Br. J. Nutr.* **2007**, *98*, 416–421. [CrossRef] [PubMed]

21. Ambrosini, G.L.; Emmett, P.M.; Northstone, K.; Jebb, S.A. Tracking a dietary pattern associated with increased adiposity in childhood and adolescence. *Obesity (Silver Spring)* **2014**, *22*, 458–465. [CrossRef] [PubMed]

22. Kim, W.Y.; Cho, M.S.; Lee, H.S. Development and validation of mini dietary assessment index for Koreans. *Korean J. Nutr.* **2003**, *36*, 82–92.

23. Park, S.; Cho, S.C.; Hong, Y.C.; Oh, S.Y.; Kim, J.W.; Shin, M.S.; Kim, B.N.; Yoo, H.J.; Cho, I.H.; Bhang, S.Y. Association between dietary behaviors and attention-deficit/hyperactivity disorder and learning disabilities in school-aged children. *Psychiatry Res.* **2012**, *198*, 468–476. [CrossRef] [PubMed]

24. Gorgulho, B.M.; Pot, G.K.; Sarti, F.M.; Marchioni, D.M. Indices for the assessment of nutritional quality of meals: A systematic review. *Br. J. Nutr.* **2016**, *115*, 2017–2024. [CrossRef] [PubMed]

25. Alissa, E.M.; Ferns, G.A. Dietary fruits and vegetables and cardiovascular diseases risk. *Crit. Rev. Food Sci. Nutr.* **2015**. [CrossRef] [PubMed]

26. Hung, H.C.; Joshipura, K.J.; Jiang, R.; Hu, F.B.; Hunter, D.; Smith-Warner, S.A.; Colditz, G.A.; Rosner, B.; Spiegelman, D.; Willett, W.C. Fruit and vegetable intake and risk of major chronic disease. *JNCI J. Natl. Cancer Inst.* **2004**, *96*, 1577–1584. [CrossRef] [PubMed]

27. Jang, Y.A.; Lee, H.S.; Kim, B.H.; Lee, Y.; Lee, H.J.; Moon, J.J.; Kim, C.I. Revised dietary guidelines for Koreans. *Asia Pac. J. Clin. Nutr.* **2008**, *17*, 55–58.

28. Im, J.G.; Kim, S.H.; Lee, G.Y.; Joung, H.; Park, M.J. Inadequate calcium intake is highly prevalent in Korean children and adolescents: The Korea National Health and Nutrition Examination Survey (KNHANES) 2007–2010. *Public Health Nutr.* **2014**, *17*, 2489–2495. [CrossRef] [PubMed]

29. Kim, S.; Moon, S.; Popkin, B.M. The nutrition transition in South Korea. *Am. J. Clin. Nutr.* **2000**, *71*, 44–53. [PubMed]

30. Woo, H.D.; Shin, A.; Kim, J. Dietary patterns of Korean adults and the prevalence of metabolic syndrome: A cross-sectional study. *PLoS ONE* **2014**, *9*, e111593. [CrossRef] [PubMed]

31. Striegel-Moore, R.H.; Thompson, D.; Affenito, S.G.; Franko, D.L.; Obarzanek, E.; Barton, B.A.; Schreiber, G.B.; Daniels, S.R.; Schmidt, M.; Crawford, P.B. Correlates of beverage intake in adolescent girls: The National Heart, Lung, and Blood Institute Growth and Health Study. *J. Pediatr.* **2006**, *148*, 183–187. [CrossRef] [PubMed]

32. Demory-Luce, D.; Morales, M.; Nicklas, T.; Baranowski, T.; Zakeri, I.; Berenson, G. Changes in food group consumption patterns from childhood to young adulthood: The Bogalusa Heart Study. *J. Am. Diet. Assoc.* **2004**, *104*, 1684–1691. [CrossRef] [PubMed]

33. Northstone, K.; Emmett, P. Multivariate analysis of diet in children at four and seven years of age and associations with socio-demographic characteristics. *Eur. J. Clin. Nutr.* **2005**, *59*, 751–760. [CrossRef] [PubMed]

34. Béghin, L.; Dauchet, L.; De Vriendt, T.; Cuenca-García, M.; Manios, Y.; Toti, E.; Plada, M.; Widhalm, K.; Repasy, J.; Huybrechts, I.; et al. Influence of parental socio-economic status on diet quality of European adolescents: Results from the HELENA study. *Br. J. Nutr.* **2014**, *111*, 1303–1312. [CrossRef] [PubMed]

35. Darmon, N.; Drewnowski, A. Does social class predict diet quality? *Am. J. Clin. Nutr.* **2008**, *87*, 1107–1117. [PubMed]

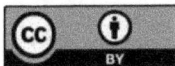

nutrients

MDPI

Article

Dietary Patterns of European Children and Their Parents in Association with Family Food Environment: Results from the I.Family Study

Antje Hebestreit [1,*,†], Timm Intemann [1,†], Alfonso Siani [2], Stefaan De Henauw [3], Gabriele Eiben [4], Yiannis A. Kourides [5], Eva Kovacs [6,7], Luis A. Moreno [8], Toomas Veidebaum [9], Vittorio Krogh [10], Valeria Pala [10], Leonie H. Bogl [1,11,12], Monica Hunsberger [4], Claudia Börnhorst [1] and Iris Pigeot [1] on behalf of the I.Family Consortium

[1] Leibniz-Institute for Prevention Research and Epidemiology—BIPS, 28359 Bremen, Germany; intemann@leibniz-bips.de (T.I.); leonie-helen.bogl@helsinki.fi (L.H.B.); boern@leibniz-bips.de (C.B.); pigeot@leibniz-bips.de (I.P.)
[2] Institute of Food Sciences, National Research Council, 83100 Avellino, Italy; asiani@isa.cnr.it
[3] Department of Public Health, Ghent University, 9000 Ghent, Belgium; stefaan.dehenauw@ugent.be
[4] Department of Public Health and Community Medicine, University of Gothenburg, 40530 Gothenburg, Sweden; gabriele.eiben@medfak.gu.se (G.E.); monica.hunsberger@gu.se (M.H.)
[5] Research and Education Institute of Child Health, 2035 Strovolos, Cyprus; kourides@cytanet.com.cy
[6] Institute for Medical Information Processing, Biometrics and Epidemiology, Ludwig-Maximilians-Universität München, 81377 Munich, Germany; eva.kovacs@med.uni-muenchen.de
[7] German Center for Vertigo and Balance Disorders, Ludwig-Maximilians-Universität München, 81377 Munich, Germany
[8] GENUD (Growth, Exercise, Nutrition and Development) Research Group, Instituto Agroalimentario de Aragón (IA2), Instituto de Investigación Sanitaria Aragón (IIS Aragón), Centro de Investigación Biomédica en Red Fisiopatología de la Obesidad y Nutrición (CIBERObn), University of Zaragoza, 50009 Zaragoza, Spain; lmoreno@unizar.es
[9] Department of Chronic Diseases, National Institute for Health Development, 11619 Tallinn, Estonia; toomas.veidebaum@tai.ee
[10] Department of Preventive and Predictive Medicine, Fondazione IRCCS Istituto Nazionale dei Tumori, 20133 Milan, Italy; Vittorio.Krogh@istitutotumori.mi.it (V.K.); Valeria.Pala@istitutotumori.mi.it (V.P.)
[11] Department of Public Health, University of Helsinki, 00014 Helsinki, Finland
[12] Finnish Institute of Molecular Medicine, University of Helsinki, 00014 Helsinki, Finland
* Correspondence: hebestr@leibniz-bips.de; Tel.: +49-421-2185-6849
† Shared first authorship.

Received: 18 November 2016; Accepted: 3 February 2017; Published: 10 February 2017

Abstract: The aim of this study was to determine whether an association exists between children's and parental dietary patterns (DP), and whether the number of shared meals or soft drink availability during meals strengthens this association. In 2013/2014 the I.Family study cross-sectionally assessed the dietary intakes of families from eight European countries using 24-h dietary recalls. Usual energy and food intakes from six- to 16-year-old children and their parents were estimated based on the NCI Method. A total of 1662 child–mother and 789 child–father dyads were included; DP were derived using cluster analysis. We investigated the association between children's and parental DP and whether the number of shared meals or soft drink availability moderated this association using mixed effects logistic regression models. Three DP comparable in children and parents were obtained: Sweet & Fat, Refined Cereals, and Animal Products. Children were more likely to be allocated to the Sweet & Fat DP when their fathers were allocated to the Sweet & Fat DP and when they shared at least one meal per day (OR 3.18; 95% CI 1.84; 5.47). Being allocated to the Sweet & Fat DP increased when the mother or the father was allocated to the Sweet & Fat DP and when soft drinks were available (OR 2.78; 95% CI 1.80; 4.28 or OR 4.26; 95% CI 2.16; 8.41, respectively). Availability of soft drinks and negative parental role modeling are important predictors of children's dietary patterns.

Keywords: food consumption; family resemblance; cluster analysis; shared meals; soft drink; childhood obesity

---

1. Introduction

Family members share similar eating habits that are affected by individual factors and the family food environment [1]. Parental role modeling and perception of adequacy of their child's diet are important predictors for the child's current dietary behavior [2] and watching the parents eat raises the children's awareness of their parents' eating behaviors [3,4]. Despite the fact that fathers and mothers were found to influence the child's eating behavior [5,6], the influence differs for mothers compared to fathers [7,8]. Paternal dietary influence was identified for fruit but also for fat-and energy-dense, nutrient-poor foods [9,10], whereas positive child–mother correlations have been reported for fruit and vegetable intake [11] and soft drinks [12]. Thus, parents build their children's food environment by making healthy foods [13] or unhealthy foods [14] available. Accordingly the children's food consumption was associated with healthy foods (so-called core foods, e.g., cereals, dairy, fruit, and vegetables) or with unhealthy non-core foods (e.g., snack foods, fats, and oils) [5]. As an example, adolescents were more likely to consume fruit and vegetables when parents made those foods available [15,16]. It has been observed that the person who prepares the majority of family meals largely influences the consumption of fruit and vegetables but also high-fat foods; this association increases with increasing numbers of shared meals [17].

Previous research has demonstrated that the association between parental and child intake increased with an increasing number of family meals at home [18] and that the number of family meals was positively associated with the consumption of healthier foods [19]. Family mealtimes provide structure and a regular opportunity for developing emotional connections among family members and therefore help children to monitor their mood and learn healthy dietary behaviors [20]. Accordingly, higher family meal frequency was found to be associated with significantly fewer weekly servings of sweets and sugar-sweetened beverages [21]; however, the consumption of those non-core foods (e.g., sugar sweetened beverages) was found to be higher when their home availability was higher [5]. Consumption of sugar-sweetened beverages is one epidemiological key health indicator of the European Core Health Indicators [22] and is frequently used in public health monitoring, especially when addressing socioeconomic determinants of eating behavior in European children and adolescents [23,24]. Investigations in low-income parent–child dyads found that soft drink availability at home was a strong influencing factor for the children's soft drink intake [25], identifying parents as gatekeepers for the family food environment.

Apart from this literature, it is striking that there is little knowledge about the resemblance of entire dietary patterns among children and their parents across Europe, which was described in the present study. The previous literature mainly investigated parental influence on the children's intake of particular food groups such as fruit and vegetables or sugar-sweetened beverages. We therefore aimed at adding knowledge on the influence of the entire parental DP on the children's DP. Besides parental intake, home availability has also been found to predict children's intake of core-food and non-core foods. Thus, we aimed at determining whether the family food environment (operationalized as the number of shared meals and availability of soft drinks during meals) moderated the association between children's DP and parental DP. Understanding to what extent the family food environment, along with the parental DP, influences children's eating behavior has important public health implications, because in this age children and adolescents mostly still live with their parents and potentially eat up to three meals a day at home. Development of intervention strategies to improve children's dietary patterns is likely to be more successful if supported by an understanding not only healthy but also unhealthy food intake.

2. Materials and Methods

2.1. Study Participants

Data from this investigation were obtained from the I.Family cohort. In 2013/2014 the I.Family study cross-sectionally examined children and parents from Sweden, Germany, Hungary, Italy, Cyprus, Spain, Belgium, and Estonia in order to investigate associations between eating habits and lifestyle factors leading to overweight and obesity [26]. For this investigation children and adolescents from six years to approximately 16 years who lived with their families were invited to the examination, together with the person having the care and custody of the child (hereinafter named parents). In the present analysis we included children and parents providing at least one 24HDR (N = 4816). In the final mixed effects logistic regression model, we included 1662 child–mother dyads (with 1269 mothers) and 789 child–father dyads (with 566 fathers); of those, 516 families provided information from siblings and 362 families provided information from the mother and father. Information on the availability of soft drinks during meals was provided for 1607 child–mother dyads and 763 child–father dyads.

Parents and children older than 16 years provided written informed consent. Younger children gave oral consent for examinations and sample collection. Study subjects and their parents could consent to single components of the study while abstaining from others. Study participants did not undergo any procedures unless they (and their parents) had given consent for examinations, collection of samples, subsequent analysis, and storage of personal data and collected samples. All applicable institutional and governmental regulations concerning the ethical use of human volunteers were followed during this research. Each participating center obtained ethical approval from the local responsible authorities in accordance with the ethical standards of the 1964 Declaration of Helsinki and its later amendments.

2.2. Questionnaires and Anthropometric Measurements

Questionnaires were developed in English, translated into local languages, and then back-translated to check for translation errors. Parents reported the age and sex of their children and themselves in addition to their highest educational level according to the International Standard Classification of Education (ISCED) [27], which was used as a proxy indicator for the socioeconomic status (SES) of the family. Additionally, parents reported if soft drinks are available at home during meals (answer options: Yes, often or always; No or rarely).

The field methods comprised anthropometric measurements of standing height (cm) using a Seca 225 stadiometer (Seca GmbH & KG, Birmingham, UK) in accordance with international standards for anthropometric assessment and weight (kg) [28]. Body weight was assessed in fasting status using a prototype of the TANITA BC 420 SMA digital scale for children and a TANITA BC 418 MA for adolescents and adults (TANITA Europe GmbH, Sindelfingen, Germany). All measurements were performed in light clothing (e.g., underwear) [29].

The BMI of the participants was calculated by dividing body weight in kilograms by squared body height in meters. The BMI of children was transformed to an age- and sex-specific z-score according to Cole et al. [30]. Weight groups (thin/normal and overweight/obese) of children were categorized using age- and sex-specific cutoff values based on the extended IOTF criteria [31]. Weight groups of adolescents and parents above 18 years were calculated using WHO cutoffs [32]. Even though weight status was not a focus of this investigation, it was calculated for a better characterization of the study population.

2.3. Dietary Information

Dietary intake of the previous 24 h was assessed using an online 24-h dietary recall (24HDR) assessment program, called 'Self-Administered Children, Adolescents and Adult Nutrition Assessment' (SACANA), based on the validated SACINA offline version [33]. The instrument has been validated and results supported the validity of SACANA as a self-reporting instrument for assessing intakes in children (publications in progress).

Children and parents were asked to recall their diet and to enter the type and amount (g) of all drinks and foods consumed during the previous day, starting with the first intake after waking up in the morning. Children under 11 years were advised to ask their parents for help [34]. Study participants above 11 years of age could ask for assistance from a dietician or trained study nurse during the survey examinations, but the majority of participants had no questions since they already participated in the IDEFICS study and were therefore familiar with the recall procedures and software structure used. Standardized photographs were used to assist with accurate estimation of portion size [35]. In the present study, participants were asked to complete at least three 24HDR during the upcoming four weeks. However, the availability of repeated 24HDR varied among individuals from one to four recalls. For 43% of parents (39% of children), three repeated 24HDR were available.

The total number of main meals (breakfast, lunch, and dinner) per participant was calculated. Breakfast was defined as "shared" if the total number of shared breakfasts (parent with child) divided by the number of all reported breakfasts of the respective parent was at least 0.5. Shared lunches and dinners were categorized accordingly. The sum of all shared main meals per parent was calculated and the following categories were derived: (1) <1 shared meal per day and (2) ≥1 shared meal per day.

2.4. Dietary Data Analysis

Missing or implausible values for intake of single food items that could not be corrected were imputed by country, food group, and age-specific median intakes (0.15% of the entries). Incomplete 24HDR (recalls that have not been completed throughout) and those with more than four imputed values were excluded from the analysis.

Age- and sex-specific Goldberg cutoffs were applied to classify each recall day as under-reported, plausibly reported, and over-reported energy intake, as described elsewhere [36].

In total, we excluded 955 participants classified as misreporters from the analysis: 484 children and 471 adults; among those 95% and 99% were under-reporters, and 5% and 1% were over-reporters, respectively.

Each food recorded by SACANA was assigned to one of 15 dietary categories: healthy and unhealthy cereals and cereal products, unhealthy sugar and sugar products, healthy and unhealthy fat and fat savory sauces, healthy fruit and vegetables, healthy and unhealthy meat and meat products, healthy meat alternatives, healthy and unhealthy milk and dairy products, healthy and unhealthy non-alcoholic beverages, healthy and unhealthy mixed dishes (Table 1). Foods were categorized as "healthy" when they contained less energy, less sugar, less (unhealthy) fat, or more fiber than the unhealthy food alternative, e.g., table water (healthy beverage) vs. juice (unhealthy beverage), plain yogurt (healthy) vs. full fat and sweetened yogurt (unhealthy). Consumption of unhealthy mixed dishes was so rare that this category was not included in further analysis.

After food categorization, individual usual daily energy intake (EI, kcal/day) and individual usual intakes of dietary categories (kcal/day, healthy non-alcoholic beverages: g/day) were estimated based on the U.S. National Cancer Institute Method [37,38]. This method allows the inclusion of covariates like age and additional food frequency information, accounts for different intake on weekend vs. work days, and corrects for the variance inflation caused by the daily variation in diet. Usual intakes were estimated for children as well as for their parents, stratified by sex (all participants with at least one plausible 24HDR). Age was considered as a covariate in all models. When estimating usual food intakes, the corresponding food consumption frequency obtained from the I.Family food frequency questionnaire was also used as a covariate to improve estimates (except for mixed dishes, as this food group was not queried in the food frequency questionnaire but was a generic category in SACANA food groups). The I.Family food frequency questionnaire was built on the valid and reproducible IDEFICS study food frequency questionnaire, which was described in detail previously [39–41]. The FFQ contained 59 food items comparable to those in the SACANA web tool, thus allowing categorizing the food items according to the 15 dietary categories mentioned above. The answer possibilities in the FFQ were "never/less than once a week", "1–3 times a week", "4–6 times a week", "1 time/day", "2 times a day", "3 times a day", and "I have no idea". All participants were asked to complete one FFQ for the four weeks prior to the survey examination.

Table 1. Food groups and healthy/unhealthy dietary categories.

Food Group	Healthy Alternative	Unhealthy Alternative
Cereals & cereal products	Low sugar content (<15%), low fat content (<20%) and high fiber content (≥5%)	≥15% sugar, ≥20% fat, and <5% fiber content
Sugar & sweets	-	Sugar, sweets, candies, marzipan, chocolate, nut spreads, jam, honey, ice cream, canned/sugared fruit, etc.
Fats & oils	From mainly plant origin, and for sauces <40% fat content	Mainly animal and processed origin and ≥40% fat for sauces
Non-alcoholic beverages	Non-caloric and non-processed beverages such as table water, plain herbal teas, plain coffee	Sweetened and processed beverages: manufactured juices, sodas, ice tea, energy drinks, coffee/tea with milk/sugar, broth
Meat	Containing <10% fat, and meat products with <20% fat from poultry, rabbit or game	Meat from all other origins than poultry, including offal, with ≥10% fat and meat products containing ≥20% fat
Meat alternative	Soy products, meat and dairy substitutes from soy, vegetarian burgers, tempeh, tofu, seitan and lean prepared fish and eggs	-
Milk & dairy products	Low fat and unsweetened	Full fat and sweetened, flavored
Fruit & vegetables	Fresh fruit and vegetables, their fresh juices/smoothies, or lean preparation, without added sugars	-
Mixed dishes	Based on cereals, legumes, vegetables/potatoes with small amounts of fish, egg or dairy, soups, veloutés, mixed salad	Based on meat; fried foods (also fried vegetables), fast food, snack foods (not included in the final cluster analysis)

The individual percentage of energy contribution from all dietary categories was calculated to correct for individual total EI. For children and adults separately, these percentages were transformed into z-scores using sample means and sample standard deviations. The z-score represents the distance between the percentage of energy contribution and the corresponding population mean in units of the standard deviation. This procedure was not applied for usual EI and usual intake of non-alcoholic beverages (g/day) since EI correction is neither reasonable for EI itself nor for the calorie-free dietary category. Therefore, age-dependent z-scores were derived for these variables with the Generalized Additive Models for Location, Scale, and Shape (this procedure is described in detail in Appendix A).

2.5. Statistical Analysis

K-means clustering was applied for children and parents separately to identify distinct clusters of participants with similar dietary patterns. In this procedure the previously derived z-scores were taken into account. Details of this procedure are described in Appendix A. As clusters were comparable between children and parents, the same cluster names were used. Three clusters representing the DP (Figure 1) were obtained: Sweet and Fat cluster, Refined Cereals cluster, and Animal Products cluster. Each participant was allocated to exactly one DP and corresponding indicator variables were derived (participant is in the respective cluster versus participant is not in the respective cluster).

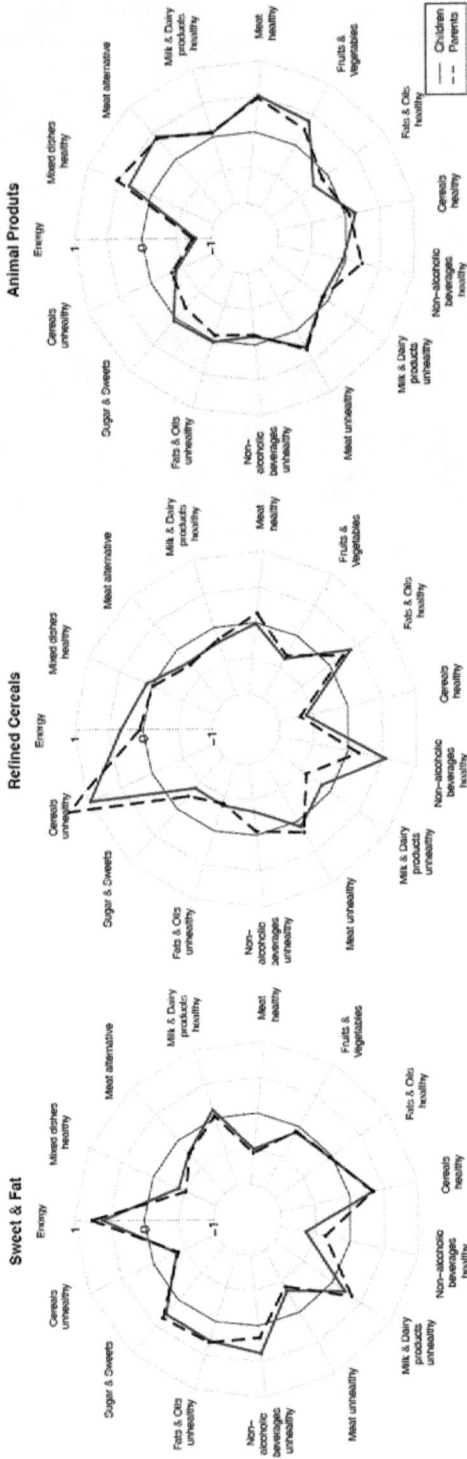

Figure 1. Dietary patterns of children and their parents: Sweet and Fat, Refined Cereals, and Animal Products. Mean z-scores of percentage of energy intake of different food groups in the three clusters for children and parents are shown (for details, see Table 2). The scale ranges from -1 to 1 with tick lines for -0.5, 0 (solid line) and 0.5.

Family food environment was operationalized using the number of shared meals (<1 or ≥1 shared meal per day) as an indicator of parental role modeling and the availability of soft drinks during meals as an indicator of home food availability. As a first step, we investigated associations between the outcome children's DP (indicator variable) and the exposure parental DP (indicator variable) and the number of shared meals using mixed effects logistic regression. To examine whether the number of shared meals strengthened the associations between parental and children's DP, an interaction term was included (number of shared meal × parental DP). For each of the three DP, we conducted a regression analysis separately for fathers and mothers (six models). Accordingly, we investigated in a second step the associations between children's DP and the exposure parental DP and availability of soft drinks during meals. To examine whether the availability of soft drinks during meals strengthened the associations between parental DP and children's DP, an interaction term (availability of soft drinks during meals × parental DP) was included. The models were adjusted for sex, age and BMI z-score of the children, ISCED, country, and BMI of the respective parent. In order to account for dependencies between siblings, a random effect was added for family membership. Based on the mixed effects logistic regression models, odds ratios (OR) and confidence intervals (95%CI) were calculated for a child being allocated to the DP corresponding to the parental DP depending on the number of shared meals and availability of soft drinks during meals. The analysis was performed using the procedure PROC GLIMMIX of the statistical software SAS (version 9.3; SAS Institute, Cary, NC, USA).

3. Results

The aims of the present study were to investigate the resemblance of children's DP and their parents' DP as well as to determine whether structural conditions of the family food environment moderated the association between children's DP and parental DP.

3.1. Dietary Clusters

Based on dietary categories (Table 1) and usual EI, the three-cluster solutions were derived. For comparable clusters of children and parents, the following labels were assigned: Sweet and Fat (*N* = 697 for children and *N* = 728 for parents), Refined Cereals (*N* = 563 for children and *N* = 410 for parents), and Animal Products (*N* = 716 for children and *N* = 747 for parents).

Table 2 presents the mean z-scores and standard deviations of usual intake for all dietary categories in the three clusters for children and parents.

In general, we observed a resemblance of children's dietary patterns to parents' dietary pattern; details of these analyses can be found in Appendix A. The overall agreement between cluster allocation of children and mothers was 52% (for fathers, 53%).

In particular, we observed the following characteristics for the three clusters representing dietary patterns (DP).

Sweet and Fat: Children and adults allocated to this cluster reported higher-than-mean intake of sugar and sweets (children's mean 0.27; parents' mean 0.34), unhealthy fats and oils (children's mean 0.29; parents' mean 0.31), unhealthy (sweetened) non-alcoholic beverages (children's mean 0.39; parents' mean 0.17) and unhealthy milk and dairy products (children's mean 0.22; parents' mean 0.34) (Figure 1). Cereals were categorized as healthy in case of low sugar content and low fat content and high fiber content (Table 1), such as whole-grain breads, plain breakfast cereals, or crispbread (children's mean 0.34; parents' mean 0.33). Family members allocated to this DP reported the highest EI (children's mean 0.60; parents' mean 0.75).

Refined Cereals: Children and parents from this cluster reported higher-than-mean intake of unhealthy cereals (e.g., white breads, refined and/or sugared breakfast cereals, pasta from refined wheat, refined rice, sweet and/or fatty bakery products (biscuits, cakes, fritters, etc.; children's mean 0.96; parents' mean 1.32) and healthy fats and oils (children's mean 0.36; parents' mean 0.23). Both children and parents also consumed more healthy non-alcoholic beverages (children's mean 0.54; parents' mean 0.15).

Table 2. z-scores of usual intake in the three clusters for children and for parents (mean values and standard deviations).

Children	Sweet & Fat (N = 697; 35%)		Ref. Cereals (N = 563; 28%)		Animal Products (N = 716; 36%)	
	Mean	SD	Mean	SD	Mean	SD
Energy	0.60 [a]	0.82	0.32	0.83	−0.78 [b]	0.79
Non-alcoholic beverages—healthy	−0.64 [b]	0.89	0.54 [a]	0.81	−0.04	1.01
Non-alcoholic beverages—unhealthy	0.39 [a]	1.24	−0.33 [b]	0.67	−0.12	0.82
Cereals—unhealthy	−0.37	0.7	0.96 [a]	1.06	−0.40 [b]	0.61
Cereals—healthy	0.34 [a]	1.05	−0.61 [b]	0.64	0.14	0.97
Sugar & Sweets	0.27 [a]	0.94	−0.39 [b]	0.94	0.05	1.00
Fats & Oils—unhealthy	0.29 [a]	1.21	−0.38 [b]	0.61	0.02	0.93
Fats & Oils—healthy	−0.03	1.03	0.36 [a]	1.18	−0.25 [b]	0.69
Fruit & Vegetables	−0.09	0.96	−0.37 [b]	0.87	0.39 [a]	1.00
Meat—unhealthy	−0.35 [b]	0.88	0.09	1.02	0.27 [a]	1.00
Meat—healthy	−0.51 [b]	0.73	−0.01	0.96	0.51 [a]	1.01
Milk & Dairy products—unhealthy	0.22 [a]	1.13	−0.15 [b]	0.91	−0.1	0.89
Milk & Dairy products—healthy	0.12 [a]	1.09	−0.22 [b]	0.82	0.05	1.02
Meat alternative	−0.24	0.78	−0.25 [b]	0.71	0.42 [a]	1.22
Mixed dishes—healthy	−0.41 [b]	0.89	0.08	0.97	0.34 [a]	0.98
Parents	Sweet & Fat (N = 728; 39%)		Ref. Cereals (N = 410; 22%)		Animal Products (N = 747; 40%)	
	Mean	SD	Mean	SD	Mean	SD
Energy	0.75 [a]	0.76	0.05	0.83	−0.73 [b]	0.75
Non-alcoholic beverages—healthy	−0.36 [b]	1.01	0.15	0.87	0.23 [a]	0.96
Non-alcoholic beverages—unhealthy	0.17 [a]	1.12	−0.05	1.03	−0.14 [b]	0.82
Cereals—unhealthy	−0.40 [b]	0.59	1.32	1.09	−0.34	0.55
Cereals—healthy	0.33 [a]	1.02	−0.69 [b]	0.58	0.06	0.97
Sugar & Sweets	0.34 [a]	0.96	−0.24 [b]	0.93	−0.20	0.99
Fats & Oils—unhealthy	0.31 [a]	1.17	−0.41 [b]	0.66	−0.08	0.87
Fats & Oils—healthy	−0.03	1.04	0.23 [a]	1.11	−0.09 [b]	0.87
Fruit & Vegetables	−0.08	0.94	−0.32 [b]	0.95	0.25 [a]	1.02
Meat—unhealthy	−0.41 [b]	0.87	0.18	0.91	0.30 [a]	1.03
Meat—healthy	−0.56 [b]	0.74	0.13	0.84	0.48 [a]	1.03
Milk & Dairy products—unhealthy	0.34 [a]	1.14	−0.42 [b]	0.72	−0.09	0.87
Milk & Dairy products—healthy	0.03	1.02	−0.18 [b]	0.93	0.07 [a]	1.00
Meat alternative	−0.25	0.77	−0.29 [b]	0.65	0.40 [a]	1.21
Mixed dishes—healthy	−0.53 [b]	0.91	−0.01	0.84	0.52 [a]	0.89

[a] The highest mean value within a row; [b] The lowest mean value within a row.

Animal Products: Children and parents who were allocated to this cluster reported higher intake of all types of meat (children's mean for meat unhealthy 0.27, meat healthy 0.51; parents' mean 0.30 and 0.48, respectively) and meat alternatives (children's mean 0.42; parents' mean 0.40) as well as of healthy mixed dishes (children's mean 0.34; parents' mean 0.52). Healthy mixed dishes were mainly based on cereals, legumes, and vegetables/potatoes, with small proportions of fish, egg, or dairy. Children and parents further reported higher-than-mean intakes of fruit and vegetables (children's mean 0.39; parents' mean 0.25). Parents reported a higher-than-mean intake for healthy non-alcoholic beverages (mean 0.23). The energy intake of children and parents was lowest in this DP (children's mean −0.78; parents' mean −0.73).

3.2. Participant Characteristics

The largest proportion of children (36%) and parents (40%) was allocated to the Animal Products cluster (Table 3). The mean age of children (11.4 years) and parents (44.2 years) was highest in the

Refined Cereals cluster. Girls (39%) and mothers (44%) were mainly found in the Sweet and Fat cluster, whereas most boys and men were found in the Animal Products cluster (38% and 44%, respectively).

Table 3. Characteristics of the study population, including plausible reporters stratified by cluster membership and misreporters (number and percentages).

Covariates	Plausible Reporters												Misreporters			
	Children, Adolescents						Parents						Children, Adolescents		Parents	
	Sweet & Fat (N = 697; 35%)		Ref. Cereals (N = 563; 28%)		Animal Products (N = 716; 36%)		Sweet & Fat (N = 728; 39%)		Ref. Cereals (N = 410; 22%)		Animal Products (N = 747; 40%)		(N = 484)		(N = 471)	
Age mean (SD)	10.9 (2.1)		11.4 (2.1)		11.2 (2.1)		41.8 (5.4)		44.2 (5.8)		41.8 (5.4)		12.2 (1.9)		42.3 (5.7)	
Age range (min; max)	6.0; 15.8		6.0; 16.0		6.0; 16.0		28.1; 58.5		30.3; 65.4		27.0; 63.0		6.5; 15.7		27.8; 58.7	
Sex (N, %)																
Male	322	32	311	30	387	38	149	26	173	30	257	44	238	49	139	30
Female	375	39	252	26	329	34	579	44	237	18	490	38	246	51	332	71
Weight group (N, %N) [a]																
Normal weight	588	37	403	25	613	38	428	43	175	18	388	39	310	64	159	34
Overweight	93	32	115	39	84	32	209	34	157	25	255	41	123	25	156	33
Obese	16	20	45	56	19	24	91	33	78	29	104	38	51	11	156	33
ISCED-Level of parents [b] (N, %)																
Low Education	5	12	31	76	5	12	1	3	24	71	9	26	26	5	31	7
Medium Education	200	31	245	38	207	32	185	30	190	31	234	38	227	47	235	50
High Education	482	39	271	22	491	39	529	44	182	15	488	41	226	47	199	42
Missing ISCED [c]	10	26	16	41	13	33	13	30	14	33	16	37	5	1	6	1
County (N, %)																
Italy	8	3	232	85	32	12	14	6	179	77	38	16	59	12	77	16
Estonia	275	50	29	5	246	45	341	56	28	5	244	40	148	31	82	17
Cyprus	28	17	66	39	75	44	33	21	40	26	81	53	27	6	41	9
Belgium	67	44	14	9	73	47	66	55	14	12	39	33	24	5	18	4
Sweden	133	39	120	35	89	26	113	40	58	20	113	40	55	11	66	14
Germany	149	49	40	13	113	37	133	47	39	14	114	40	143	30	147	31
Hungary	29	32	38	42	23	26	11	12	41	45	39	43	17	4	25	5
Spain	8	8	24	25	65	67	17	16	11	10	79	74	11	2	15	3

[a] Weight categories according to Cole et al. [30] for children and according to WHO for adults; [b] International Standard Classification of Education Maximum (ISCED); maximum of both parents (0, 1, 2 = low education; 3, 4 = medium education; 5, 6 = high education); [c] Those individuals with missing ISCED information were excluded from mixed effects logistic regression models.

Most normal weight children were allocated to the Animal Products cluster (38%), whereas most overweight (39%) and obese (56%) children were allocated to the Refined Cereals cluster. Most normal weight adults (43%) were in the Sweet and Fat cluster; most overweight (41%) and obese (38%) adults were found in the Animal Products cluster.

Children and adults from low SES families mainly belonged to the Refined Cereals cluster (76% and 71%, respectively). Children from high SES families were equally allocated to the Sweet and Fat and the Animal Products clusters (both 39%).

In all countries—except Belgium—those cluster memberships with the highest proportion of children and parents were comparable. In Italy and Hungary most children and parents shared the Refined Cereals cluster; in Estonia, Sweden and Germany most shared the Sweet and Fat cluster; and in Cyprus and Spain most shared the Animal Products cluster. In Belgium 47% of children were found in the Animal Products cluster, but 55% of their parents in the Sweet and Fat cluster.

3.3. Family Food Environment

Shared meals: Resemblance was observed between parental DP and children's DP: the chance of the child being allocated to the Sweet and Fat DP, the Refined Cereals DP, and the Animal Products DP is higher if the mother was allocated to the same DP, independently of the number of shared meals, compared to the chance if the mother was in a different DP (Table 4). Overall, children were more likely to be allocated to the Sweet and Fat DP if the father was allocated to the same DP; the odds ratio increased with an increase in the number of shared meals from <1 to ≥1 (OR 2.30; 95% CI 1.15; 4.57 or OR 3.18; 95% CI 1.84; 5.47, respectively).

Soft drink availability during meals: The child was more likely to be allocated to the Sweet and Fat DP if soft drinks were available during meals, even if the mother was not allocated to the Sweet and Fat DP (OR 1.97; 95% CI 1.20; 3.25, Table 5). The chance of being allocated to the Sweet and Fat DP was highest if the mother was allocated to the Sweet and Fat DP and soft drinks were available during meals (OR 2.78; 95% CI 1.80; 4.28). The child was more likely to be allocated to the Refined Cereals DP or the Animal Products DP if the mother was allocated to the same DPs and if no soft drinks were available during meals (OR 2.48; 95% CI 1.43 and 4.27; OR 2.16;1.59; 2.92, respectively). The child was most likely to be allocated to the Sweet and Fat DP, the Refined Cereals DP, and the Animal Products DP if the father was allocated to the respective DP and if soft drinks were not available during meals (OR 2.48; 95% CI 1.58; 3.87, OR 2.05; 95% CI 1.22; 3.45 and OR 2.48; 95% CI 1.62; 3.79, respectively). The chance of the child sharing the father's Sweet and Fat DP is higher if soft drinks are available during meals (OR 4.26; 95% CI 2.16; 8.41).

Table 4. Odds Ratios (OR) and confidence intervals (CI) for a child being allocated to a dietary pattern depending on parental dietary pattern and number of shared daily meals, given by sex of parents; all models were adjusted for age and BMI z-score of child, parental BMI, highest ISCED of family, and country of residence.

Parental Dietary Pattern	Children's Dietary Pattern								
	Sweet & Fat			Ref. Cereals			Animal Products		
	N	OR	95%CI	N	OR	95%CI	N	OR	95%CI
Maternal dietary pattern (N = 1662)									
Different & <1 shared meal (reference)	132	1.00		265	1.00		183	1.00	
Different & ≥1 shared meals	771	0.97	0.59; 1.58	1096	1.20	0.70; 2.07	877	1.06	0.70; 1.60
Identical & <1 shared meal	158	2.12	1.18; 3.81	25	5.70	1.51; 21.48	107	2.18	1.21; 3.92
Identical & ≥1 shared meals	601	1.91	1.17; 3.13	276	2.70	1.34; 5.45	495	2.19	1.41; 3.40
Paternal dietary pattern (N = 789)									
Different & <1 shared meal (reference)	149	1.00		153	1.00		112	1.00	
Different & ≥1 shared meals	430	1.31	0.82; 2.09	396	0.83	0.45;1.54	338	0.55	0.32; 0.92
Identical & <1 shared meal	58	2.30	1.15; 4.57	54	1.66	0.68;4.06	95	1.45	0.78; 2.71
Identical & ≥1 shared meals	152	3.18	1.84; 5.47	186	1.99	0.98;4.08	244	1.54	0.91; 2.59

Table 5. Odds Ratios (OR) and confidence intervals (CI) for a child being allocated to a dietary pattern depending on parental dietary pattern and availability of soft drinks during meals, given by sex of parents; all models were adjusted for age and BMI z-score of child, parental BMI, highest ISCED of family, and country of residence.

Parental Dietary Pattern	Children's Dietary Pattern								
	Sweet & Fat			Ref. Cereals			Animal Products		
	N	OR	95%CI	N	OR	95%CI	N	OR	95%CI
Maternal dietary pattern (N = 1607)									
Different & soft drink not available (reference)	742	1.00		1017	1.00		767	1.00	
Different & soft drink is available	138	1.97	1.20; 3.25	294	0.46	0.25; 0.84	256	0.95	0.65; 1.38
Identical & soft drink not available	521	2.04	1.49; 2.80	246	2.48	1.43; 4.27	496	2.16	1.59; 2.92
Identical & soft drink is available	206	2.78	1.80; 4.28	50	1.67	0.66; 4.22	88	1.42	0.82; 2.47
Paternal dietary pattern (N = 763)									
Different & soft drink not available (reference)	465	1.00		407	1.00		360	1.00	
Different & soft drink is available	92	1.55	0.90; 2.68	122	0.43	0.18; 1.04	80	0.83	0.45; 1.52
Identical & soft drink not available	151	2.48	1.58; 3.87	209	2.05	1.22; 3.45	256	2.48	1.62; 3.79
Identical & soft drink is available	55	4.26	2.16; 8.41	25	1.97	0.61; 6.39	67	1.80	0.96; 3.36

4. Discussion

The present study suggests important similarities between children's and parental DP. Three DP were obtained in this multi-country study: Animal Products, Refined Cereals, and Sweet and Fat. To our knowledge, this is the first study presenting the resemblance of the DP of pan-European children and their parents using cluster analysis. The study was further able to describe how the family food environment (operationalized as the number of shared meals and the availability of soft drinks during meals) moderated the association between children's DP and parental DP.

Resemblance of dietary patterns between children and parents: Previously, maternal consumption of core foods (e.g., cereals, dairy, fruit, and vegetables) and non-core foods (e.g., snack foods, fats, and oils) has been shown to be associated with a child's higher intake of the same foods [5]. Mothers tend to be the person habitually preparing the family meals [17] and mothers reported greater perceived responsibility for feeding their children [18]. Women are known to exert positive influence on children's food consumption [42] because they are more likely to adhere to dietary guidelines [43]. This is in line with our findings that identified the influencing nature of the maternal Animal Products DP per se and when the mother was eating with the child: in our study the Animal Products DP was characterized through the above-the-mean intake of healthy food alternatives such as fruit vegetables, healthy alternatives for meat, meat substitutes, milk and dairy products, cereals, and mixed dishes (Figure 1). Reported EIs were lowest in the Animal Products DP and we observed the highest proportion of normal weight children in this DP but the highest proportion of overweight parents. Fathers' influence on the child's food choices was highest for the foods of the Sweet and Fat DP including all types of sugar and sweets, unhealthy fats and oils, unhealthy beverages, and unhealthy milk and dairy products. In particular, the z-scores for non-alcoholic unhealthy beverages (including also soft drinks) were highest in the Sweet and Fat DP compared to the other two DP. Likewise, previous studies have reported that fathers have primary influence on the children's intake of non-core foods [8].

Dietary patterns and shared meals: In our study associations were found between children's DP and maternal DP independently of the number of shared meals and in particular between children's DP and fathers' Sweet and Fat DP if ≥1 meal was eaten together. Also in previous studies, paternal influence has been found to predict child's food intake in that fathers used pressure tactics whereas mothers praised children for eating certain things [44]. In particular, Robinson et al. [7] observed strong correlations for foods typically eaten at breakfast such as grains and fruit in child–father dyads for families with working mothers, indicating that fathers have breakfast with their children when mothers leave home early. Children and adolescents sharing three or more meals per week with the family had healthier dietary patterns compared to those who share fewer than three family meals [45]. This is in contrast to our findings, where children who eat together with their fathers at least once a day were more likely to share the Sweet and Fat DP with their fathers than sharing the generally healthier Animal Products DP.

Dietary patterns and the availability of soft drinks during meals: Although the mechanisms for how family meals facilitate healthy eating behaviors have not been empirically explained, different approaches are currently discussed. Eating together is an important ritual for interacting with family members and offers opportunities for children to learn about eating by watching others [3]. Also, low availability and consumption of convenient foods or sodas during family meals can contribute to healthy dietary intake patterns [46]. On the other hand, the availability of soft drinks during shared meals and parental soft drink consumption were associated with the child's soft drink consumption (Sweet and Fat DP) in our study. This is in line with earlier findings from U.S. studies where parental food choices [3] and soft drink availability were strong influencing factors for the children's intake [25], identifying parents as gatekeepers for the family food environment and as role models. Those foods (preferred and) consumed by the parents were the foods to which children were routinely exposed and shaped the children's food preferences and consumption [47,48]. It is not surprising that the availability of soft drinks and chips has been observed to be greater in families who frequently consumed fast food during family meals [49]. We therefore suggest that home availability of foods is an important predictor for children's preferences, even more so if parents choose the same foods during meals [50]. Making healthy foods available and also eating those foods may enhance children's understanding and acceptance of a healthy diet [51].

Limitations and Strengths

In the I.Family study dietary information was mainly given by self-respondents. Self-reporting can be susceptible to reporting bias [52]. We therefore followed a rigorous approach in order to reduce errors due to portion size estimation, incomplete recalls, misreporting, or daily variations in intake. Firstly, the development of the SACANA computer-assisted assessment tool with standardized photographs, multiple plausibility checks, and reminding questions facilitated the reporting of accurate portion sizes and complete recall. Secondly, as a first step in the data analysis, the exclusion of incomplete recalls and recalls with implausible energy reporting helped to correct for reporting bias. Individuals with misreported EI (under-reporters: 462 children, 465 adults; over-reporters: 22 children, six adults) were more likely to be female, from medium educated families, and from Estonia or Germany. They were more often overweight and obese (66% of adults; 36% of children) compared to plausible reporters (16% adults, 4% children). In a separate analysis we derived the clusters including the 955 misreporters in order to compare cluster memberships of the plausible reporters sample (1662 child–mother dyads and 789 child–father dyads) with the cluster memberships of the full study sample (2269 child–mother dyads and 1058 child–father dyads). After comparing the cluster membership of the full sample (also including misreporters) with the final study sample (plausible reporters only) we observed that the three DP remained comparable, except that EI was found to be lower in the Animal Products cluster when misreporters were included. As the Animal Products cluster included 58% of misreporting children and 83% of misreporting parents, including misreporters would overestimate intake (particularly in the Animal Product cluster) and underestimate the intake of plausible reporters (particularly in the Refined Cereals and Sweet and Fat clusters), given that we consider the percentage of energy contribution from dietary categories. We therefore decided to exclude the misreporters from the analysis. However, the question of how to handle possibly implausible interviews has not been answered conclusively: the inclusion of misreports may obscure or even inverse diet–disease relationships, as recently reported, and adjustment for the reporting group may also lead to bias [53]. Finally, deriving the usual intake based on the NCI method [37] and accounting for day-to-day variation in intake is a clear strength of this study.

As might be expected, we observed a resemblance between the parental DP and children's DP. These improved relations do not reflect reporting bias (due to proxy-reporting of dietary intake), as reported in other studies [18]. In the present study, participants personally reported dietary intake; thus the strength of association between child–mother dyads and child–father dyads truly reflect the environmental influence of parents on the child's DP and can be seen as an additional strength of this study. In general, the I.Family study allows a deep insight into the resemblance of DP among family members across Europe and the influence of parental DP on their child's DP when eating together or not. The large sample size comprises data from eight European countries; the strictly standardized data assessment, documentation, and data cleaning processing guarantee the highest possible data quality.

5. Conclusions

Using cluster analysis to derive dietary patterns allowed us to compare groups of European children and their parents with different dietary profiles and to examine the effect of daily number of shared meals and soft drink availability during meals on the association between child's and parental DP. The availability of soft drinks during meals and negative parental role modeling are important predictors for intake of sweet and fat foods in children. Intervention strategies should focus on healthy shopping choices. Parents as gatekeepers for home food availability and as role models for children's eating behavior should be counseled in which foods should be consumed on a regular basis and which foods should be avoided at home. Not purchasing unhealthy foods will decrease their availability at home and during meals; thus, their consumption may be hampered and may decline in parents and their children.

Acknowledgments: We gratefully acknowledge the financial support of the European Community within the Seventh RTD Framework Program Contract No. 266044. We thank the I.Family children and their parents for participating in this extensive examination. We are grateful for the support from school boards, headmasters, and communities. The publication of this article was funded by the Open Access Fund of the Leibniz Association.

Author Contributions: The authors' responsibilities were as follows—Antje Hebestreit had the idea for the analysis and wrote the paper; Antje Hebestreit and Timm Intemann had primary responsibility for the final content; Claudia Börnhorst and Timm Intemann performed the data analysis; Alfonso Siani, Stefaan De Henauw, Gabriele Eiben, Yiannis A. Kourides, Eva Kovacs, Luis A. Moreno, Toomas Veidebaum, Vittorio Krogh, Valeria Pala, Leonie H. Bogl, Monica Hunsberger, and Iris Pigeot participated in the coordination of the data collection. All authors were responsible for critical revisions and final approval of the manuscript. This manuscript represents original work that has not been published previously and is not currently being considered by another journal. If accepted, it will not be published elsewhere, including electronically in the same form, in English or in any other language, without the written consent of the copyright holder.

Conflicts of Interest: The authors declare no conflict of interest.

Appendix A

In the appendix we give details on (1) the derivation of z-scores of usual energy intake and z-scores of healthy non-alcoholic beverages and (2) on the clustering procedure. Both were conducted with the statistical software R (version 3.1.0) [54].

Appendix A.1. Derivation of z-Scores

In contrast to the intake of the food groups (measured in kcal/day) the usual energy intake (kcal/day) and usual intake of healthy non-alcoholic beverages (g/day) cannot be reasonably adjusted for total energy intake. Therefore, we decided to adjust energy intake and the percentage of intake contribution from healthy non-alcoholic beverages for age and sex as a surrogate for adjustment for total energy intake, since age and sex are strongly associated with total energy intake. We applied the Generalized Additive Models for Location, Scale, and Shape (GAMLSS) [55] in order to derive sex- and age-specific z-scores for these variables. GAMLSS allows for deriving sex- and age-specific percentile curves. Stratified by sex and separately for children and parents, such curves were estimated. By default, we used a GAMLSS model consisting of Box–Cox power exponential distribution.

The distribution parameters were modeled with penalized B-splines depending on age. If this default model did not converge or provided inadequate results, we used the Box–Cox Cole and Green distribution (BCCG) and/or cubic splines instead: For energy intake in men and intake of healthy non-alcoholic beverages in women, we used the BCCG distribution; for healthy non-alcoholic beverages in boys we used cubic splines. According to the estimated curves, values of usual energy intake and intake of healthy non-alcoholic beverages were transformed into individual z-scores.

The interpretation of the z-scores derived by GAMLSS differs slightly from the common z-scores of the food groups (measured in kcal/day): For the common z-score, a positive (negative) value indicates a value above (below) the mean percentage of energy from the specific food group, whereas for the z-scores derived by GAMLSS, a positive (negative) value indicates a value above (below) the sex- and age-specific mean. However, for both types of z-scores, the mean is zero and the standard deviation is one.

Appendix A.2. Clustering Procedure

Cluster analysis using the k-means approach by Hartigan and Wong [56] was applied to identify clusters of children and clusters of parents with similar dietary patterns. The usual intake variables (sex- and age-adjusted z-scores and energy-adjusted z-scores) were used in the cluster analysis to find clusters of children and adults with distinct dietary patterns.

Since the true number of clusters is unknown and k-means only converge to a local minimum, the k-means algorithm was applied with 50 random starts for each number of clusters from two to eight. Accordingly, out of these 50 solutions the one with the lowest total within cluster sum of squares was chosen. For these solutions the convergence criterion was reached in fewer than nine iterations. To decide on the appropriate number of clusters, all final two to eight cluster solutions were examined: since silhouette coefficients [57] and the total within cluster sum of squares did not give a clear indication for an appropriate number of clusters, the interpretability of the clusters was used as the decision criterion. The three-cluster solution was favored. To evaluate the reproducibility of the cluster solutions, we conducted a cluster analysis in a randomly chosen subsample containing 85% of subjects [58]. This was repeated 10 times for children and adults separately. Compared to the whole sample solutions, the percentage of agreement and the adjusted Rand Index (ARI) [59] were calculated for the three-cluster solutions, leading to a mean agreement of 97% (95%) and a mean ARI of 0.92 (0.87) for adults (children).

Since the dietary patterns of children and parents were very similar, the same cluster names were used. The Euclidian distances between cluster centroids among children and adults were calculated (Table A1), showing that the distances between same labeled clusters were lowest. Two examples illustrating the Euclidean distances between children's and parents' DP are given: a constant difference of 0.1 between children's and parents' z-scores leads to a distance of 0.39; a constant difference of 0.6 leads to a distance of 2.32.

Table A1. Cross-tabulation of Euclidean distances between the cluster means of children and parents.

Parents	Children, Adolescents Sweet & Fat	Ref. Cereals	Animal Products
Sweet & Fat	0.45	2.54	2.45
Ref. Cereals	2.7	0.77	2.51
Animal Products	2.48	2.25	0.49

References

1. Patrick, H.; Nicklas, T.A. A review of family and social determinants of children's eating patterns and diet quality. *J. Am. Coll. Nutr.* **2005**, *24*, 83–92. [CrossRef] [PubMed]
2. Campbell, K.J.; Crawford, D.A.; Ball, K. Family food environment and dietary behaviors likely to promote fatness in 5–6 year-old children. *Int. J. Obes. (Lond.)* **2006**, *30*, 1272–1280. [CrossRef] [PubMed]

3. Draxten, M.; Fulkerson, J.A.; Friend, S.; Flattum, C.F.; Schow, R. Parental role modeling of fruits and vegetables at meals and snacks is associated with children's adequate consumption. *Appetite* **2014**, *78*, 1–7. [CrossRef] [PubMed]
4. Brown, R.; Ogden, J. Children's eating attitudes and behaviour: A study of the modelling and control theories of parental influence. *Health Educ. Res.* **2004**, *19*, 261–271. [CrossRef] [PubMed]
5. Johnson, L.; van Jaarsveld, C.H.; Wardle, J. Individual and family environment correlates differ for consumption of core and non-core foods in children. *Br. J. Nutr.* **2011**, *105*, 950–959. [CrossRef] [PubMed]
6. Freeman, E.; Fletcher, R.; Collins, C.E.; Morgan, P.J.; Burrows, T.; Callister, R. Preventing and treating childhood obesity: Time to target fathers. *Int. J. Obes. (Lond.)* **2012**, *36*, 12–15. [CrossRef] [PubMed]
7. Robinson, L.N.; Rollo, M.E.; Watson, J.; Burrows, T.L.; Collins, C.E. Relationships between dietary intakes of children and their parents: A cross-sectional, secondary analysis of families participating in the family diet quality study. *J. Hum. Nutr. Diet.* **2014**, *28*, 443–451. [CrossRef] [PubMed]
8. Raynor, H.A.; Van Walleghen, E.L.; Osterholt, K.M.; Hart, C.N.; Jelalian, E.; Wing, R.R.; Goldfield, G.S. The relationship between child and parent food hedonics and parent and child food group intake in children with overweight/obesity. *J. Am. Diet. Assoc.* **2011**, *111*, 425–430. [CrossRef] [PubMed]
9. Hall, L.; Collins, C.E.; Morgan, P.J.; Burrows, T.L.; Lubans, D.R.; Callister, R. Children's intake of fruit and selected energy-dense nutrient-poor foods is associated with fathers' intake. *J. Am. Diet. Assoc.* **2011**, *111*, 1039–1044. [CrossRef] [PubMed]
10. Wang, Y.; Beydoun, M.A.; Li, J.; Liu, Y.; Moreno, L.A. Do children and their parents eat a similar diet? Resemblance in child and parental dietary intake: Systematic review and meta-analysis. *J. Epidemiol. Community Health* **2011**, *65*, 177–189. [CrossRef] [PubMed]
11. Fisher, J.O.; Mitchell, D.C.; Smiciklas-Wright, H.; Birch, L.L. Parental influences on young girls' fruit and vegetable, micronutrient, and fat intakes. *J. Am. Diet. Assoc.* **2002**, *102*, 58–64. [CrossRef]
12. Grimm, G.C.; Harnack, L.; Story, M. Factors associated with soft drink consumption in school-aged children. *J. Am. Diet. Assoc.* **2004**, *104*, 1244–1249. [CrossRef] [PubMed]
13. Hanson, N.I.; Neumark-Sztainer, D.; Eisenberg, M.E.; Story, M.; Wall, M. Associations between parental report of the home food environment and adolescent intakes of fruits, vegetables and dairy foods. *Public Health Nutr.* **2005**, *8*, 77–85. [CrossRef] [PubMed]
14. Martens, M.K.; van Assema, P.; Brug, J. Why do adolescents eat what they eat? Personal and social environmental predictors of fruit, snack and breakfast consumption among 12–14-year-old dutch students. *Public Health Nutr.* **2005**, *8*, 1258–1265. [CrossRef] [PubMed]
15. Ray, C.; Roos, E.; Brug, J.; Behrendt, I.; Ehrenblad, B.; Yngve, A.; Te Velde, S.J. Role of free school lunch in the associations between family-environmental factors and children's fruit and vegetable intake in four european countries. *Public Health Nutr.* **2013**, *16*, 1109–1117. [CrossRef] [PubMed]
16. Pearson, N.; Biddle, S.J.; Gorely, T. Family correlates of breakfast consumption among children and adolescents. A systematic review. *Appetite* **2009**, *52*, 1–7. [CrossRef] [PubMed]
17. Hannon, P.A.; Bowen, D.J.; Moinpour, C.M.; McLerran, D.F. Correlations in perceived food use between the family food preparer and their spouses and children. *Appetite* **2003**, *40*, 77–83. [CrossRef]
18. Oliveria, S.A.; Ellison, R.C.; Moore, L.L.; Gillman, M.W.; Garrahie, E.J.; Singer, M.R. Parent-child relationships in nutrient intake: The framingham children's study. *Am. J. Clin. Nutr.* **1992**, *56*, 593–598. [PubMed]
19. Neumark-Sztainer, D.; Story, M.; Resnick, M.D.; Blum, R.W. Correlates of inadequate fruit and vegetable consumption among adolescents. *Prev. Med.* **1996**, *25*, 497–505. [CrossRef] [PubMed]
20. Fiese, B.H.; Hammons, A.; Grigsby-Toussaint, D. Family mealtimes: A contextual approach to understanding childhood obesity. *Econ. Hum. Biol.* **2012**, *10*, 365–374. [CrossRef] [PubMed]
21. Welsh, E.M.; French, S.A.; Wall, M. Examining the relationship between family meal frequency and individual dietary intake: Does family cohesion play a role? *J. Nutr. Educ. Behav.* **2011**, *43*, 229–235. [CrossRef] [PubMed]
22. Expert Group on Health Information. The European Core Health Indicators Shortlist. Available online: http://ec.europa.eu/health/indicators/docs/echi_shortlist_by_policy_area_en.pdf (accessed on 7 February 2017).
23. Fismen, A.; Smith, O.R.F.; Torsheim, T.; Rasmussen, M.; Pagh, T.P.; Augustine, L.; Ojala, K.; Samdal, O. Trends in food habits and their relation to socioeconomic status among nordic adolescents 2001/2002-2009/2010. *PLoS ONE* **2016**, *11*. [CrossRef] [PubMed]
24. Mathieson, A.; Koller, T. *Addressing the Socioeconomic Determinants of Healthy Eating Habits and Physical Activity Levels among Adolescents*; World Health Organization: Geneva, Switzerland, 2005.

25. Pinard, C.A.; Davy, B.M.; Estabrooks, P.A. Beverage intake in low-income parent-child dyads. *Eat. Behav.* **2011**, *12*, 313–316. [CrossRef] [PubMed]

26. Ahrens, W.; Siani, A.; de Henauw, S.; Eiben, G.; Gwozdz, W.; Hebestreit, A.; Hunsberger, M.; Kaprio, J.; Krogh, V.; Lissner, L.; et al. Cohort profile: The transition from childhood to adolescence in european children-how I.Family extends the IDEFICS cohort. *Int. J. Epidemiol.* **2016**. [CrossRef] [PubMed]

27. UNESCO. International Standard Classification of Education. Available online: http://www.uis.unesco.org/Education/Documents/isced-2011-en.pdf (accessed on 7 February 2017).

28. Stomfai, S.; Ahrens, W.; Bammann, K.; Kovacs, E.; Marild, S.; Michels, N.; Moreno, L.A.; Pohlabeln, H.; Siani, A.; Tornaritis, M.; et al. Intra- and inter-observer reliability in anthropometric measurements in children. *Int. J. Obes. (Lond.)* **2011**, *35* (Suppl. S1), S45–S51. [CrossRef] [PubMed]

29. Suling, M.; Hebestreit, A.; Peplies, J.; Bammann, K.; Nappo, A.; Eiben, G.; Alvira, J.M.; Verbestel, V.; Kovacs, E.; Pitsiladis, Y.P.; et al. Design and results of the pretest of the IDEFICS study. *Int. J. Obes. (Lond.)* **2011**, *35* (Suppl. S1), S30–S44. [CrossRef] [PubMed]

30. Cole, T.J.; Freeman, J.V.; Preece, M.A. British 1990 growth reference centiles for weight, height, body mass index and head circumference fitted by maximum penalized likelihood. *Stat. Med.* **1998**, *17*, 407–429. [CrossRef]

31. Cole, T.J.; Lobstein, T. Extended international (IOTF) body mass index cut-offs for thinness, overweight and obesity. *Pediatr. Obes.* **2012**, *7*, 284–294. [CrossRef] [PubMed]

32. World Health Organization. The International Classification of Adult Underweight, Overweight and Obesity according to BMI. Available online: http://apps.who.int/bmi/index.jsp?introPage=intro_3.html (accessed on 7 February 2017).

33. Hebestreit, A.; Börnhorst, C.; Barba, G.; Siani, A.; Huybrechts, I.; Tognon, G.; Eiben, G.; Moreno, L.A.; Fernandez Alvira, J.M.; Loit, H.M.; et al. Associations between energy intake, daily food intake and energy density of foods and BMI z-score in 2–9-year-old european children. *Eur. J. Nutr.* **2014**, *53*, 673–681. [CrossRef] [PubMed]

34. Livingstone, M.B.; Robson, P.J. Measurement of dietary intake in children. *Proc. Nutr. Soc.* **2000**, *59*, 279–293. [CrossRef] [PubMed]

35. Hebestreit, A.; Barba, G.; De Henauw, S.; Eiben, G.; Hadjigeorgiou, C.; Kovacs, E.; Krogh, V.; Moreno, L.A.; Pala, V.; Veidebaum, T.; et al. Cross-sectional and longitudinal associations between energy intake and BMI z-score in european children. *Int. J. Behav. Nutr. Phys. Act.* **2016**, *13*, 23. [CrossRef] [PubMed]

36. Börnhorst, C.; Huybrechts, I.; Ahrens, W.; Eiben, G.; Michels, N.; Pala, V.; Molnar, D.; Russo, P.; Barba, G.; Bel-Serrat, S.; et al. Prevalence and determinants of misreporting among european children in proxy-reported 24 h dietary recalls. *Br. J. Nutr.* **2012**, *109*, 1257–1265. [CrossRef] [PubMed]

37. Tooze, J.A.; Midthune, D.; Dodd, K.W.; Freedman, L.S.; Krebs-Smith, S.M.; Subar, A.F.; Guenther, P.M.; Carroll, R.J.; Kipnis, V. A new statistical method for estimating the usual intake of episodically consumed foods with application to their distribution. *J. Am. Diet. Assoc.* **2006**, *106*, 1575–1587. [CrossRef] [PubMed]

38. Kipnis, V.; Midthune, D.; Buckman, D.W.; Dodd, K.W.; Guenther, P.M.; Krebs-Smith, S.M.; Subar, A.F.; Tooze, J.A.; Carroll, R.J.; Freedman, L.S. Modeling data with excess zeros and measurement error: Application to evaluating relationships between episodically consumed foods and health outcomes. *Biometrics* **2009**, *65*, 1003–1010. [CrossRef] [PubMed]

39. Lanfer, A.; Hebestreit, A.; Ahrens, W.; Krogh, V.; Sieri, S.; Lissner, L.; Eiben, G.; Siani, A.; Huybrechts, I.; Loit, H.M.; et al. Reproducibility of food consumption frequencies derived from the children's eating habits questionnaire used in the IDEFICS study. *Int. J. Obes. (Lond.)* **2011**, *35* (Suppl. S1), S61–S68. [CrossRef] [PubMed]

40. Bel-Serrat, S.; Mouratidou, T.; Pala, V.; Huybrechts, I.; Bornhorst, C.; Fernandez-Alvira, J.M.; Hadjigeorgiou, C.; Eiben, G.; Hebestreit, A.; Lissner, L.; et al. Relative validity of the children's eating habits questionnaire-food frequency section among young european children: The IDEFICS study. *Public Health Nutr.* **2014**, *17*, 266–276. [CrossRef] [PubMed]

41. Huybrechts, I.; Bornhorst, C.; Pala, V.; Moreno, L.A.; Barba, G.; Lissner, L.; Fraterman, A.; Veidebaum, T.; Hebestreit, A.; Sieri, S.; et al. Evaluation of the children's eating habits questionnaire used in the IDEFICS study by relating urinary calcium and potassium to milk consumption frequencies among european children. *Int. J. Obes. (Lond.)* **2011**, *35* (Suppl. S1), S69–S78. [CrossRef] [PubMed]

42. Drucker, R.R.; Hammer, L.D.; Agras, W.S.; Bryson, S. Can mothers influence their child's eating behavior? *J. Dev. Behav. Pediatr.* **1999**, *20*, 88–92. [CrossRef] [PubMed]

43. Turrell, G. Compliance with the australian dietary guidelines in the early 1990's: Have population-based health promotion programs been effective? *Nutr. Health* **1997**, *11*, 271–288. [CrossRef] [PubMed]

44. Orrell-Valente, J.K.; Hill, L.G.; Brechwald, W.A.; Dodge, K.A.; Pettit, G.S.; Bates, J.E. "Just three more bites": An observational analysis of parents' socialization of children's eating at mealtime. *Appetite* **2007**, *48*, 37–45. [CrossRef] [PubMed]

45. Hammons, A.J.; Fiese, B.H. Is frequency of shared family meals related to the nutritional health of children and adolescents? *Pediatrics* **2011**, *127*, e1565–e1574. [CrossRef] [PubMed]

46. Gillman, M.W.; Rifas-Shiman, S.L.; Frazier, A.L.; Rockett, H.R.; Camargo, C.A., Jr.; Field, A.E.; Berkey, C.S.; Colditz, G.A. Family dinner and diet quality among older children and adolescents. *Arch. Fam. Med.* **2000**, *9*, 235–240. [CrossRef] [PubMed]

47. Cullen, K.W.; Baranowski, T.; Rittenberry, L.; Olvera, N. Social-environmental influences on children's diets: Results from focus groups with african-, euro- and mexican-american children and their parents. *Health Educ. Res.* **2000**, *15*, 581–590. [CrossRef] [PubMed]

48. Birch, L.L. Children's preferences for high-fat foods. *Nutr. Rev.* **1992**, *50*, 249–255. [CrossRef] [PubMed]

49. Boutelle, K.N.; Fulkerson, J.A.; Neumark-Sztainer, D.; Story, M.; French, S.A. Fast food for family meals: Relationships with parent and adolescent food intake, home food availability and weight status. *Public Health Nutr.* **2007**, *10*, 16–23. [CrossRef] [PubMed]

50. Trofholz, A.C.; Tate, A.D.; Draxten, M.L.; Neumark-Sztainer, D.; Berge, J.M. Home food environment factors associated with the presence of fruit and vegetables at dinner: A direct observational study. *Appetite* **2016**, *96*, 526–532. [CrossRef] [PubMed]

51. Hebestreit, A.; Keimer, K.M.; Hassel, H.; Nappo, A.; Eiben, G.; Fernandez, J.M.; Kovacs, E.; Lasn, H.; Shiakou, M.; Ahrens, W. What do children understand? Communicating health behavior in a european multicenter study. *J. Public Health* **2010**, *18*, 391–400. [CrossRef]

52. Subar, A.F.; Freedman, L.S.; Tooze, J.A.; Kirkpatrick, S.I.; Boushey, C.; Neuhouser, M.L.; Thompson, F.E.; Potischman, N.; Guenther, P.M.; Tarasuk, V.; et al. Addressing current criticism regarding the value of self-report dietary data. *J. Nutr.* **2015**, *145*, 2639–2645. [CrossRef] [PubMed]

53. Greenland, P.; Robins, J.M. Confounding and misclassification. *Am. J. Epidemiol.* **1985**, *122*, 495–506. [PubMed]

54. R Core Team. *R: A Language and Environment for Statistical Computing*; R Foundation for Statistical Computing: Vienna, Austria, 2014.

55. Stasinopoulos, D.M.; Rigby, R.A. Generalized additive models for location scale and shape (GAMLSS) in R. *J. Stat. Softw.* **2007**, *23*, 1–46. [CrossRef]

56. Hartigan, J.A.; Wong, M.A. Algorithm AS 136: A k-means clustering algorithm. *Appl. Stat.* **1979**, *28*, 100–108. [CrossRef]

57. Rousseeuw, P.J. Silhouettes: A graphical aid to the interpretation and validation of cluster analysis. *J. Compl. Appl. Math.* **2015**, *20*, 53–65. [CrossRef]

58. Lo, S.G.; Yasui, Y.; Csizmadi, I.; McGregor, S.E.; Robson, P.J. Exploring statistical approaches to diminish subjectivity of cluster analysis to derive dietary patterns: The Tomorrow Project. *Am. J. Epidemiol.* **2011**, *173*, 956–967.

59. Hubert, L.; Arabie, P. Comparing partitions. *J. Classif.* **1985**, *2*, 193–218. [CrossRef]

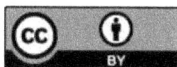

![nutrients logo] *nutrients*

MDPI

Review

Relationship between Long Chain *n*-3 Polyunsaturated Fatty Acids and Autism Spectrum Disorder: Systematic Review and Meta-Analysis of Case-Control and Randomised Controlled Trials

Hajar Mazahery [1], Welma Stonehouse [2], Maryam Delshad [1], Marlena C. Kruger [3], Cathryn A. Conlon [1], Kathryn L. Beck [1] and Pamela R. von Hurst [1,*]

[1] Massey Institute of Food Science and Technology, School of Food and Nutrition, Massey University, Auckland 0745, New Zealand; h.mazahery@massey.ac.nz (H.M.); delshad.maryam@yahoo.com (M.D.); c.conlon@massey.ac.nz (C.A.C.); k.l.beck@massey.ac.nz (K.L.B.)
[2] Commonwealth Scientific Industrial Research Organisation (CSIRO) Food, Nutrition and Bioproducts, Adelaide SA 5000, Australia; welma.stonehouse@csiro.au
[3] Massey Institute of Food Science and Technology, School of Food and Nutrition, Massey University, Palmerston North 4410, New Zealand; m.c.kruger@massey.ac.nz
* Correspondence: p.r.vonhurst@massey.ac.nz; Tel.: +64-9-213-6657

Received: 9 December 2016; Accepted: 13 February 2017; Published: 19 February 2017

Abstract: Omega-3 long chain polyunsaturated fatty acid supplementation (*n*-3 LCPUFA) for treatment of Autism Spectrum Disorder (ASD) is popular. The results of previous systematic reviews and meta-analyses of *n*-3 LCPUFA supplementation on ASD outcomes were inconclusive. Two meta-analyses were conducted; meta-analysis 1 compared blood levels of LCPUFA and their ratios arachidonic acid (ARA) to docosahexaenoic acid (DHA), ARA to eicosapentaenoic acid (EPA), or total *n*-6 to total *n*-3 LCPUFA in ASD to those of typically developing individuals (with no neurodevelopmental disorders), and meta-analysis 2 compared the effects of *n*-3 LCPUFA supplementation to placebo on symptoms of ASD. Case-control studies and randomised controlled trials (RCTs) were identified searching electronic databases up to May, 2016. Mean differences were pooled and analysed using inverse variance models. Heterogeneity was assessed using I^2 statistic. Fifteen case-control studies ($n = 1193$) were reviewed. Compared with typically developed, ASD populations had lower DHA (-2.14 [95% CI -3.22 to -1.07]; $p < 0.0001$; $I^2 = 97\%$), EPA (-0.72 [95% CI -1.25 to -0.18]; $p = 0.008$; $I^2 = 88\%$), and ARA (-0.83 [95% CI, -1.48 to -0.17]; $p = 0.01$; $I^2 = 96\%$) and higher total *n*-6 LCPUFA to *n*-3 LCPUFA ratio (0.42 [95% CI 0.06 to 0.78]; $p = 0.02$; $I^2 = 74\%$). Four RCTs were included in meta-analysis 2 ($n = 107$). Compared with placebo, *n*-3 LCPUFA improved social interaction (-1.96 [95% CI -3.5 to -0.34]; $p = 0.02$; $I^2 = 0$) and repetitive and restricted interests and behaviours (-1.08 [95% CI -2.17 to -0.01]; $p = 0.05$; $I^2 = 0$). Populations with ASD have lower *n*-3 LCPUFA status and *n*-3 LCPUFA supplementation can potentially improve some ASD symptoms. Further research with large sample size and adequate study duration is warranted to confirm the efficacy of *n*-3 LCPUFA.

Keywords: meta-analysis; omega-3; long chain polyunsaturated fatty acids; concentration; intervention; autism; symptoms

---

1. Introduction

The prevalence of Autism Spectrum Disorder (ASD) has dramatically increased over the past few years. While previous prevalence studies of ASD identified less than 10 in 10,000 individuals [1], recent estimates suggest rates of 90 to 250 in 10,000 individuals [2–5]. ASD is a life-long neurodevelopment disorder that appears during the first years of life [6]. Depending on the child's predominant symptomatology, children with ASD exhibit difficulties with expressing and understanding certain emotions, understanding others' mood, expressive language, and maintaining normal eye contact, as well as preference for minimal changes to routine, restricted ways of using toys and isolated play, all of which make it difficult for individuals to establish relationships with others, to act in an appropriate way and to live independently [6]. In addition, children with ASD frequently experience behaviour problems and medical conditions, including inflammation, oxidative stress, and autoimmune disorders [7–12], and altered brain structure and function (in a subset of individuals) [13,14]. The rising ASD rates are ascribed, in part, to a complex interaction between multiple genes and environmental risk factors [15], among which omega-3 long chain polyunsaturated fatty acids (*n*-3 LCPUFAs) is a strong candidate. LCPUFAs and their metabolic products have been implicated in ASD via their roles in brain structure and function, neurotransmission, cell membrane structure and microdomain organisation, inflammation, immunity and oxidative stress [16–20].

Blood polyunsaturated fatty acids (plasma, serum, red blood cell (RBC), and whole blood) levels are considered reliable biomarkers of their status [21]. Abnormality in blood levels of *n*-3 LCPUFA has been reported in psychiatric disorders including, but not limited to, attention deficit hyperactivity disorder (ADHD) and ASD [22–24]. Explanations for such abnormalities have been suggested to be lower dietary intake of *n*-3 LCPUFAs, and disturbances in fatty acid metabolism and incorporation of these fatty acids into cellular membranes in autistic populations compared to healthy controls [24–26]. A smattering of reports indicate differences in *n*-3 LCPUFAs, *n*-6 LCPUFAs and/or *n*-6 to *n*-3 LCPUFA ratios between populations with autism and healthy controls [14,26], but a few also failed to show any differences [27,28]. The reason for such discrepancies is not well examined, and there have been no attempts to systematically compare these studies. Hence, systematic analysis and synthesis of the evidence are warranted to determine if there are any differences in these blood fatty acids levels among healthy and individuals with ASD, and if so, whether *n*-3 LCPUFA supplementation may be beneficial in reducing symptoms in ASD.

To our knowledge, the efficacy of *n*-3 LCPUFA supplementation in ASD has been investigated by six open-label trials [29–34] and one case study [35], the majority of which (six out of seven studies) showed significant improvement in symptoms of ASD (Table S1). Despite this promising evidence, randomised controlled trials (RCTs) examining the beneficial effect of *n*-3 LCPUFAs in reducing symptoms of ASD have yielded inconclusive results. For example, Amminger et al. (2007) showed that supplementation with *n*-3 LCPUFA (EPA + DHA) was superior over placebo in reducing stereotypy, inappropriate speech and hyperactivity [36], while Mankad et al. (2015) failed to show any effect of *n*-3 LCPUFA supplementation on autism severity symptoms, adaptive functioning, externalizing behaviour or verbal ability [37].

To date, two systematic reviews of interventions with *n*-3 LCPUFA in ASD have been published [38,39]. In the review by Bent et al., published in 2009, authors set broad inclusion criteria and included all intervention trials of *n*-3 LCPUFAs of any type, dose, and duration addressing core and associated symptoms of ASD [38]. They identified six studies; one randomised controlled trial, four open-label trials and one case-study and concluded that the evidence was insufficient to support clinical recommendations [38].

Two years later, James, Montgomery and Williams (2011) published a Cochrane review including only two RCTs and performing meta-analyses on three primary outcomes (social interaction, communication and stereotypy) and one secondary outcome (hyperactivity) [39]. The authors reached the same conclusion as the Bent et al. review [38], and identified four ongoing studies. At the time of writing this review, the findings of one trial was published [37], one was terminated in 2014 (NCT01248130), and no information was available regarding the recruitment status or the availability of data for two trials (NCT00467818 and NCT01260961).

An updated systematic review is timely; more studies are now available, the prevalence of ASD is increasing together with a greater interest in the medical community (health professionals) on the beneficial effect of *n*-3 LCPUFA in the treatment of neurodevelopment disorders, as well as an increasing interest in using complementary and alternative medication in this population [40]. We aimed to conduct a current examination of evidence. We designed two systematic reviews and meta-analyses;

- Meta-analysis 1: a meta-analysis of evidence regarding blood *n*-3 LCPUFA levels in populations with ASD compared to typically developing counterparts (with no neurodevelopmental disorders) of any age and sex. A secondary aim for meta-analysis 1 was to perform a priori subgroup analysis to investigate the influence of ASD on fatty acid composition across different age groups (studies including only young children vs. studies also including children, teenagers, and adults).
- Meta-analysis 2: a meta-analysis of randomised controlled trials of *n*-3 LCPUFA supplementation (of any type, dose and duration) in ASD populations (of any age and sex) to assess the clinical efficacy of *n*-3 LCPUFAs treatment in reducing core symptoms of ASD and co-existing conditions.

2. Materials and Methods

All study procedures for both meta-analyses were pre-defined, but have not been registered or published elsewhere.

2.1. Eligibility Criteria

For meta-analysis 1, we included case-control observational studies that examined the differences in blood fatty acid levels between populations with ASD and healthy typically developing controls (with no neurodevelopmental disorders) of any age and sex. Studies were excluded it they included non-typically developing controls, were non-English or unpublished. Because DHA, EPA and ARA are amongst the most reported fatty acids of *n*-3 LCPUFAs and *n*-6 LCPUFAs categories, respectively, and have been shown to be more biologically active in the brain and been linked to neurodevelopment disorders, we focused on these fatty acids as well as the ratio of ARA to EPA and DHA and the ratio of *n*-6 LCPUFA to *n*-3 LCPUFA [41,42]. We included studies that reported LCPUFA in various blood fractions expressed as either % of total fatty acids or in concentration units, including RBC, serum, plasma, plasma phospholipids and whole blood [21]. These fractions have been shown to be reliable markers for the general fatty acid pool [21].

For meta-analysis 2, we included RCTs of any dose, type, and duration of *n*-3 LCPUFAs in participants with ASD of any age and sex who were randomised to receive either intervention or placebo, and reporting one of the following outcome measures: core symptoms of ASD including social interaction, communication, and repetitive restrictive behaviours or interests (RRB), and symptoms or behaviours associated with ASD including hyperactivity, irritability, sensory issues, and gastrointestinal symptoms. Unpublished and non-English studies were excluded.

Meta-analyses were performed if at least two studies employed the same assessment tool to measure the outcome of interest. There is a large variability in outcome assessment methods in ASD studies [43]. This use of different tools not only compromises the validity of a study by increasing the likelihood of type 1 error [44], but also complicates an effective comparison across studies.

2.2. Search Methods for Identification of Studies

We searched PubMed, MEDLINE, Web of Science, CINAHL, PsycINFO, PsycARTICLES and PsycNET up to May, 2016 to identify relevant studies in English. We employed broad search terms to include all potential studies that may fall within each of the mentioned reviews. The search strategy used the following terms: ("omega 3" OR "omega3" OR "omega-3" OR "polyunsaturated fatty acids" OR "polyunsaturated fatty acid" OR "essential fatty acids" OR "essential fatty acid") AND ("autism" OR "autistic" OR "autism spectrum disorder" OR "Asperger"). We also reviewed the reference lists of all identified studies to identify additional studies. Results from each database were downloaded into EndNote (version X6, 2012, Thomson Reuters, Philadelphia, PA, USA). Duplicates were removed and abstracts were screened. When an abstract met the eligibility requirements, it was assigned to one of two meta-analyses and the full article was read to ensure the inclusion and exclusion criteria were met. The study identification was done by one investigator (H.M.).

2.3. Data Extraction, Management, and Quality Assessment

Two reviewers (H.M. and M.D.) independently performed data extraction from each study into pre-piloted extraction tables. Discrepancies in the data extraction were resolved by discussion and reaching consensus.

The following data were extracted for both meta-analyses: author, date of publication and setting, sources of funding, conflict of interest, aims, objectives and hypothesis, and population characteristics while extractions specific to each meta-analyses are described below.

For meta-analysis 1, the following data were also extracted: the mean and SD for blood *n*-3 LCPUFAs (DHA, EPA or total), *n*-6 LCPUFAs (ARA or total), and for *n*-6 to *n*-3 LCPUFA ratios (ARA to DHA, ARA to EPA, or total *n*-6 to total *n*-3 LCPUFA), fatty acid analysis method, the body tissue in which the fatty acid was measured, the unit of measure, and the significance value. If a study reported LCPUFA in two different blood tissues, the priority was given to RBC, followed by plasma phospholipids, serum/plasma, and whole blood. While RBC and plasma phospholipids LCPUFA reflects long-term fatty acid intake, serum/plasma or whole blood LCPUFA are influenced by recent intake of these fatty acids [21,45]. If a study reported both relative and absolute measures, the former measures were included in the meta-analysis to limit the methodological heterogeneity. The method by which blood fatty acid composition is expressed (relative vs. absolute) has been shown to modify the LCPUFA—disease relationship [46]. Inter-study variation in extraction and separation efficiencies in fatty acid analyses can be overcome by relative expression of fatty acids (expressed as a percentage of a fatty acid normalised to the total amount of all measured fatty acids in a sample) [46]. If more than two groups were included, only relevant groups were selected. A quality appraisal was performed in duplicate by two investigators (H.M. and M.D.) using the "Health Canada Quality Appraisal Tools for Observational Studies" [47]. A quality score of ≤ 6 was considered lower quality [47]. No studies were excluded based on quality scores, but sensitivity analysis was performed to assess the impact of these studies on the overall results.

For meta-analysis 2, study design, intervention (the dose of intervention was converted, where required, to gram from milligram for easy comparison), delivery method, compliance, intervention period, outcome measures, assessment tools, results, conclusion, potential confounders and assessment of bias risk following Cochrane bias risk assessment including selection, performance, detection, attrition, reporting and commercial bias were also extracted [48]. A further quality appraisal was performed in duplicate by two investigators (H.M. and M.D.) using the "Health Canada Quality Appraisal Tools for Randomised Controlled Trials" to assess the quality of the individual studies [47]. A quality score of ≤ 7 was considered lower quality [47].

2.4. Statistical Analysis

Both meta-analyses were performed using Review Manager (RevMan, version 5.3, The Nordic Cochrane Centre, Copenhagen, Denmark).

2.4.1. Meta-Analysis 1

For each outcome, the mean and SD for each study group (cases and controls) was entered into Review Manager. If *n*-3 to *n*-6 fatty acid (total *n*-3 to *n*-6 LCPUFA, EPA to ARA or DHA to ARA) was reported, the ratio was converted to *n*-6/*n*-3 (1/ratio). The Review Manager calculator (between group differences) was employed to calculate the SD for these reverse ratios. The reverse ratio and SD were calculated for five studies [49–53].

The primary meta-analysis compared mean differences (95% confidence intervals (CI)) in outcomes across study groups. Due to significant heterogeneity a random effects model was used to calculate the forest plots with standardised mean differences and 95% CI. Standardised mean differences were calculated because blood levels of LCPUFA were measured and reported in different ways. A combination of Chi^2-statistic ($p < 0.1$), I^2 statistics (I^2 0%–40%, low; 30%–60%, moderate; 50%–90%, substantial; 75%–100%, considerable heterogeneity), and considering the variation of point estimates and the overlap of CIs across different studies was performed to measure heterogeneity [48].

To avoid false positive or negative results, we limited the number of subgroup analyses to one (stratified by age) and sensitivity analyses to three (blood tissue type, study quality, and author's calculations). Then a priori subgroup analysis was performed using Chi^2-statistic with a p value of <0.05 taken to indicate statistical significance [48]. We could not conduct meta-regression to investigate the impact of the potential mediators (location, sex, and the way by which fatty acid composition is expressed) due to the limited study numbers. To include one mediator in the analysis, at least 10 studies are required [48]. These variables were however carefully examined when the results were interpreted. Publication bias was examined using funnel plots in which the SE of the studies were plotted against their corresponding effect sizes.

2.4.2. Meta-Analysis 2

For each outcome, the mean change and SD of change from baseline to endpoint for each intervention group (n-3 LCPUFA and placebo) was entered into Review Manager. If only baseline and end data were available the mean change was calculated by deducting the baseline from the end value, and the SD was then imputed from a mean correlation coefficient for an outcome from other studies in the meta-analysis. Standard deviations were calculated for one study [54]. Study authors were contacted for missing data, and if no response was received the data was not included in the meta-analysis. Data was unable to be retrieved for three studies [55–57].

The primary meta-analyses compared mean (95% CI) differences (net change in scores) in each domain between n-3 LCPUFA and control groups. Heterogeneity between studies was small hence a fixed-effects model was used to calculate forest plots with mean differences and 95% CI. Heterogeneity between studies was indicated using the same analyses employed in meta-analysis 1. No subgroup analyses or meta-regression were performed due to limited number of studies included in the meta-analysis. However, one sensitivity analysis was performed to evaluate the impact of calculations (SDs) and major methodological differences on heterogeneity and the overall results. Publication bias was not assessed due to the small number of studies included in this meta-analysis.

3. Results

From the initial searches, 510 articles and from the cross-reference check, five articles were retrieved. Titles and abstracts of 254 articles were screened after non-English and duplicates were removed. At this level, 216 were excluded as not relevant to the current topic. The remaining 38 articles were read and categorised into two groups; 24 articles into the case-control studies group and 15 into the intervention group (Figure 1, PRISMA Flow Diagram).

3.1. Systematic Review and Meta-Analysis 1

Of the 24 articles identified for meta-analysis 1, 15 were included in the meta-analysis. Reasons for exclusion were: not a case-control design [58,59], inappropriate control [25], the data not reported in a form suitable for analysis [26,60–62], and double-reporting [63,64]. Characteristics of included studies can be found in Table 1.

The majority of studies were conducted in the Middle East (n = 5; 2 Saudi Arabia (from one study group), 1 Oman, 2 Egypt) and Europe (n = 4; 2 UK, 1 Belgium, 1 Italy), with others conducted in the US (n = 2), Latin America (n = 1), Canada (n = 1), Asia (Japan, n = 1), and Australia (n = 1).

The 15 studies included 623 children and young people with ASD and 570 controls. Most studies included children under the age of 12, while a few included teenagers and adults also (n = 3) [24,49,53]. One study included adults up to age 22 years [49]. Cases and controls were matched on both age and sex (*n* = 8), two of which included other attributes such as IQ, home environment and dietary intake (*n* = 1) or geographical region (*n* = 1). Others matched two groups on either age (*n* = 3) or sex (*n* = 1), and one study included only males. Matching of cases and controls was not reported in two studies. In those studies including both sexes and reporting the sex distribution, the male/female ratio ranged from 2/1 to 12/1.

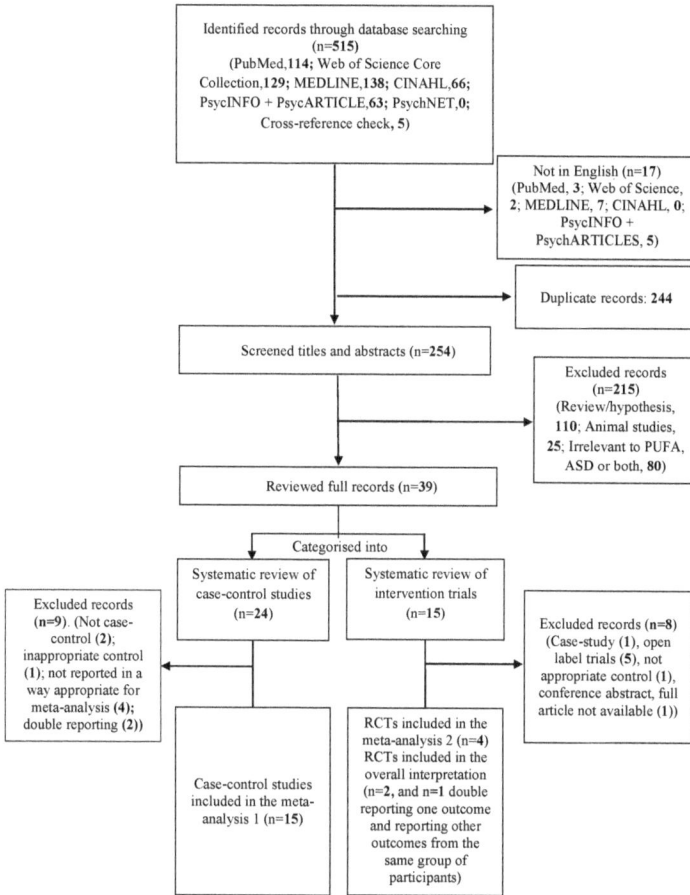

Figure 1. Flow diagram for selection of studies (PRISMA flow diagram).

Most studies did not report the fasting state of blood samples while one study analysed non-fasting blood samples, and five studies fasting blood sample (ranging from 2 h to overnight fasting) [28,49–51,65]. Fasting state is considered to affect fatty acid composition measured in plasma/serum but not in RBC [21,45]. While most studies reported serum/plasma fatty acid composition, four studies reported RBC levels [24,28,52,66] and two reported both [27,51]. Most studies reported relative levels while five studies reported absolute levels (all from the Middle East) [26,30,50,65,67], and one both levels [53]. Sensitivity analysis showed no impact of blood tissue type and the way by which fatty acid composition is expressed on the heterogeneity. However, the way by which fatty acid composition is expressed affected the overall effect size for some measures (Refer to the next section).

Table 1. Characteristics of case-control studies included in meta-analysis 1.

Reference and Setting	Cases Characteristics				Controls Characteristics					Blood Tissue Type	Outcome		FA and Ratios Compared and the Direction of Difference	Quality Score [†]
	N	Condition, Classification System, Tools [δ]	Age (Years) *	Sex (M, F)	N	Health Condition	Age (Years) *	Sex (M, F)	Matching		Fasting State (Length)	Values Reported as		
Al-Farsi (2013) [67] Oman	40	Autism, based on DSM-IV, NR	4.1 (0.9)	NR	40	Healthy and TD	4.1 (0.8)	NR	Age Sex	Serum	NR	μg/mL	DHA ↓	6
Bell (2004) [66] UK	29	11 classical autism and 18 regressive autism, NR, NR	NR	NR	55	Healthy and TD	NR	NR	None	RBC	NR	% of total FA	Total n3 ↓ DHA ↓ EPA ↓ Total ↔ ARA ↔ ARA/EPA ↑	4
Bell (2010) [27] UK	45	Autism, based on DSM-IV and ICD-10, ADI-R	7.5 (3.5)	39 M, 5 F	52	Healthy and TD	7.5 (3.6)	49 M, 3 F	Age Sex (45 pairs matched)	RBC Plasma	NR	% of total FA	Total n3 ↑ ↔ DHA ↔ EPA ↔ Total ↔ ARA ↔ Total n6/n3 2↑ ARA/EPA ↑	8
Brigandi (2015) [24] US	121	Autism (but not Asperger or PDD-NOS), based on DSM-IV, CARS	3–17 **	NR	110	Non autistic and developmentally delayed	3–17 **	NR	NR	RBC	No	% of total FA	Total n3 ↓ DHA ↓ EPA ↔ Total n6 ↓ ARA ↓ Total n6/n3 2↑	6
Bu (2006) [28] US	40	Autism and regressive autism, based on DSM-IV and ICD-10, ADI-R and ADOS	3.6 ***	37 M, 3 F	20	TD	3.5 ***	16 M, 4 F	Age Sex Geographical residential area	RBC	Yes (2 h)	% of total FA	Total n3 ↔ DHA ↔ EPA ↔ Total ↔ ARA ARA/EPA ↔	8
El-Ansari (2011a) [50] Saudi	25	Autism, NR, ADI-R, ADOS, 3di	4–12 **	NR	16	Healthy and TD	4–11 **	NR	Age	Plasma	Yes (10 h)	mmol/L	ARA/DHA ↓	7
El-Ansari (2011b) [65] Saudi Arabia	22	Autism, NR, ADI-R, ADOS, 3di	4–12 **	NR	26	Healthy and TD	4–11 **	NR	Age	Plasma	Yes (10 h)	mmol/L	DHA ↓ EPA ↔ ARA ↓	7
Ghezz (2013) [14] Italy	21	Autism, DSM-IV, ADOS and CARS	6.8 (2.2)	17 M, 4 F	20	Healthy and TD	7.6 (1.9)	14 M, 6 F	Age Sex	Serum	NR	% of total FA	DHA ↓ EPA ↓ ARA ↔ Total n6/n3 ↑	11
Jory (2016) [51] Canada	11	Autism, DSM (version NR), NR	3.9 (1.7)	8M, 3F	15	Healthy and TD	3.9 (1.1)	6 M, 9 F	Age	RBC Serum	Yes (NR)	% of total FA	DHA ↑ EPA ↓ ARA ↓ Total n6/n3 ↑ ARA/DHA ↔ ARA/EPA ↔	7
Meguid (2008) [30] Egypt	30	Autism, DSM-IV, clinical evaluations and CARS	3–11 **	18 M, 12 F	30	Healthy and TD	NR	NR	Age Sex	Whole blood	NR	μg/mL	DHA ↓ ARA ↓ ARA/DHA ↓	7

Table 1. Cont.

Reference and Setting	Cases Characteristics				Controls Characteristics				Matching	Outcome				Quality Score †
	N	Condition, Classification System, Tools δ	Age (Years) *	Sex (M, F)	N	Health Condition	Age (Years) *	Sex (M, F)		Blood Tissue Type	Fasting State (Length)	Values Reported as	FA and Ratios Compared and the Direction of Difference	
Mostafa (2015) [26] Egypt	80	Autism, DSM-IV, clinical evaluation and CARS	7.4 (3.3)	66 M, 14 F	80	Healthy and TD	7.3 (3.1)	66 M, 14 F	Age Sex	Plasma	NR	mmol/L	DHA ↓ ARA ↓ ARA/DHA ↓	8
Parletta (2016) [52] Australia	85	Autism, clinical evaluation and CARS	5.3 (2.1) ˄	68 M, 17 F	79	Healthy and TD	8.3 (2.5) ˄	61 M, 18 F	Sex	RBC	NR	% of total FA	DHA ↓ EPA ↓ ARA ↓ Total n6/n3 ↑ ARA/EPA ↑	9
Sliwinski (2006) [49] Belgium	18	Autism with IQ > 55 and post pubertal, DSM-IV, ADI-R	12–20 **	Only male	22	TD post pubertal	12–22	Only male	None	Plasma	Yes (overnight)	% of total FA	Total n3 ↑ DHA ↑ EPA ↔ Total n6 ↔ ARA ↔ Total n6/n3 ↓	8
Tostes (2013) [68] Brazil	24	Autism, DSM-IV, clinical evaluation	7.4 (2.9)	18M, 6F	24	Healthy and TD	7.2 (1.8)	18 M, 6 F	Age sex	Plasma	NR	% of total FA	DHA ↓ EPA ↓ ARA ↑ ARA/DHA 3 ↑ ARA/EPA 3 ↑	9
Yui (2016) [53] Japan	28	Autism with IQ/70, DSM-IV, ADI-R	13.5 (4.7)	20M, 8F	21	Healthy and TD	13.9 (5.7)	15 M, 6 F	Age Sex IQ Eating habit Home environment	Plasma	NR	% of total FA and μg/mL	DHA 4 ↑ EPA ↑ ARA ↓ ARA/DHA ↓ ARA/EPA ↓	8

δ Psychological assessment tools used to confirm ASD diagnosis. * Reported as mean (SD) unless otherwise stated. † Health Canada Quality Appraisal Tool for Observational Studies; A quality score of ≥7 was considered higher quality [47]. ** Inclusion criteria. *** Median. ˄ Significantly different. ↓ Cases had lower levels than controls (p < 0.05). ↑ Cases had higher levels than controls (p < 0.05). ↔ No difference across groups (p > 0.05). 1 RBC values are reported. 2 A borderline significance. 3 The significance was not reported. 4 % of total fatty acids is reported. ADI-R, Autism Diagnostic Interview-Revised; ADOS, Autism Diagnostic Observation Schedule; ARA, arachidonic acid; CARS, Childhood Autism Rating Scale; DHA, docosahexaenoic acid; DSM-IV, Diagnostic and Statistical Manual of Mental Disorder-Fourth Edition; EPA, eicosapentaenoic acid; F, female; FA, fatty acids; M, male; N, number of participants; NR, not reported; RBC, red blood cell; TD, typically developing; 3di, the Developmental, Dimensional, and Diagnostic Interview.

The majority of studies reported DHA, EPA and ARA levels while two studies did not report levels of EPA [26,67], and one ARA [67]. Five studies reported both total *n*-3 LCPUFA and total *n*-6 LCPUFA levels. One study did not report either of the mentioned measures but the ratio of ARA to DHA and ARA to EPA [50]. Total *n*-6/*n*-3 LCPUFA ratio was reported in six studies, of which two reported ARA/EPA ratio [27,52], and one reported both ARA/EPA and ARA/DHA also [51]. Of the remaining studies, two reported the ratio of ARA/EPA [28,66] and ARA/DHA each [26,30], one both [53], and three no ratios [65,67,68]. Reverse ratios and SDs were calculated in five studies ([50] (only the ARA to EPA) and [49,51–53]). With the exception of one study [50] (refer to the next section), sensitivity analysis showed no impact of calculation on the overall results.

All studies included in the review scored between four and nine points out of a possible 11 in our quality assessment tool, with three studies scoring ≤ 6 [24,66,67] (Table S2). It should be noted that the maximum score for the "Health Canada Quality Appraisal Tools for Observational Studies" is 12 [47] but because "measuring the exposure in duplicate or more" is of no relevance for case-control studies and all studies received a score of "0" for this criterion, the maximum score adds up to 11 for this review. Studies with scores of ≥7 are considered having higher quality. Sensitivity analysis showed no impact of removing studies with a quality score ≤6 on the heterogeneity or overall results.

The quality criteria failed by most studies were attrition and the reasons for attrition. Although attrition is not important for case-control studies, it could be of relevance to ASD clinical studies. Drop out of some populations with particular characteristics such as high anxiety levels or sensory issues (a distinct criterion under RRB domain in ASD diagnosis [6]) that are associated with fear of blood test and consequently inability to obtain a blood sample or withdrawal from a study could affect the external validity of a study. The most prevalent confounding factors that were not controlled for in statistical analysis were dietary intake of LCPUFA and medication use. No conflict of interest that may have affected study outcomes was apparent in any study.

3.1.1. Individual *n*-3 LCPUFA (DHA, EPA, and ARA) and Their Ratios (ARA to DHA and ARA to EPA)

Significant differences were seen between those studies that recruited children only vs. those that also included teenagers and adults for blood levels of DHA and EPA (Chi^2 = 11.78, *p* = 0.0006 and Chi^2 = 7.02, *p* = 0.008, respectively) but not ARA (Chi^2 = 1.49, *p* = 0.22) (Figure 2). Hence results for DHA and EPA for these subgroups were described separately. For ARA, the results described are from all studies combined.

Overall, in the younger age group studies, ASD children had significantly lower DHA and EPA levels than typically developing controls (standardised mean difference (95% CI) −2.14 [−3.22, −1.07], Z = 3.91, *p* < 0.0001 and −0.72 [−1.25, −0.18], Z = 2.64, *p* = 0.008, respectively). Considerable heterogeneity was seen for DHA (I^2 = 97%, *p* < 0.00001) and EPA (I^2 = 88%, *p* < 0.00001). Heterogeneity for DHA was not altered by removing any studies. Heterogeneity for EPA reduced slightly by removing the Parletta, 2016 study [52] (I^2 = 74%, *p* = 0.0008). Removal of this study together with the Tostes, 2013 study [68] significantly reduced heterogeneity for EPA (I^2 = 0%, *p* = 0.78) that was accompanied by a reduction in the difference between cases and controls (−0.30 [−0.51, −0.08], Z = 2.73, *p* = 0.006, *n* = 356). These two studies were different with respect to some characteristics that may affect outcomes compared to other studies; children with ASD were significantly younger than typically developing children in the Parletta, 2016 study [52], and 88% of children with ASD in the Tostes, 2013 study were on psychotropic drugs [68].

In studies including all age groups (children, teenagers, and adults), no significant differences were seen in DHA and EPA levels between cases and controls (0.28 [−0.59, 1.16] and 0.27 [−0.23, 0.76], respectively). Heterogeneity for DHA and EPA was substantial (I^2 = 90%, *p* = 0.0001 and I^2 = 68%, *p* = 0.04, respectively). Removal of the Brigandi, 2015 study [24] reduced the heterogeneity significantly for DHA (I^2 = 0%, *p* = 0.65) and slightly for EPA (I^2 = 64%, *p* = 0.10). Removal of this study resulted in children with ASD having significantly higher DHA (0.69 [0.26, 1.12], Z = 3.13, *p* = 0.002, *n* = 89) levels than typically developing controls but no impact on EPA. The Brigandi, 2015 study [24] was different from the other two studies in this subgroup in that both classic and regressive type ASD were included, cases and controls were not matched by any attributes, intellectual functioning of patients was not considered, and this study had a low quality appraisal score. The Sliwinski, 2006 [49] and Yui, 2016 [53] studies included ASD patients with a borderline or normal intellectual functioning (IQ > 70). The results should be interpreted with caution because the number of studies included is small ($n = 3$).

With regard to ARA, children with ASD had significantly lower ARA levels than typically developing controls (-0.83 [-1.48, -0.17], $Z = 2.48$, $p = 0.01$), but heterogeneity between studies was substantial ($I^2 = 96\%$, $p = 0.00001$). Heterogeneity was not reduced by excluding any single study. However, removing studies that reported absolute levels [26,30,65] resulted in a smaller overall effect estimate (-0.24 [-0.88, 0.41], $Z = 0.71$, $p = 0.48$, $n = 840$).

Only one study that included all age groups (children, teenagers, and adults) reported either ARA/DHA or ARA/EPA [53] thus the combined results of older and younger children are described (Figure 3). The ratio of ARA/DHA and ARA/EPA did not differ significantly between ASD populations and typically developing controls ($p = 0.94$ and $p = 0.09$, respectively). The heterogeneity was considerably high for both ratios. Heterogeneity was not reduced by excluding any studies (both ARA/DHA and ARA/EPA). With regard to ARA/EPA, however, the overall effect estimate changed considerably by the removal of El-Ansary, 2011a study [50] (0.99 [0.32, 1.67], $Z = 2.88$, $p = 0.004$, $I^2 = 91\%$). Cases and controls were not matched on sex in this study, the reverse ratio and SD was calculated, and the absolute level was reported.

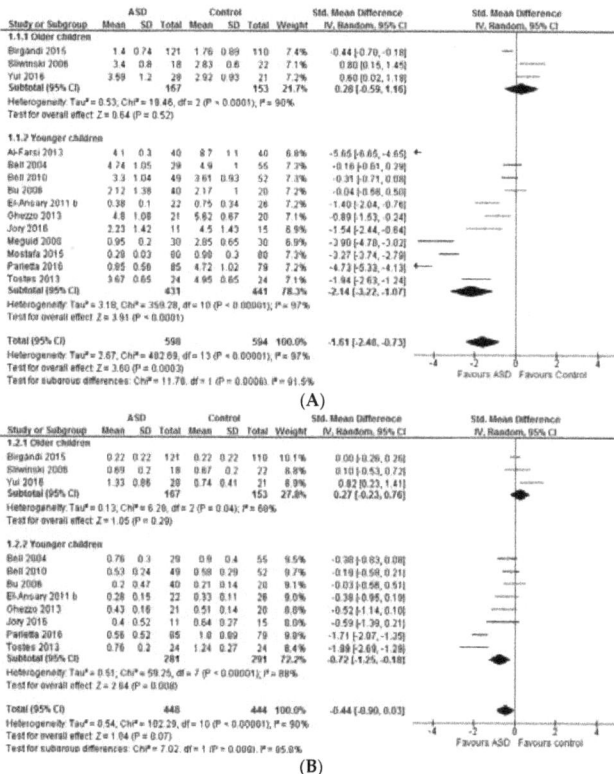

(A)

(B)

Figure 2. *Cont.*

(C)

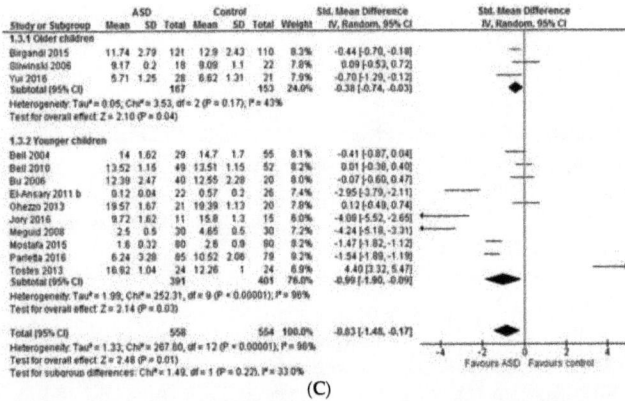

Figure 2. Forest plots of mean (95% confidence interval (CI)) weighted difference in blood levels of docosahexaenoic acid (DHA) (**A**); eicosapentaenoic acid (EPA) (**B**); and arachidonic acid (ARA) (**C**) between populations with Autism Spectrum Disorder (ASD) and typically developing controls stratified for subgroups with studies including all age groups (children, teenagers, and adults) vs. those including children only. Direction of effect (negative, lower mean in ASD group; positive, lower mean in control group; zero, no difference between groups).

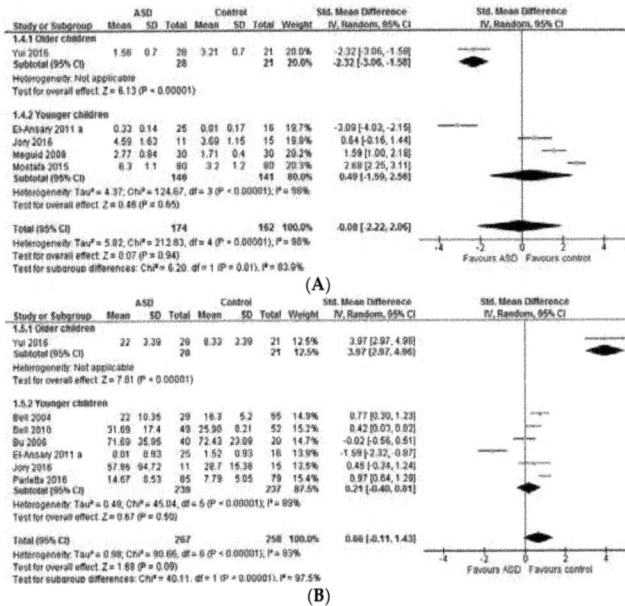

(A)

(B)

Figure 3. Forest plots of mean (95% confidence interval (CI)) weighted difference in the ratio of arachidonic acid (ARA) to docosahexaenoic acid (DHA) (**A**) and the ratio of ARA to eicosapentaenoic acid (EPA) (**B**) between populations with Autism Spectrum Disorder (ASD) and typically developing children stratified for subgroups with studies including all age groups (children, teenagers, and adults) vs. young children only. Direction of effect (negative, lower mean in ASD group; positive, lower mean in control group; zero, no difference between groups).

3.1.2. Total *n*-3 and *n*-6 LCPUFA and Their Ratios

No significant differences were observed in total *n*-3 and *n*-6 LCPUFA between studies including young children only and those including all age groups (children, teenagers, and adults) (Chi^2 = 0.70, *p* = 0.40 and Chi^2 = 3.84, *p* = 0.05, respectively) thus the results for the combined groups are described (Figure 4).

The pooled standard mean differences for the total *n*-3 LCPUFA and total *n*-6 LCPUFA between ASD and typically developing children were −0.16 [−0.54, 0.21] (I^2 = 73%, substantial heterogeneity) and 0.57 [−0.19, 1.33] (I^2 = 93%, considerable heterogeneity), respectively. Both were not statistically significant. Excluding comparisons that included teenagers and adults also [24,49] reduced heterogeneity in total *n*-3 LCPUA (I^2 = 42%, *p* = 0.18) (−0.34 [−0.68, 0.01], *Z* = 1.88, *p* = 0.06, *n* = 245). Heterogeneity was reduced to an acceptable level when the Sliwinski, 2006 study [49] only was removed (I^2 = 14%, *p* = 0.32) (−0.36 [−0.56, −0.15], *Z* = 3.40, *p* = 0.0007, *n* = 472). The Sliwinski, 2006 study [49] was different from other studies with respect to several characteristics; it included post pubertal youngsters up to age 22 years, it was a male-only study, and included those with an IQ > 55. Heterogeneity in total *n*-6 LCPUFA was not altered by the removal of any studies.

The ratio of total *n*-6 LCPUFA to *n*-3 LCPUFA did not differ significantly between studies including young children only and those including all age groups (children, teenagers, and adults) (Chi^2 = 3.04, *p* = 0.08) thus the overall results are described here (Figure 5). Children with ASD had a significantly higher *n*-6 LCPUFA to *n*-3 LCPUFA ratio (0.42 [0.06, 0.78], *Z* = 2.27, *p* = 0.02). The heterogeneity was substantial and was decreased by the exclusion of comparisons that also included teenagers and adults [24,49] (I^2 = 29%, *p* = 0.24). The difference between cases and controls as well as the effect size increased considerably, 0.65 [0.36, 0.94], *Z* = 4.43, *p* < 0.00001, *n* = 328.

The funnel plots for DHA and ARA, indicated publication bias with a lack of smaller studies [studies with larger standard errors (SEs)] reporting negative results. Examination of funnel plot for EPA indicated no evidence of publication bias.

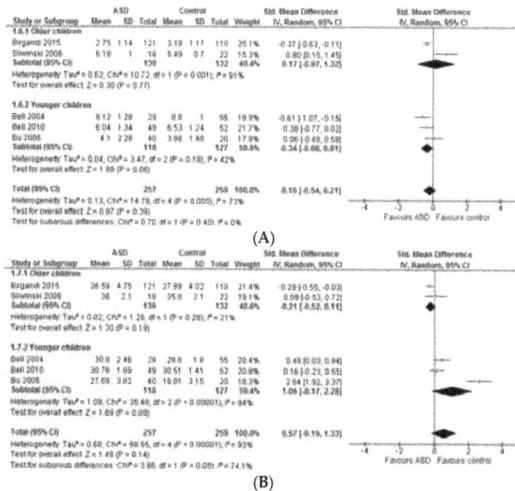

Figure 4. Forest plots of mean (95% confidence interval (CI)) weighted difference in the total *n*-3 long chain polyunsaturated fatty acids (*n*-3 LCPUFA) (**A**) and total *n*-6 long chain polyunsaturated fatty acids (*n*-6 LCPUFA) (**B**) between populations with Autism Spectrum Disorder (ASD) and typically developing children stratified for subgroups with studies including all age groups (children, teenagers, and adults) vs. young children only. Direction of effect (negative, lower mean in ASD group; positive, lower mean in control group; zero, no difference between groups).

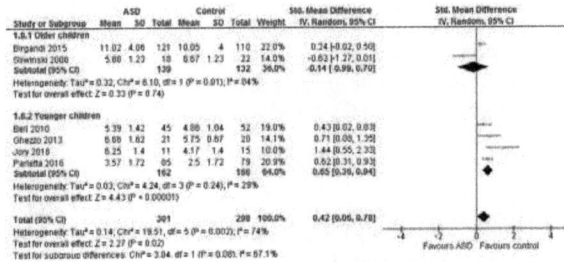

Figure 5. Forest plot of mean (95% confidence interval (CI)) weighted difference in the ratio of total *n*-6 long chain polyunsaturated fatty acids (*n*-6 LCPUFA) to total *n*-3 long chain polyunsaturated fatty acids (*n*-3 LCPUFA) between populations with Autism Spectrum Disorder (ASD) and typically developing children stratified for subgroups with studies including all age groups (children, teenagers, and adults) vs. young children only. Direction of effect (negative, lower mean in ASD group; positive, lower mean in control group; zero, no difference between groups).

3.2. Systematic Review and Meta-Analysis 2

Of the 15 RCTs identified for systematic review and meta-analysis 2, four were included in the meta-analysis [36,54,69,70], two were included in the overall interpretation but not included in the meta-analysis [37,55], one was a double-reporting of one outcome [54] and reporting other outcomes from the same group of participants [57], and eight were excluded (Figure 1). Reasons for not being included in the meta-analysis 2 but being included in the overall interpretation were: data not reported in a format suitable for analysis [55], and use of an assessment tool not used by others [37]. Reasons for complete exclusion were: a conference paper with unpublished results at the time of writing this review [56], one open label randomised parallel intervention trial including a low sugar healthy diet as the control [29], and not being a RCT (*n* = 6, one case-study and 5 open label trials [30–35]). Characteristics of included studies can be found in Table 2 and of excluded studies in Table S1.

Of those included in the meta-analysis 2, two were conducted in the US [69,70], one in Austria [36], and one in Japan [54]. In the four studies, 55 participants with ASD received *n*-3 LCPUFA supplements and 52 received placebo. The Bent, 2011 and 2014 studies included children under the age of 8 years [69,70], the Amminger, 2007 study included children under 17 years [36], and the Yui, 2011 study included children older than 6 years and adults up to 28 years [54].

Of the two studies that could not be included in the meta-analysis, one study was from the US [55] and one from Canada [37] together including 37 and 34 individuals in the intervention and placebo groups, respectively. Children under the age of 5 and 10 years were included in the Mankad, 2015 and Voigt, 2014 studies, respectively [37,55].

All but one (the Amminger, 2007 study included only males [36]) included both males and females. Study groups were not matched on sex in these trials. The male to female ratio ranged from 3/1 to 12/1.

Of the RCTs included in the meta-analysis 2, the severity of autism at baseline was not considered in two trials [36,70], and the other two included patients with pre-defined severity (moderate severity and ABC social withdrawal subscale of >10 in the Bent, 2011 and Yui, 2011 studies, respectively) and IQ level (>50 and >80 in the Bent, 2011 and Yui, 2011 studies, respectively [54,69]). Of those included in the overall interpretation, the Voigt, 2014 study included patients with pre-defined severity (CARS score of >30 [55] and the Mankad, 2015 study equally distributed the severity across groups [37]. Co-existing problem behaviour was an inclusion criteria in two trials entered the meta-analysis 2 (hyperactivity in the Amminger, 2007 [36] and Bent, 2014 studies [70]).

Study length ranged from 6–16 weeks in RCTs included in the meta-analysis 2 and was 26 weeks in RCTs included in the overall interpretation. The majority of participants were supplemented with both EPA and DHA. The Yui, study (2011 and 2012) [54,57] used a combination of DHA and AA and the Voigt, 2014 study used only DHA [55]. Intake of EPA and DHA ranged from 0.70 to 0.84 g/day and 0.24

to 0.70 g/day, respectively, with the Yui, 2011 (and 2012) and Voigt, 2014 studies having the lowest DHA dose [54,55,57]. The Mankad, 2015 study reported an initial total dose of EPA and DHA of 0.75 g/day for two weeks which was doubled when tolerability to that dose was determined [37]. Placebos used were olive oil [37,54,57], safflower oil [69,70], corn oil + soybean oil [55], and coconut oil [36].

Behaviours were assessed using a variety of assessment tools (ranging from one to six tools used in each study) including, Aberrant Behaviour Checklist (ABC) ([36,54,55,69,70] but the outcome was not reported), Social Responsiveness Scale (SRS) [57,69,70], Behaviour Assessment System for Children (BASC) [37,55,69], Clinical Global Impression (CGI) [37,55,69,70], and further several tools that were used in isolation. Of these, full data was available for only four studies using the same assessment tool (ABC) [36,54,69,70].

All studies included in the review were of good quality, scoring 11–14 points out of a possible 15 (Table S3). Studies with scores of >7 are considered as having higher quality.

The quality criteria failed by most studies were whether intention-to-treat or per-protocol analysis was conducted (though according to final sample size analysed—larger than the sample size with drop outs deducted—it was apparent that the majority employed intention-to-treat analysis), and controlling for potential confounders. The most prevalent potential confounding factors that were not reported or reported but not considered in statistical analysis were dietary intake of LCPUFA or baseline LCPUFA status (as a measure of LCPUFA status, either dietary intake or blood level of LCPUFA needs to be reported).With the exception of the Bent, 2011 study [69] which investigated the impact of baseline LCPUFA status on behavioural changes in response to supplementation, the majority of studies failed to examine such a relationship while assessing baseline LCPUFA status [37,54,55,57]. Further factors were compliance (not reported in most studies) and medical regimen (most studies recruited patients on a stable medical regimen but did not report the type of regimen and its distribution across groups). It is also worth noting that a small number of females were included in these studies (with a male/female ratio ranging from 1/3 to 1/12) which could be a limitation in terms of generalisability, though reflecting the gender distribution of ASD.

The risk of bias for each study is summarized in Figure S1. Participants in the Amminger, 2007 and Yui 2011 (and 2012) studies were reported to be randomised but no details were available for random sequence generation [36,54,57]. Other studies used computer generated number [69,70] and block randomisation stratified by attributes including severity [37] and sex [55]. With the exception of the Amminger, 2007 study [36], randomisation was prepared by a third party in all trials [37,54,55,57,69,70]. The Amminger, 2007 provided no details regarding who performed the randomization [36]. All studies were reported as double-blinded (both researchers/assessors and participants) [37,54,55,57,69,70]. However, in the Amminger, 2007 study it is unclear if the researchers/assessors were blinded [36]. It is also unclear when researchers/assessors and participants were unblinded in the Amminger, 2007, Yui, 2011 (and 2012), and Mankad, 2015 studies [36,37,54,57]. The blinding was kept for the entire study (including data analyses) in the Bent, 2011, Bent 2014, and Voigt, 2014 studies [55,69,70]. With the exception of the Yui, 2011 (and 2012, no drop outs) [54,57] and Bent, 2014 (all included in the final analyses) [70] studies, participants were lost to follow up in the Amminger, 2007 (one individual from control) [36], Mankad, 2015 (one individual from *n*-3 LCPUFA group) [37], Bent 2011 (two individuals; one from each arm) [69], and Voigt, 2014 (five from *n*-3 LCPUFA and nine from control) [55] studies. The reason for drop outs in the Voigt, 2014 study were difficulty with participation (four from *n*-3 LCPUFA and three from control), trouble taking the supplements (one from *n*-3 LCPUFA and three from control), and concerns about supplement side effects (three from control) [55]. Regarding the latter concern, it is not clear if participants withdrew due to worsening behaviour, not observing any improvement, or because of an actual side effect during the intervention. With the exception of the Voigt, 2014 study [55], all outcomes in all trials were reported. The Voigt, 2014 study examined 52 behavioural subscales but only three outcomes were reported [55]. It is worth noting that the primary outcome was the measure of CGI which was completely reported. Other sources of bias including commercial bias were not apparent in any study.

Table 2. Study characteristics of randomised controlled trials (RCTs) included in systematic literature review.

Reference and Setting	Age (Years)	Sex Distribution (M, F)	Sample size	Intervention Active	Placebo	Duration	Outcome Measure	Outcome	Quality Score †
				RCTs included in Meta-Analysis 2 (n = 4)					
Amminger (2007) [36] Austria Pilot	5–17	All male	Intervention (n = 7) Placebo (n = 6, 1 lost)	0.84 g/day EPA 0.7 g/day DHA	7 g/day coconut oil	6 weeks	ABC	No significant differences between groups at 6 weeks, but a greater change in hyperactivity and stereotypy subscale with a large effect size in the omega-3 group than placebo (7 and 2.4 units, effect size of 0.71 and 0.72, respectively). Well tolerated and safe.	10
Ben (2011) [69] US Pilot	3–8	24 M, 3 F	Intervention (n = 14, 1 lost and 4discontinued) Placebo (n = 13, 1 lost and 2 discontinued)	0.7 g/day EPA 0.46 g/day DHA	Orange flavoured pudding containing safflower oil	12 weeks	ABC PPVT EVT BASC SRS CGI-S	Significant increase in the percentage of serum omega-3 fatty acids. No significant differences in all measure across groups. Non-significant greater improvement in hyperactivity subscale in omega-3 group than placebo (2.7 vs. 0.3 units, effect size of 0.38). Decreases in some fatty acids correlated with decreased in hyperactivity. Well tolerated and safe.	13
Bent (2014) [70] US Internet-based	5–8	50 M, 7 F	Intervention (n = 29, 8 discontinued and 2 improper enrolment) Placebo (n = 28, 4 discontinued and 1 improper enrolment)	0.7 g/day EPA 0.46 g/day DHA	Orange flavoured pudding containing safflower oil	6 weeks	ABC-(parent and teacher) SRS CGI-I	No significant differences in changes in SRS and CGI-I between groups. Non-significant greater improvement in hyperactivity subscale in omega-3 group than placebo (−5.3 vs. −3.4, effect size of 0.26). Significantly greater improvements in stereotypy and lethargy subscales (p = 0.05 and 0.01, respectively). Well tolerated and safe.	13
Yui (2011 and 2012) * [54,57] Japan Pilot	6–28	12 M, 1 F	Intervention (n = 7) Placebo (n = 6)	0.24 g/day DHA 0.24 g/day AA	Olive oil	16 weeks	ABC ADI-R SRS	Significant increase in plasma AA. No differences in plasma DHA and EPA. Significant improvement in social withdrawal subscale of ABC (p = 0.04) and stereotyped and repetitive behaviours of ADI-R (p = 0.04). Significant improvement in communication subscale of SRS reported in both treatment and placebo groups, though the effect size was more favourable for the treatment group than placebo group (0.87 vs. 0.44, respectively). Safe.	10

Table 2. *Cont.*

RCTs Not included in the Meta-Analysis 2 but included in the Overall Interpretation (*n* = 2)

Reference and Setting	Age (Years)	Sex Distribution (M, F)	Sample Size	Intervention Active	Placebo	Duration	Outcome Measure	Outcome	Quality Score †
Mankad (2015) [37] Canada	2–5	27 M, 10 F	Intervention (*n* = 19, 4 drop outs) Placebo (*n* = 19, 2 drop outs) Stratified by severity	1.5 g/day EPA + DHA	Refined olive oil in medium chain triglyceride	6 months	PDDBI BASC-2 CGI-I VABS-II PLS-4	No significant differences between groups in all measures at 6 months, but mild improvement in BASC-2 externalising subscale in placebo but worsening in omega-3 group (−3 vs. 3, respectively; *p* = 0.02) Relatively well tolerated and safe.	13
Voigt (2014) [55] US	3–10	40 M, 8 F	Intervention (*n* = 24, 5 discontinued) Placebo (*n* = 24, 9 discontinued) Stratified by age	0.2 g/day DHA	0.25 g/day corn oil + 0.25 g/day soybean oil	6 months	CGI-I CDI ABC BASC	431% increase in plasma phospholipid DHA No significant differences in the percentage with a positive response (CGI-I) across groups and in all other measures across groups. Well tolerated and safe.	13

† Health Canada Quality Appraisal Tool for Experimental Studies; A quality score of ≥8 was considered higher quality [47]. * Different outcomes from the same group of participants were reported in two different papers. AA, arachidonic acid; ABC, Aberrant Behaviour Checklist; ADI-R, Autism Diagnostic Interview-Revised; BASC, Behaviour Assessment System for Children; CDI, Child Development Inventory; CGI-I, Clinical Global Impression-Improvement; CGI-S, Clinical Global Impression-Severity; DHA, docosahexanoic acid; EPA, eicosapentanoic acid; EVT, Expressive Vocabulary Test; F, Female; M, Male; n, Number; PDDBI, Pervasive Developmental Disorders Behavioural Inventory; PLS-4, Preschool Language Scale; PPVT, Peabody Picture Vocabulary Test; SRS, Social Responsiveness Scale; US, United States; VABS-II, Vineland Adaptive Behaviour Scale.

3.2.1. Effect of *n*-3 LCPUFA on Core Symptoms of ASD

Social interaction: The fixed mean difference for social interaction (assessed using ABC) significantly favoured *n*-3 LCPUFA with small effect (−1.96 [−3.5, −0.34], Z = 2.37, *p* = 0.02) and no heterogeneity (I^2 = 0%, *p* = 0.92) (Figure 6A). Removing the Yui, 2011 study [54] did not change the results. The Yui, 2011 study [54] differs from others in that their sample included older participants (2–28 years) and those with IQ > 50, the daily dose of DHA was lower (0.24 g/day) and ARA (0.24 g/day) was added to the supplement, they used different dosing regimens for different age groups (half a dose for children aged 6–10 years) and SD was imputed resulting in a substantially greater SD in the *n*-3 LCPUFA group compared to the placebo group and other studies. Using SRS social interaction sub-domains (social motivation, social cognition, and social awareness), the Bent, 2014 study [70] found no effect of *n*-3 LCPUFA on social interaction (all domains > 0.05). Similarly, the Yui, 2012 study [57] did not find any effect of *n*-3 LCPUFA on any sub-domains of social interaction (measured by SRS, all *p* > 0.05). The social interaction in response to intervention did not differ across groups in the Mankad, 2015 study [37] where the authors used other assessment tools. The mean change scores decreased (showing an improvement) in both treatment groups in these studies. Voigt et al. (2014) found a significant difference in BASC social skills, favouring *n*-3 LCPUFA (−0.2 vs. 3.0, *p* = 0.04), which disappeared after correction for multiple comparisons [55].

Communication: Communication scores (assessed using ABC) did not differ between *n*-3 LCPUFA and placebo groups (−0.38 [−1.33, 0.56], *p* = 0.42) (Figure 6B). Moderate heterogeneity was seen in the meta-analysis for communication (I^2 = 51%, *p* = 0.11). Removing the Yui, 2011 study [54] reduced the heterogeneity to 0% but had no impact on the overall result. Bent et al. (2011) and Bent et al. (2014) also used other tools including Peabody Picture Vocabulary Test (PPVT), Expressive Vocabulary Test (EVT) and the communication sub-domain of SRS, respectively [69,70]. Neither study found any effect of *n*-3 LCPUFA on communication. Similarly, the Mankad, 2015 study [37] did not find any differences across groups and the Voigt, 2014 study [55] reported worsened outcome (reported by teachers) in response to *n*-3 LCPUFA supplementation compared to placebo that showed improvement (1.4 vs. −4.5, *p* = 0.02). However, the Yui, 2012 study [57] found greater improvements in SRS communication sub-scale scores in *n*-3 LCPUFA group than the placebo group (−23.6 vs. −20.6, *p* = 0.03).

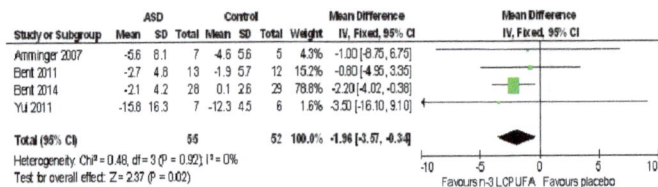

(A)

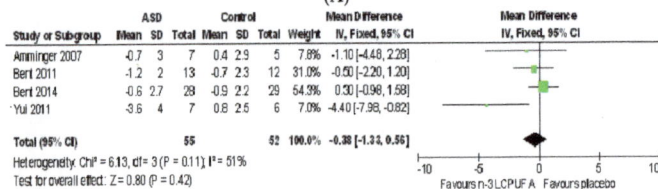

(B)

Figure 6. *Cont.*

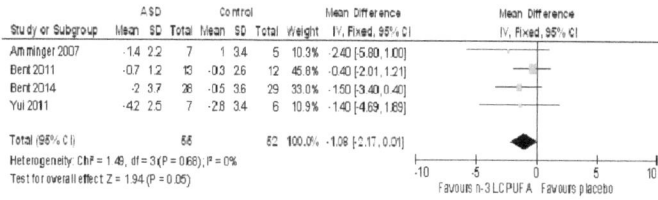

	ASD			Control				Mean Difference	Mean Difference
Study or Subgroup	Mean	SD	Total	Mean	SD	Total	Weight	IV, Fixed, 95% CI	IV, Fixed, 95% CI
Amminger 2007	-1.4	2.2	7	1	3.4	5	10.3%	-2.40 [-5.80, 1.00]	
Bent 2011	-0.7	1.2	13	-0.3	2.6	12	45.8%	-0.40 [-2.01, 1.21]	
Bent 2014	-2	3.7	28	-0.5	3.6	29	33.0%	-1.50 [-3.40, 0.40]	
Yui 2011	-4.2	2.5	7	-2.8	3.4	6	10.9%	-1.40 [-4.69, 1.89]	
Total (95% CI)			55			52	100.0%	-1.09 [-2.17, -0.01]	

Heterogeneity: Chi² = 1.49, df = 3 (P = 0.68); I² = 0%
Test for overall effect: Z = 1.94 (P = 0.05)

Favours n-3 LCPUFA   Favours placebo

(C)

Figure 6. Forest plot of mean (95% confidence interval (CI)) fixed difference in change in social interaction (ABC) (**A**); communication (ABC) (**B**); and repetitive and restricted interests and behaviours (ABC) (**C**) in populations with Autism Spectrum Disorder (ASD) receiving *n*-3 long chain polyunsaturated fatty acid supplementation (LCPUFA) and placebo. Direction of effect (negative, more improvement in *n*-3 LCPUFA groups; positive, more improvement in placebo group; zero, no difference between groups).

Repetitive and restricted interests and behaviours: The fixed mean difference for RRB (assessed using ABC) favoured *n*-3 LCPUFA with small effect (-1.08 [-2.17, -0.01], $Z = 1.94$, $p = 0.05$) (Figure 6C) and nil heterogeneity ($I^2 = 0\%$, $p = 0.68$). Removing the Yui, 2011 study [54] removed the significance ($p = 0.08$) perhaps due to low statistical power. Using the Autism Diagnostic Interview-Revised (ADI-R) scale, Yui et al. (2011) also reported a significant improvement in one of four RRB sub-domains, stereotyped and repetitive motor movement (-1.7 vs. -0.7, $p = 0.04$). However, Bent et al. (2014), using the RRB sub-domain of SRS, reported a trend favouring placebo, -2.9 ± 12.0 (placebo) vs. -8.6 ± 11.4 (*n*-3 LCPUFA), $p = 0.08$ [70]. Neither Yui et al. (2012) (using SRS RRB subscale) nor Mankad et al. (using Pervasive Developmental Disorders Behavioural Inventory (PDDBI) resistance to change subscale) showed an effect of *n*-3 LCPUFA intervention on RRB ($p > 0.05$) [37,57]. The mean scores improved in both treatment groups in these studies.

3.2.2. Effect of LCPUFA on Co-Existing Conditions

Hyperactivity: Hyperactivity scores (assessed using ABC) did not differ between treatment groups (-2.13 [-4.89, 0.62], $p = 0.13$) (Figure 7A) and heterogeneity was nil ($I^2 = 0\%$, $p = 0.98$). Sensitivity analysis by removing studies including older participants [36,54] had no effect on the overall result. Similarly, using BASC hyperactivity sub-domain, the Bent, 2011 study [69] did not find any difference between groups ($p = 0.83$). Using the BASC externalizing behaviour scale, Mankad et al. (2015) reported a significantly worsened outcome in response to *n*-3 LCPUFA supplementation compared to placebo (3.2 vs. -3.0, $p = 0.02$) [37]. It should be noted that BASC externalizing behaviour is a composite measure of hyperactivity, aggression and conduct problem. The authors suggested that greater pre-existing gastrointestinal distress at baseline (8/19 vs. 1/19, in the *n*-3 LCPUFA group vs. placebo group) may have predisposed the *n*-3 LCPUFA group to higher externalizing behaviour.

Irritability: Irritability scores (assessed using ABC) did not differ between groups (0.13 [-2.08, 2.34], $p = 0.91$) (Figure 7B) and heterogeneity was nil ($I^2 = 0\%$, $p = 1.00$). Sensitivity analysis by removing studies including older participants [36,54] had no effect on the overall result.

Sensory issues: The Mankad, 2015 study [37] was the only study that assessed the effect of *n*-3 LCPUFA supplementation on sensory issues (using sensory/perceptual approach behaviour domain of PDDBI). Sensory symptoms comparably improved in both study groups. It should be noted that this domain has five clusters, all of which tap into a variety of repetitive behaviours.

Gastrointestinal symptoms: The Mankad, 2015 study [37] was the only study that assessed the effect of the intervention on gastrointestinal distress and found no differences across treatment groups ($p > 0.9$) (assessed using CGI-I).

Publication bias could not be determined for any outcome measures due to small number of studies included in the meta-analysis (*n* = 4).

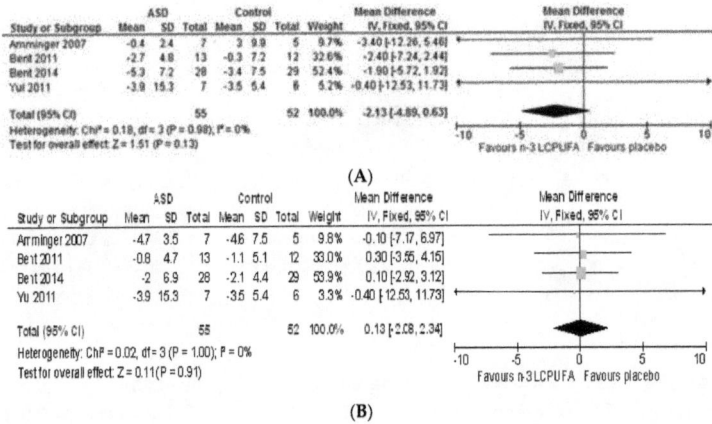

Study or Subgroup	ASD Mean	SD	Total	Control Mean	SD	Total	Weight	Mean Difference IV, Fixed, 95% CI
Amminger 2007	-0.4	2.4	7	3	9.9	5	9.7%	-3.40 [-12.26, 5.46]
Bent 2011	-2.7	4.8	13	-0.3	7.2	12	32.6%	-2.40 [-7.24, 2.44]
Bent 2014	-5.3	7.2	28	-3.4	7.5	29	52.4%	-1.90 [-5.72, 1.92]
Yui 2011	-3.9	15.3	7	-3.5	5.4	6	5.2%	-0.40 [-12.53, 11.73]
Total (95% CI)			55			52	100.0%	-2.13 [-4.89, 0.63]

Heterogeneity: Chi² = 0.18, df = 3 (P = 0.98); I² = 0%
Test for overall effect: Z = 1.51 (P = 0.13)

Favours n-3 LCPUFA   Favours placebo

(**A**)

Study or Subgroup	ASD Mean	SD	Total	Control Mean	SD	Total	Weight	Mean Difference IV, Fixed, 95% CI
Amminger 2007	-4.7	3.5	7	-4.6	7.5	5	9.8%	-0.10 [-7.17, 6.97]
Bent 2011	-0.8	4.7	13	-1.1	5.1	12	33.0%	0.30 [-3.55, 4.15]
Bent 2014	-2	6.9	28	-2.1	4.4	29	53.9%	0.10 [-2.92, 3.12]
Yu 2011	-3.9	15.3	7	-3.5	5.4	6	3.3%	-0.40 [-12.53, 11.73]
Total (95% CI)			55			52	100.0%	0.13 [-2.08, 2.34]

Heterogeneity: Chi² = 0.02, df = 3 (P = 1.00); I² = 0%
Test for overall effect: Z = 0.11 (P = 0.91)

Favours n-3 LCPUFA   Favours placebo

(**B**)

Figure 7. Forest plot of mean (95% confidence interval (CI)) fixed difference in change in hyperactivity (ABC) (**A**) and irritability (ABC) (**B**) in populations with Autism Spectrum Disorder (ASD) receiving *n*-3 long chain polyunsaturated fatty acid supplementation (*n*-3 LCPUFA) and placebo. Direction of effect (negative, more improvement in *n*-3 LCPUFA group; positive, more improvement in placebo group; zero, no difference between groups).

3.2.3. Tolerability and Safety of LCPUFA Supplementation

All RCTs included in this review concluded that LCPUFA supplementation was well tolerated and safe. Adverse effects reported were not serious and were comparable across treatment groups.

4. Discussion

The findings of each meta-analysis are individually discussed (starting with a discussion of findings of meta-analysis 1 and then meta-analysis 2) followed by a discussion on potential mechanistic pathways that might underlie the relationship between LCPUFA and ASD.

4.1. Systematic Review and Meta-Analysis 1

The current study (meta-analysis 1), to our knowledge, is the first meta-analysis of case control studies of blood fatty acid levels in populations with ASD. The findings of this study were that children with ASD had lower levels of DHA, EPA, and higher total *n*-6 LCPUFA to *n*-3 LCPUFA ratio, but not ARA to DHA and ARA to EPA ratios, compared to typically developing children. However, the differences were only evident in studies that included children only and not in studies with wide age ranges that also included adolescents and adults. One should be cautious to make conclusions regarding the modulating effect of age on the relationship since the number of studies including homogenous samples of adolescents and homogenous samples of adults are limited.

Herein we compare the findings of the current study with those of meta-analyses in ADHD because there is an overlap in symptoms between ASD and ADHD. Our results are in agreement with recently published meta-analyses showing lower *n*-3 LCPUFA levels, with larger effect size when DHA and EPA within each study were pooled than when these fatty acids were separately considered [71], and higher ratios of *n*-6 LCPUFA to *n*-3 LCPUFA [42] in patients with ADHD compared with healthy controls.

Another finding of the current study is that while the majority of included studies were of high quality, there was large methodological and clinical heterogeneity between studies, highlighting the importance of discussing the results in light of the study and population characteristics. The type of blood tissue in which the fatty acid composition is analysed has been suggested to affect the findings of case-control studies [27,51]. Bell et al. (2010) and Jory (2016) compared plasma/serum fatty acid composition with those of RBC [27,51]. The authors found significantly lower LA [27], ARA, DHA, and EPA [51] and higher *n*-6 LCPUFA to *n*-3 LCPUFA ratio [51] in RBC of autistic children compared with healthy controls. No polyunsaturated fatty acids in Bell et al.'s study [27] and only DHA in Jory's study [51] were found to be significantly different across groups when plasma/serum were compared. However, sensitivity analysis in the current study revealed no effect of removing studies that reported RBC fatty acids on heterogeneity.

The method by which blood fatty acid composition is expressed (relative vs. absolute) has also been shown to alter the findings of case-control studies investigating the fatty acid composition across groups and to modify the LCPUFA—disease relationship [46,53]. Yui et al. (2016) compared relative levels of plasma fatty acids with the same fatty acids expressed as absolute [53]. The authors found a significant difference in DHA, EPA, DPA, and arachidic acid, and the ratios of ARA to DHA and ARA to EPA (the reverse ratios were reported) across groups when relative levels were expressed. However, the significance disappeared for DHA and arachidic acid when absolute levels were compared. Although the removal of those studies reporting absolute levels had no impact on the heterogeneity, it resulted in the loss of significance across groups for ARA and in a significantly higher ARA to EPA in populations with ASD than typically developing controls. These findings highlight the importance of taking the method by which blood fatty acid composition is expressed into account when blood fatty acid profile is investigated. A potential explanation for such findings could be the inter-study variation in extraction and separation efficiencies in fatty acid analysis [46].

The high heterogeneity reported in this meta-analysis could also be explained by populations' characteristics. The role of age and sex on fatty acid status has been well documented [60,72,73]. Using a linear model, Wiest et al. (2009) demonstrated that ARA level was modified by sex; while ARA level did not differ between male autistic children and healthy controls, female autistic children had significantly lower ARA than healthy controls [60]. Thus, an uneven distribution of age (particularly if a wide age range is included) and sex across groups could alter the results in different ways; mask the difference, change the effect direction, or influence the effect size, all of which may contribute to heterogeneity seen in this study. Lack of effect in the Bell, 2004 study (EPA, DHA, and ARA) [66], change of direction in the El-Ansary, 2011a (ARA/EPA and ARA/DHA ratios) and 2011b (ARA), and Sliwinski, 2006 studies (total *n*-3 LCPUFA, DHA, and total *n*-6/*n*-3 LCPUFA ratio) [49,50,65], and the large effect size in the Parletta, 2016 study (EPA, DHA, ARA and their ratios) [52] may be explained by such characteristics.

The use of psychotropic medication can be another modifier. Psychotropic medications such as rispiradone may affect RBC fatty acid composition through their effect on oxidative stress and lipid peroxidation [23,74]. The Parletta, 2016 study [52] together with the Tostes, 2013 study [68] resulted in high levels of heterogeneity in EPA. ASD children in the former study were significantly younger than typically developing children [52], and approximately 88% of children with ASD in the Tostes, 2013 study were on psychotropic medication [68].

Location is another factor that may modify the fatty acid composition–autism relationship. With reference to those studies included in this meta-analysis, the Yui, 2016 [53] and Sliwinski, 2006 [49] were conducted in Japan and Belgium (among European countries) where the habitual dietary intake of fish and fish products are potentially high [75]. Both studies reported the autistic population having significantly higher DHA and EPA levels and lower *n*-6 to *n*-3 LCPUFA ratio than healthy controls, and both affected heterogeneity largely [49,53]. High consumption of *n*-3 LCPUFA rich foods can mask the difference, and in populations who are potentially prone to disturbances in fatty acid metabolism can alter the effect direction [49,53].

Altered fatty acid composition in ASD has been suggested to be, in part, due to low dietary intake of LCPUFA. Children with ASD have very limited food preferences that may result in these children having limited intake of LCPUFA rich foods [67]. Only three studies included in this meta-analysis assessed the dietary intake of fatty acids [14,53,67]. Al-Farsi, 2013 reported a lower intake of ALA, assessed using a semi-quantitative food frequency questionnaire, in children with ASD than healthy controls [0.8 (0.2) vs. 1.2 (0.4) g/day, $p = 0.001$] [67]. However, Ghezzo et al. (2013) [14] and Yui et al. (2016) [53] found no difference in LCPUFA intake across groups, pointing to the facts that these abnormalities could be due to disturbances in fatty acid metabolism rather than intake. For a brief discussion on the potential mechanistic pathways of LCPUFA in ASD refer to Section 4.3 (Potential mechanistic pathways).

4.2. Systematic Review and Meta-Analysis 2

Few RCTs have been completed and reported to date on *n*-3 LCPUFA supplementation for ASD; only six trials were included in this review (four included in the meta-analysis and two in the overall interpretation), with a total of 178 participants. In this meta-analysis, a small but significant benefit of *n*-3 LCPUFA supplementation was found for social interaction and RRB but not communication and co-existing behaviours and conditions. No evidence of significant heterogeneity between trials were found.

Four trials included in the present meta-analysis with a total of 107 participants are however insufficient to provide robust evidence. Furthermore, the findings cannot be generalised to all children on the autism spectrum because the included children predominantly comprised males, were of different age groups (less than eight years and up to 28 years), displayed moderate to severe symptoms [54,69] or high hyperactivity level [36,70].

The findings of this review to some extent contradict the results of previous systematic reviews and meta-analysis [38,39]. These reviews did not find any statistically significant improvement in behaviour, but reported a larger positive effect on hyperactivity [38,39] while the present review found a significant improvement in social interaction and no improvement in hyperactivity. Our results, however, are in line with those of previous reviews [38,39] in that no improvement was identified in communication and irritability. With respect to RRB, sensory issues and gastrointestinal symptoms, no comparison can be made because they were not considered by these reviews. It should be noted that the small number of RCTs included in the review by Bent et al. (*n* = 1) [38] and James et al. (*n* = 2) [39] could have compromised the statistical power to detect any difference across groups.

Although case-control and open label studies provided evidence for a role of *n*-3 LCPUFA in ASD, RCTs of supplementation with *n*-3 LCPUFA yielded mixed results. One reason for such inconsistencies between studies may result from inadequately controlling for age, trial duration, habitual dietary intake of *n*-3 LCPUFA and levels of these fatty acids in the circulation over the course of trial, participants' general health conditions at the baseline and over the course of study, and outcome tools assessing behaviour. Response to *n*-3 LCPUFA supplementation has been shown to be predicted by body weight adjusted dose, baseline omega-3 index (RBC DHA + EPA), sex, age, and physical activity level; with populations receiving larger doses, having lower starting omega-3 index, older population, females and those with higher physical activity level experiencing a greater increase in the omega-3 index in response to supplementation [76].

Dietary intake of *n*-3 LCPUFA rich foods in children with autism is low [67]. However, omega-3 fatty acid supplements are among the most commonly used complementary and alternative medication in ASD [40]. It is plausible to suggest that even though the mentioned trials excluded participants that used *n*-3 LCPUFA supplements on their own initiatives at baseline, participants may have had high habitual dietary intake of these fatty acids due to their popularity, therefore responding differently to supplements which leads to diminishing the differences across treatment groups. An example of such implication could be the Voigt, 2014 study [55]; all children in this study had baseline LCPUFA levels above paediatric reference ranges for nutritional deficiencies and metabolic disorders (established at the Mayo Clinic [77]), and despite an increase of 431% in plasma DHA level, no improvement in behaviour was reported. Bent et al. (2011), on the other hand, showed that higher baseline level of some *n*-6 and *n*-3 polyunsaturated fatty acids including eicosadienoic acid ($r = -0.79$, $p = 0.02$), docosadienoate acid ($r = -0.65$, $p = 0.03$), and ALA ($r = -0.64$, $p = 0.03$) were associated with reduction in hyperactivity [69]. In an open label trial of *n*-3 LCPUFA in 41 autistic children aged 7–18 years, Ooi et al. (2015) showed an inverse correlation between autism mannerism severity and change in RBC fatty acids after 12 weeks of intervention and the severity was associated with baseline EPA level [32]. Unfortunately, the number of trials included in this review was inadequate to provide data on the effect of baseline *n*-3 LCPUFA intake or status on behavioural changes in response to supplementation.

The sex differences in ASD might be partly explained by sex differences in fatty acid metabolism; males may be more vulnerable than females to deficiencies in LCPUFA because of hormonal reasons [78], and thus may respond poorly to supplements [76]. With the exception of one study [36], no trials included in this review stratified the randomisation by sex. Unfortunately, no analysis could be performed for subgroups stratified by sex in this review because far more males than females were included and no studies reported behavioural changes in response to supplementation for males and females separately. With regard to the potential effect of age, three out of six studies included a wide age range (children and young people up to 28 years) which may have resulted in greater response variability. Due to the small number of studies included in this review, we could not perform subgroup analysis for different age bands to examine the effect of age on behavioural change in response to omega-3 supplementation.

The trial duration varied widely in studies included in this review (6–26 weeks). Evidence suggests that PUFA erythrocyte membrane reaches a steady state after 6 months [79] and at least 4 months is needed to demonstrate an effect on cognitive performance [41]. It has also been suggested that longer study periods of one year might be needed to demonstrate behavioural changes in response to *n*-3 LCPUFA supplementation [80]. Furthermore, the majority of outcome assessment tools are retrospectively completed (and duration over which behaviour is assessed varies depending on the assessment tool used); for example, parents are required to consider the behaviour over the past four weeks when completing ABC questionnaire while the timeframe for SRS is the past six months. It is of importance to avoid assessing and considering behaviour when the LCPUFA erythrocyte membrane has not yet reached its steady state. Therefore, wide variation and insufficient trial duration could explain the inconsistencies. Due to the small number of studies included in this review, we could not perform subgroup analysis for different intervention lengths to examine the effect of duration on behavioural change in response to omega-3 supplementation.

Gastrointestinal symptoms are highly prevalent in populations with ASD [81–83]. Mazurek et al. (2013) reported that of 2973 children with ASD, 24.7% had at least one chronic gastrointestinal symptom [83]. Compared to typically developing children, developmentally delayed and ASD children were more likely to have at least one frequent gastrointestinal symptom [83]. ASD children with frequent abdominal pain, gaseousness, diarrhea, constipation or pain on stooling had worse scores in four (irritability, social withdrawal, stereotypy, and hyperactivity) out of five ABC subscales than ASD children with no frequent gastrointestinal symptoms [84]. The pain and discomfort caused by gastrointestinal distress can worsen the behaviour in people with ASD, more particularly in non-verbal individuals who cannot express their feelings. Mankad et al. (2015) reported significantly worsened externalizing behaviours in response to *n*-3 LCPUFA supplementation which could be attributed to higher gastrointestinal distress reported in the active treatment group compared with the placebo (8/19 vs. 1/19, respectively) [37]. Thus, it is important to consider the potential modulating effect of gastrointestinal symptoms over the course of study on behavioural changes in response to supplementation.

Additionally, a variety of assessment tools (ranging from one to six tools) were used in each study which complicated effective comparisons across studies resulting in the exclusion of three studies from the meta-analysis, and potentially compromised the validity of a study by increasing the likelihood of type 1 error [44]. With the exception of ABC, a widely-used tool to assess problem behaviours in pharmacological trials in ASD, the majority of assessment tools have been designed for diagnostic purposes and there is a lack of evidence regarding the sensitivity of these tools to slight changes in behaviour in response to intervention in ASD populations. It is also worth noting that the inappropriate speech subscale of ABC is not a comprehensive measure of communication compared to other tools like SRS (inappropriate speech subscale of ABC comprises of four questions while the SRS communication subscale consists of 22 questions). Thus, findings regarding communication (measured by ABC) should be interpreted with caution.

It is also worth noting that the small or lack of effect reported here could be due to large placebo response in many trials included in this review. The large placebo response may have limited our capacity to identify any differences in some behaviour across groups. It is documented that different factors [e.g., raters of outcome assessment tools (clinicians vs. parents), increased response to active intervention, location, pharmacological and adjunctive intervention, participants' age (younger vs. older), study duration (shorter vs. longer), and severity of condition (lower baseline severity vs. higher severity)] are associated with the increased placebo response in ASD and other neurodevelopment and psychiatric disorders [85–87]. However, the reason for observed improvement in placebo groups included in this review is unclear and could not be determined due to small number of studies included.

4.3. Potential Mechanistic Pathways

There are, though not very well understood, several potential biological pathways for a role of LCPUFA in ASD [88,89]. Approximately 60% of the brain's dry weight is fat, with DHA comprising 60% and 40% of the PUFA in the retina and brain, respectively [90], suggesting that it is structurally important. Evidence suggests that some individuals with ASD have abnormalities in the gray and white matter of brain regions that are involved in social interaction, RRB, and sensory processing [13,91–93]. Ingestion of DHA (through diet or supplementation) has been shown to be positively associated with gray matter volume and its functional integrity and with white matter microstructural integrity in healthy individuals [16,17,94].

At the cellular level, PUFA interact with and influence the functioning of integral membrane proteins, including enzymes, receptors, and ion channels [95,96]. Evidence suggests that the activity of Na^+/K^+-ATPase (an enzyme that controls ion transport produced by neurotransmission) and adenylate cyclase (an enzyme that catalyses the conversion of ATP to cyclic AMP and has been shown to modulate social behaviours [97]) is disturbed in individuals with ASD [14,98]. Ghezzo et al. (2013) reported children with ASD having a significant reduction in Na^+/K^+-ATPase activity, alterations in erythrocyte fatty acid membrane (a decrease in *n*-3 LCPUFA and consequently an increase in *n*-6 LCPUFA to *n*-3 LCPUFA ratio, and an increase in monounsaturated fatty acids), and a reduction in erythrocyte membrane fluidity [14]. These alterations correlated with clinical features of ASD, particularly hyperactivity scores [14].

Further evidence for a relationship between *n*-3 LCPUFA and ASD comes from studies investigating its role in neurogenesis and several neurotransmitter systems. LCPFA, particularly *n*-3 series DHA, has been shown to favourably affect neurite survival, outgrowth and myelination in animal cultured cortical [99–101], sensory [102], and hippocampal neurons [18,103,104]. The development of axons and dentrites as well as myelination in multiple brain areas (involved in social behaviours, emotions, and RRB) has been reported to be impaired in individuals with ASD [105,106]. Similarly, an abnormal level of brain derived neurotrophic factor (BDNF, a protein that promotes the survival of neurons) in the circulation has been reported in children with ASD, which was associated with the severity of condition [88,107,108]. Docosahexaenoic acid administration normalised BDNF in the hippocampus, increased the growth of uninjured corticospinal and serotonergic fibres, and enhanced synaptic plasticity in an animal model of spinal cord injury [101,109].

Autistic children have been shown to exhibit significantly higher levels of several dopamine derivatives (in urine), dopamine transporter binding proteins, and serotonin in brain, and lower levels of serotonin transporter binding protein (in brain), glutamine signal (in basal ganglia), and oxytocin than healthy controls [110–116]. Furthermore, within the ASD populations, basal ganglia glutamine signal and plasma oxytocin negatively correlated with impaired behaviour [114,116]. In response to an n-3 PUFA limited diet in rats, dopamine levels reduced and basal synaptic release of serotonin increased while the turn over metabolites of dopamine increased and those of serotonin decreased [19,117–119]. A DHA depleted diet also altered the glutamergic system in offspring female rats [120]. This alteration was associated with anxiety-like behaviours, memory deficit and exploratory behaviours during adulthood [120]. On the other hand, DHA treatment significantly increased synaptic plasticity in hippocampal neurons and enhanced glutamatergic activity [121].

Another plausible mechanism supporting the association between LCPUFA and ASD is the anti- and pro-inflammatory properties of LCPUFA metabolic products. Eicosanoids (a collective name for prostaglandins, thromboxanes, leukotrienes and a variety of hydroxyl and hydroproxy fatty acid) are the enzymatic metabolic products of PUFA, and have important roles in inflammation [20]. While EPA or DHA derived eicosanoids have anti-inflammatory properties, those derived from ARA have pro-inflammatory properties [20]. Elevated levels of several peripheral pro-inflammatory cytokines and nuclear factor Kappa B (NF-κB, a transcription factor involved in inflammatory signaling pathways) has been reported in children with ASD [122–124]. Brigandi et al. [24] reported children with ASD having significantly higher plasma levels of PGE2 than healthy controls, a finding confirmed by El-Ansary and Al-Ayadhi (2012) [125] who also reported higher levels of leukotriene and 8-isoprostane together with PGE2 in children with ASD. In addition, lower levels of antioxidant proteins and increased levels of oxidative stress markers was associated with more severe ASD symptoms, including sensory issues [14,124,126]. Supplementation with n-3 PUFA, on the other hand, decreased the gene expression of NF-κB, IL-12 and IL-13 [127], macrophage inflammatory protein-2 (MIP2), IL-6 [128] and tumor necrosis factor-α (TNF-α) [128–130].

Decreased antioxidant capacity and increased lipid peroxidation may result in RBC LCPUFA instability and decrease these fatty acids in autism [23,74]. Instability in RBC LCPUFA composition has been shown by a great loss in PUFA levels when the blood samples of autistic children were stored at $-20\,^{\circ}$C, a finding not observed in the blood sample of healthy controls [62]. The reason for such instability could be related to cellular phospholipase activity. Tostes et al. (2013) [68] and Bell et al. (2004) [66] reported children with ASD having significantly higher phospholipase A2 (PLA2) activity than typically developing controls that was reduced by EPA supplementation [66]. PLA2 is responsible for releasing fatty acids, more particularly ARA, from phospholipids [66].

Finally, the role of LCPUFA in ASD could be explained by defects in enzymes involved in the conversion of LCPUFA from their precursors or deficits in the process of incorporation of LCPUFA into the cell membrane [24–26]. Gene variants in fatty acid desaturase (FADS)—one of the strongest genome wide associated signals—have been shown to enhance the conversion of ARA from its precursor and to be sex- and ethnicity-specific [131,132]. The effect of FADS genotype has been shown to be more pronounced in African Americans than Europeans (approximately two fold higher) [131]. The higher frequency of this genetic variant, but not the allelic effect of G allele, explained such a difference [131]. Also, while in Caucasians, one FADS2 single nucleotide polymorphism (SNP) and multiple FADS2 SNP (two SNP in males and nine SNP in females) were associated with n-6 aggregate desaturase indices, it was associated with five FADS2 SNP in East Asian Females [132]. In addition, carriers of APOE4 allele seems to have altered long chain omega-3 metabolism [133]. Compared to the non APOE4-carriers, the carriers have higher β-oxidisation rates of n-3 LCPUFA [133]. Furthermore, Shimamoto et al. (2014) showed altered mRNA gene expression levels of fatty acid binding protein 7 (FABP7) in post-mortem ASD brains, and increased hyperactivity and anxiety-related phenotype (two common features in ASD) in FABP7 knockout mice [134]. Although the modifying role of genetic variants in enzymes involved in fatty acid metabolism in the LCPUFA-disease relationship has been well documented, in the context of ASD, it warrants further investigation.

5. Conclusions

The current meta-analysis of case-controls studies, to our knowledge, is the first to investigate fatty acid composition in populations with ASD. Future observational studies of *n*-3 LCPUFA in children with ASD are encouraged while including a uniform biomarker (e.g., omega-3 index or percentage of *n*-3 LCPUFA in RBC) and reporting method (e.g., relative or absolute), collecting dietary intake of both *n*-3 and *n*-6 LCPUFA, and matching cases and controls on potential modulating attributes (e.g., age, sex, severity, genotype, and medication use). It is also critical to know whether inadequate LCPUFA status in ASD is attributed to inefficient or disrupted metabolism or other factors like LCPUFA consumption.

Based on the current evidence, *n*-3 LCPUFA supplementation cannot be recommended as an alternative to support behavioural therapies for ASD children. However, it seems prudent that *n*-3 LCPUFA could be used to complement other therapies in ASD populations given its long-term tolerability and acceptability (up to six months), potentially inefficient or disrupted LCPUFA metabolic pathways in this population, and its critical role in brain function and development, and various body processes some of which are involved in the pathobiology of ASD. It should be noted that this recommendation is made cautiously because the results of this study are based on a very small sample of studies (with methodological differences and limitations) and short duration of the interventions. Therefore, the generated statistics should not be over-interpreted but seen as indicative of the need to study the issue further (while controlling for potential modifying and confounding variables) to pursue the trends observed in this study. The effect of *n*-3 LCPUFA on behaviour may be modulated by background diet and baseline LCPUFA status, sex, age, trial duration, and gastrointestinal stress at baseline and over the study period, all of which are recommended to be considered in future research. Furthermore, an investigation of the potential modulating effect of genotype (e.g., APOE) on behavioural changes in response to LCPUFA supplementation is warranted. It is also recommended that future studies include a uniform assessment tool that is sensitive to minor behavioural changes in response to complementary/nutritional therapies. Finally, the potential placebo effect and the reasons for such effects are encouraged to be investigated and accounted for in the design stage of RCTs.

Supplementary Materials: The following are available online at http://www.mdpi.com/2072-6643/9/2/155/s1, Table S1: Study characteristics of open label trials and case-studies excluded from systematic literature review; Table S2: Quality appraisal of included case-control studies; Table S3: Quality appraisal of included RCTs; Figure S1: Risk of bias table showing judgments on each risk factor for each primary study included in both meta-analysis and overall interpretation.

Acknowledgments: No funding was received in support of this research work. Massey University provided funds for covering the costs to publish this research work in open access.

Author Contributions: H.M. conceived the manuscript idea, H.M. researched the manuscript and identified eligible studies, H.M. and M.D. extracted data and performed the quality appraisal of studies; H.M. performed the meta-analyses and drafted the manuscript, all other authors critically reviewed the manuscript.

Conflicts of Interest: The authors declare no conflict of interest.

References

1. Chakrabarti, S.; Fombonne, E. Pervasive developmental disorders in preschool children. *JAMA* **2001**, *285*, 3093–3099. [CrossRef] [PubMed]
2. New Zealand Guidelines Group. *What Does ASD Look Like? A Resource to Help Identify Autism Spectrum Disorder*; New Zealand Guidelines Group: Wellington, New Zealand, 2010.
3. Baio, J. Prevalence of Autism Spectrum Disorders—Autism and Developmental Disabilities Monitoring Network, 14 Sites, United States, 2008. *Surveill. Summ.* **2012**, *61*, 1–19.
4. Ghanizadeh, A. A preliminary study on screening prevalence of pervasive developmental disorder in schoolchildren in Iran. *J. Autism Dev. Disord.* **2008**, *38*, 759–763. [CrossRef] [PubMed]
5. Kogan, M.D.; Blumberg, S.J.; Schieve, L.A.; Boyle, C.A.; Perrin, J.M.; Ghandour, R.M.; Singh, G.K.; Strickland, B.B.; Trevathan, E.; van Dyck, P.C. Prevalence of Parent-Reported Diagnosis of Autism Spectrum Disorder Among Children in the US, 2007. *Pediatrics* **2009**, *124*, 1395–1403. [CrossRef] [PubMed]

6. Diagnostic and Statistical Manual of Mental Disorders. In *Diagnostic and Statistical Manual of Mental Disorders: DSM-5*; American Psychiatric Association: Washington, DC, USA, 2013.

7. Napolioni, V.; Ober-Reynolds, B.; Szelinger, S.; Corneveaux, J.J.; Pawlowski, T.; Ober-Reynolds, S.; Kirwan, J.; Perisco, A.M.; Melmed, R.D.; Craig, D.W.; et al. Plasma cytokine profiling in sibling pairs discordant for Autism Spectrum Disorder. *J. Neuroinflamm.* **2013**, *10*, 38. [CrossRef] [PubMed]

8. Rossignol, D.A.; Frye, R.E. Evidence linking oxidative stress, mitochondrial dysfunction, and inflammation in the brain of individuals with autism. *Front. Physiol.* **2014**, *5*, 150. [CrossRef] [PubMed]

9. Singh, V.K. Phenotypic expression of autoimmune autistic disorder (AAD): A major subset of autism. *Ann. Clin. Psychiatry* **2009**, *21*, 148–161. [PubMed]

10. Napoli, E.; Wong, S.; Hertz-Picciotto, I.; Giulivi, C. Deficits in Bioenergetics and Impaired Immune Response in Granulocytes From Children With Autism. *Pediatrics* **2014**, *133*, e1405–e1410. [CrossRef] [PubMed]

11. Rose, S.; Frye, R.E.; Slattery, J.; Wynne, R.; Tippett, M.; Pavliv, O.; Melnyk, S.; James, S.J. Oxidative Stress Induces Mitochondrial Dysfunction in a Subset of Autism Lymphoblastoid Cell Lines in a Well-Matched Case Control Cohort. *PLoS ONE* **2014**, *9*, e85436. [CrossRef] [PubMed]

12. Melnyk, S.; Fuchs, G.J.; Schulz, E.; Lopez, M.; Kahler, S.G.; Fussell, J.J.; Bellando, J.; Pavliv, O.; Rose, S.; Seidel, L.; et al. Metabolic imbalance associated with methylation dysregulation and oxidative damage in children with autism. *J. Autism Dev. Disord.* **2012**, *42*, 367–377. [CrossRef] [PubMed]

13. D'Mello, A.M.; Crocetti, D.; Mostofsky, S.H.; Stoodley, C.J. Cerebellar gray matter and lobular volumes correlate with core autism symptoms. *NeuroImage Clin.* **2015**, *7*, 631–639. [CrossRef] [PubMed]

14. Ghezzo, A.; Visconti, P.; Abruzzo, P.M.; Bolotta, A.; Ferreri, C.; Gobbi, G.; Malisardi, G.; Manfredini, S.; Marini, M.; Nanetti, L.; et al. Oxidative Stress and Erythrocyte Membrane Alterations in Children with Autism: Correlation with Clinical Features. *PLoS ONE* **2013**, *8*, e66418. [CrossRef] [PubMed]

15. Schaaf, C.P.; Zoghbi, H.Y. Solving the autism puzzle a few pieces at a time. *Neuron* **2011**, *70*, 806–808. [CrossRef] [PubMed]

16. McNamara, R.K.; Able, J.; Jandacek, R.; Rider, T.; Tso, P.; Eliassen, J.C.; Alfieri, D.; Weber, W.; Jarvis, K.; DelBello, M.P.; et al. Docosahexaenoic acid supplementation increases prefrontal cortex activation during sustained attention in healthy boys: A placebo-controlled, dose-ranging, functional magnetic resonance imaging study. *Am. J. Clin. Nutr.* **2010**, *91*, 1060–1067. [CrossRef] [PubMed]

17. Witte, A.V.; Kerti, L.; Hermannstädter, H.M.; Fiebach, J.B.; Schreiber, S.J.; Schuchardt, J.P.; Hahn, A.; Flöel, A. Long-Chain Omega-3 Fatty Acids Improve Brain Function and Structure in Older Adults. *Cereb. Cortex* **2013**, *24*, 3059–3068. [CrossRef] [PubMed]

18. Pu, H.; Guo, Y.; Zhang, W.; Huang, L.; Wang, G.; Liou, A.K.; Zhang, J.; Zhang, P.; Leak, R.K.; Wang, Y.; et al. Omega-3 polyunsaturated fatty acid supplementation improves neurologic recovery and attenuates white matter injury after experimental traumatic brain injury. *J. Cereb. Blood Flow Metab.* **2013**, *33*, 1474–1484. [CrossRef] [PubMed]

19. Tang, M.; Zhang, M.; Cai, H.; Li, H.; Jiang, P.; Dang, R.; Liu, Y.; He, X.; Xue, Y.; Cao, L.; et al. Maternal diet of polyunsaturated fatty acid altered the cell proliferation in the dentate gyrus of hippocampus and influenced glutamatergic and serotoninergic systems of neonatal female rats. *Lipids Health Dis.* **2016**, *15*, 71. [CrossRef] [PubMed]

20. Calder, P.C. *n*-3 Polyunsaturated fatty acids, inflammation, and inflammatory diseases. *Am. J. Clin. Nutr.* **2006**, *83*, S1505–S1519.

21. Serra-Majem, L.; Nissensohn, M.; Overby, N.C.; Fekete, K. Dietary methods and biomarkers of omega 3 fatty acids: A systematic review. *Br. J. Nutr.* **2012**, *107* (Suppl. 2), S64–S76. [CrossRef] [PubMed]

22. Spahis, S.; Vanasse, M.; Bélanger, S.A.; Ghadirian, P.; Grenier, E.; Levy, E. Lipid profile, fatty acid composition and pro- and anti-oxidant status in pediatric patients with attention-deficit/hyperactivity disorder. Prostaglandins Leukot. *Essent. Fatty Acids* **2008**, *79*, 47–53. [CrossRef] [PubMed]

23. Khan, M.M.; Evans, D.R.; Gunna, V.; Scheffer, R.E.; Parikh, V.V.; Mahadik, S.P. Reduced erythrocyte membrane essential fatty acids and increased lipid peroxides in schizophrenia at the never-medicated first-episode of psychosis and after years of treatment with antipsychotics. *Schizophr. Res.* **2002**, *58*, 1–10. [CrossRef]

24. Brigandi, S.; Shao, H.; Qian, S.; Shen, Y.; Wu, B.-L.; Kang, J. Autistic Children Exhibit Decreased Levels of Essential Fatty Acids in Red Blood Cells. *Int. J. Mol. Sci.* **2015**, *16*, 10061. [CrossRef]

25. Vancassel, S.; Durant, G.; Lejeune, B.; Martineau, J.; Guiloteau, D.; Andres, C.; Chalon, S. Plasma fatty acid levels of autistic children. *Prostaglandins Leukot. Essent. Fatty Acids* **2001**, *65*, 1–7. [CrossRef] [PubMed]
26. Mostafa, G.A.; Al-Ayadhi, L.Y. Reduced levels of plasma polyunsaturated fatty acids and serum carnitine in autistic children: Relation to gastrointestinal manifestations. *Behav. Brain Funct.* **2015**, *11*, 4. [CrossRef] [PubMed]
27. Bell, J.G.; Miller, D.; MacDonald, D.J.; MacKinlay, E.E.; Dick, J.R.; Cheseldine, S.; Boyle, R.M.; Graham, C.; O'Hare, A.E. The fatty acid compositions of erythrocyte and plasma polar lipids in children with autism, developmental delay or typically developing controls and the effect of fish oil intake. *Br. J. Nutr.* **2010**, *103*, 1160–1167. [PubMed]
28. Bu, B.; Ashwood, P.; Harvey, D.; King, I.B.; van de Water, J.; Jin, L.W. Fatty acid compositions of red blood cell phospholipids in children with autism. *Prostaglandins Leukot. Essent. Fatty Acids* **2006**, *74*, 215–221. [CrossRef] [PubMed]
29. Johnson, C.; Handen, B.; Zimmer, M.; Sacco, K. Polyunsaturated Fatty Acid Supplementation in Young Children with autism. *J. Dev. Phys. Disabil.* **2010**, *22*, 1–10. [CrossRef]
30. Meguid, N.A.; Atta, H.M.; Gouda, A.S.; Khalil, R.O. Role of polyunsaturated fatty acids in the management of Egyptian children with autism. *Clin. Biochem.* **2008**, *41*, 1044–1048. [CrossRef] [PubMed]
31. Meiri, G.; Bichovsky, Y.; Belmaker, R.H. Omega 3 fatty acid treatment in autism. *J. Child Adolesc. Psychopharmacol.* **2009**, *19*, 449–451. [CrossRef] [PubMed]
32. Ooi, Y.P.; Weng, S.J.; Jang, L.Y.; Low, L.; Seah, J.; Teo, S.; Ang, R.P.; Lim, C.G.; Liew, A.; Fung, D.S.; Sung, M. Omega-3 fatty acids in the management of Autism Spectrum Disorders: Findings from an open-label pilot study in Singapore. *Eur. J. Clin. Nutr.* **2015**, *69*, 969–971. [CrossRef] [PubMed]
33. Patrick, L.; Salik, R. The Effect Of Essential Fatty Acid Supplementation on Language Development and Learning Skills in Autism and Aspergers Syndrome. *Autism Asperger's Digest.* Jan-Feb **2005**, 36–37.
34. Politi, P.; Cena, H.; Comelli, M.; Marrone, G.; Allegri, C.; Emanuele, E.; Ucelli di Nemi, S. Behavioral Effects of Omega-3 Fatty Acid Supplementation in Young Adults with Severe Autism: An Open Label Study. *Arch. Med. Res.* **2008**, *39*, 682–685. [CrossRef] [PubMed]
35. Johnson, S.M.; Hollander, E. Evidence that eicosapentaenoic acid is effective in treating Autism. *J. Clin. Psychiatry* **2003**, *64*, 848–849. [CrossRef] [PubMed]
36. Amminger, G.P.; Berger, G.E.; Schäfer, M.R.; Klier, C.; Friedrich, M.H.; Feucht, M. Omega-3 Fatty Acids Supplementation in Children with Autism: A Double-blind Randomized, Placebo-controlled Pilot Study. *Biol. Psychiatry* **2007**, *61*, 551–553. [CrossRef] [PubMed]
37. Mankad, D.; Dupuis, A.; Smile, S.; Roberts, W.; Brian, J.; Lui, T.; Genore, L.; Zaghloul, D.; Iaboni, A.; Marcon, P.M.; et al. A randomized, placebo controlled trial of omega-3 fatty acids in the treatment of young children with autism. *Mol. Autism* **2015**, *6*, 18. [CrossRef]
38. Bent, S.; Bertoglio, K.; Hendren, R.L. Omega-3 fatty acids for Autistic Spectrum Disorder: A systematic review. *J. Autism Dev. Disord.* **2009**, *39*, 1145–1154. [CrossRef] [PubMed]
39. James, S.; Montgomery, P.; Williams, K. Omega-3 fatty acids supplementation for Autism Spectrum Disorders (ASD). *Cochrane Database Syst. Rev.* **2011**, *9*, CD007992.
40. Brondino, N.; Brondino, N.; Fusar-Poli, L.; Rocchetti, M.; Provenzani, U.; Barale, F.; Politi, P. Complementary and Alternative Therapies for Autism Spectrum Disorder. *Evid. Based Complement. Altern. Med. eCAM* **2015**, *2015*, 258589. [CrossRef] [PubMed]
41. Stonehouse, W. Does Consumption of LC Omega-3 PUFA Enhance Cognitive Performance in Healthy School-Aged Children and throughout Adulthood? Evidence from Clinical Trials. *Nutrients* **2014**, *6*, 2730–2758. [CrossRef] [PubMed]
42. LaChance, L.; McKenzie, K.; Taylor, V.H.; Vigod, S.N. Omega-6 to Omega-3 Fatty Acid Ratio in Patients with ADHD: A Meta-Analysis. *J. Can. Acad. Child Adolesc. Psychiatry* **2016**, *25*, 87–96. [PubMed]
43. Bolte, E.E.; Diehl, J.J. Measurement tools and target symptoms/skills used to assess treatment response for individuals with Autism Spectrum Disorder. *J. Autism Dev. Disord.* **2013**, *43*, 2491–2501. [CrossRef] [PubMed]
44. Leon, A.C. Implications of Clinical Trial Design on Sample Size Requirements. *Schizophr. Bull.* **2008**, *34*, 664–669. [CrossRef] [PubMed]
45. Sun, Q.; Ma, J.; Campos, H.; Hankinson, S.E.; Hu, F.B. Comparison between plasma and erythrocyte fatty acid content as biomarkers of fatty acid intake in US women. *Am. J. Clin. Nutr.* **2007**, *86*, 74–81. [PubMed]

46. Sergeant, S.; Ruczinski, I.; Ivester, P.; Lee, T.C.; Morgan, T.M.; Nicklas, B.J.; Mathias, R.A.; Chilton, F.H. Impact of methods used to express levels of circulating fatty acids on the degree and direction of associations with blood lipids in humans. *Br. J. Nutr.* **2016**, *115*, 251–261. [CrossRef] [PubMed]

47. Health Canada. *Guidance Document for Preparing a Submission for Food Health Claims, Bureau of Nutritional Sciences Food Directorate*; Health Products and Food Branch Health Canada: Ottawa, ON, Canada, 2009.

48. Higgins, J.P.T.; Green, S. Cochrane Handbook for Systematic Reviews of Interventions. Available online: http://training.cochrane.org/handbook (accessed on 11 February 2016).

49. Sliwinski, S.; Croonenberghs, J.; Christophe, A.; Deboutte, D.; Maes, M. Polyunsaturated fatty acids: Do they have a role in the pathophysiology of autism? *Neuro Endocrinol. Lett.* **2006**, *27*, 465–471. [PubMed]

50. El-Ansary, A.K.; Ben Bacha, A.G.; Al-Ayahdi, L.Y. Impaired plasma phospholipids and relative amounts of essential polyunsaturated fatty acids in autistic patients from Saudi Arabia. *Lipids Health Dis.* **2011**, *10*, 63. [CrossRef] [PubMed]

51. Jory, J. Abnormal fatty acids in Canadian children with autism. *Nutrition* **2016**, *32*, 474–477. [CrossRef] [PubMed]

52. Parletta, N.; Niyonsenga, T.; Duff, J. Omega-3 and Omega-6 Polyunsaturated Fatty Acid Levels and Correlations with Symptoms in Children with Attention Deficit Hyperactivity Disorder, Autistic Spectrum Disorder and Typically Developing Controls. *PLoS ONE* **2016**, *11*, e0156432. [CrossRef] [PubMed]

53. Yui, K.; Imataka, G.; Kawasak, Y.; Yamada, H. Increased omega-3 polyunsaturated fatty acid/arachidonic acid ratios and upregulation of signaling mediator in individuals with Autism Spectrum Disorders. *Life Sci.* **2016**, *145*, 205–212. [CrossRef] [PubMed]

54. Yui, K.; Koshiba, M.; Nakamura, S.; Kobayashim, Y.; Ohnishi, M. Efficacy of Adding Large Doses of Arachidonic Acid to Docosahexaenoic Acid against Restricted Repetitive Behaviors in Individuals with Autism Spectrum Disorders: A Placebo-Controlled Trial. *J. Addict. Res.Ther.* **2011**. [CrossRef]

55. Voigt, R.G.; Mellon, M.W.; Katusic, S.K.; Weaver, A.L.; Matern, D.; Mellon, B.; Jensen, C.L.; Barbaresi, W.J. Dietary docosahexaenoic acid supplementation in children with autism. *J. Pediatr. Gastroenterol. Nutr.* **2014**, *58*, 715–722. [PubMed]

56. Parellada, M.; Llorente, C.; Calvo, R.; Gutierrez, S.; Lazaro, L.; Graell, M.; Alvarez, M.; Guisasola, M.; Dulin, E.; Dorado, M.L.; et al. Double-blind crossed-over randomized controlled-trial with omega-3 fatty acids for Autism Spectrum Disorders. *Eur. Neuropsychopharmacol.* **2015**, *25*, S138. [CrossRef]

57. Yui, K.; Koshiba, M.; Nakamura, S.; Kobayashi, Y. Effects of Large Doses of Arachidonic Acid Added to Docosahexaenoic Acid on Social Impairment in Individuals With Autism Spectrum Disorders: A Double-Blind, Placebo-Controlled, Randomized Trial. *J. Clin. Psychopharmacol.* **2012**, *32*, 200–206. [CrossRef] [PubMed]

58. Esparham, A.E.; Smith, T.; Belmont, J.M.; Haden, M.; Wagner, L.E.; Evans, R.G.; Drisko, J.A. Nutritional and Metabolic Biomarkers in Autism Spectrum Disorders: An Exploratory Study. *Integr. Med.* **2015**, *14*, 40–53.

59. Wang, H.; Liang, S.; Wang, M.; Gao, J.; Sun, C.; Wang, J.; Xia, W.; Wu, S.; Sumner, S.J.; Zhang, F.; et al. Potential serum biomarkers from a metabolomics study of autism. *J. Psychiatry Neurosci.* **2016**, *41*, 27–37. [CrossRef] [PubMed]

60. Wiest, M.M.; German, J.B.; Harvey, D.J.; Watkins, S.M.; Hertz-Picciotto, I. Plasma fatty acid profiles in autism: A case-control study. *Prostaglandins Leukot. Essent. Fatty Acids* **2009**, *80*, 221–227. [CrossRef] [PubMed]

61. Pastural, É.; Ritchie, S.; Lu, Y.; Jin, W.; Kavianpour, A.; Khine, S.-M.K.; Heath, D.; Wood, P.L.; Fisk, M.; Goodenowe, D.B. Novel plasma phospholipid biomarkers of autism: Mitochondrial dysfunction as a putative causative mechanism. *Prostaglandins Leukot. Essent. Fatty Acids* **2009**, *81*, 253–264. [CrossRef] [PubMed]

62. Bell, J.G.; Sargent, J.R.; Tocher, D.R.; Dick, J.R. Red blood cell fatty acid compositions in a patient with Autistic Spectrum Disorder: A characteristic abnormality in neurodevelopmental disorders? *Prostaglandins Leukot. Essent. Fatty Acids* **2000**, *63*, 21–25. [CrossRef] [PubMed]

63. Yui, K.; Imataka, G.; Kawasaki, Y. Competitive Interaction Between Plasma Omega-3 Fatty Acids and Arachidonic Acid is Related to Down-Regulation of A Signaling Mediator. *Med. Chem.* **2016**, *12*, 318–327. [CrossRef] [PubMed]

64. Yui, K.; Imataka, G.; Kawasaki, Y.; Yamada, T. Down-regulation of Signaling Mediator in Related to Increased Ratio of Docosahexaenoic Acid/Arachidonic Acid in Individuals with Autism Spectrum Disorders. *J. Transl. Med. Dev. Disord.* **2015**, *2*, 1–9.

65. El-Ansary, A.K.; Ben Bacha, A.G.; Al-Ayahdi, L.Y. Plasma fatty acids as diagnostic markers in autistic patients from Saudi Arabia. *Lipids Health Dis.* **2011**, *10*. [CrossRef] [PubMed]

66. Bell, J.G.; MacKinlay, E.E.; Dick, J.R.; MacDonald, D.J.; Boyle, R.M.; Glen, A.C. Essential fatty acids and phospholipase A2 in Autistic Spectrum Disorders. *Prostaglandins Leukot. Essent. Fatty Acids* **2004**, *71*, 201–204. [CrossRef] [PubMed]

67. Al-Farsi, Y.M.; Waly, M.I.; Deth, R.C.; Al-Sharbati, M.M.; Al-Shafaee, M.; Al-Farsi, O.; Al-Khaduri, M.M.; Al-Adawi, S.; Hodgson, N.W.; Gupta, I.; et al. Impact of nutrition on serum levels of docosahexaenoic acid among Omani children with autism. *Nutrition* **2013**, *29*, 1142–1146. [CrossRef] [PubMed]

68. Tostes, M.H.; Polonini, H.C.; Mendes, R.; Brandao, M.A.; Gattaz, W.F.; Raposo, N.R. Fatty acid and phospholipase A2 plasma levels in children with autism. *Trends Psychiatry Psychother.* **2013**, *35*, 76–80. [CrossRef] [PubMed]

69. Bent, S.; Bertoglio, K.; Ashwood, P.; Bostrom, A.; Hendren, R.L. A pilot randomized controlled trial of omega-3 fatty acids for Autism Spectrum Disorder. *J. Autism Dev. Disord.* **2011**, *41*, 545–554. [CrossRef] [PubMed]

70. Bent, S.; Hendren, R.L.; Zandi, T.; Law, K.; Choi, J-E.; Widjaja, F.; Kalb, L.; Nestle, J.; Law, P. Internet-Based, Randomized, Controlled Trial of Omega-3 Fatty Acids for Hyperactivity in Autism. *J. Am. Acad. Child Adolesc. Psychiatry* **2014**, *53*, 658–666. [CrossRef] [PubMed]

71. Hawkey, E.; Nigg, J.T. Omega-3 fatty acid and ADHD: Blood level analysis and meta-analytic extension of supplementation trials. *Clin. Psychol. Rev.* **2014**, *34*, 496–505. [CrossRef] [PubMed]

72. Harris, W.S.; Pottala, J.V.; Varvel, S.A.; Borowski, J.J.; Ward, J.N.; McConnell, J.P. Erythrocyte omega-3 fatty acids increase and linoleic acid decreases with age: Observations from 160,000 patients. *Prostaglandins Leukot Essent Fatty Acids* **2013**, *88*, 257–263. [CrossRef] [PubMed]

73. Laryea, M.; Cieslicki, P.; Diekmann, E.; Wendel, U. Age-dependent fatty acid composition of erythrocyte membrane phospholipids in healthy children. *Z. Ernahrungswiss.* **1990**, *29*, 284–294. [CrossRef] [PubMed]

74. Evans, D.R.; Parikh, V.V.; Khan, M.M.; Coussons, C.; Buckley, P.F.; Mahadik, S.P. Red blood cell membrane essential fatty acid metabolism in early psychotic patients following antipsychotic drug treatment. *Prostaglandins Leukot. Essent. Fatty Acids* **2003**, *69*, 393–399. [CrossRef] [PubMed]

75. Castano, A.; Cutanda, F.; Esteban, M.; Part, P.; Navarro, C.; Gomez, S.; Rosado, M.; Lopez, A.; Lopez, E.; Exley, K.; et al. Fish consumption patterns and hair mercury levels in children and their mothers in 17 EU countries. *Environ. Res.* **2015**, *141*, 58–68. [CrossRef] [PubMed]

76. Flock, M.R.; Skulas-Ray, A.C.; Harris, W.S.; Etherton, T.D.; Fleming, J.A.; Kris-Etherton, P.M. Determinants of erythrocyte omega-3 fatty acid content in response to fish oil supplementation: A dose-response randomized controlled trial. *J. Am. Heart Assoc.* **2013**, *2*, e000513. [CrossRef] [PubMed]

77. Lagerstedt, S.A.; Hinrichs, D.R.; Batt, S.M.; Magera, M.J.; Rinaldo, P.; McConnell, J.P. Quantitative determination of plasma c8-c26 total fatty acids for the biochemical diagnosis of nutritional and metabolic disorders. *Mol. Genet. Metab.* **2001**, *73*, 38–45. [CrossRef] [PubMed]

78. Alessandri, J.M.; Extier, A.; Al-Gubory, K.H.; Harbeby, E.; Lallemand, M.S.; Linard, A.; Lavialle, M.; Guesnet, P. Influence of gender on DHA synthesis: The response of rat liver to low dietary alpha-linolenic acid evidences higher omega3 4-desaturation index in females. *Eur. J. Nutr.* **2012**, *51*, 199–209. [CrossRef] [PubMed]

79. Katan, M.B.; Deslypere, J.P.; van Birgelen, A.P.; Penders, M.; Zegwaard, M. Kinetics of the incorporation of dietary fatty acids into serum cholesteryl esters, erythrocyte membranes, and adipose tissue: An 18-month controlled study. *J. Lipid Res.* **1997**, *38*, 2012–2022. [PubMed]

80. Raine, A.; Portnoy, J.; Liu, J.; Mahoomed, T.; Hibbeln, J.R. Reduction in behavior problems with omega-3 supplementation in children aged 8–16 years: A randomized, double-blind, placebo-controlled, stratified, parallel-group trial. *J. Child Psychol. Psychiatry* **2015**, *56*, 509–520. [CrossRef] [PubMed]

81. Sun, C.; Xia, W.; Zhao, Y.; Li, N.; Zhao, D.; Wu, L. Nutritional status survey of children with autism and typically developing children aged 4–6 years in Heilongjiang Province, China. *J. Nutr. Sci.* **2013**, *2*, e16.

82. Wang, L.W.; Tancredi, D.J.; Thomas, D.W. The prevalence of gastrointestinal problems in children across the United States with Autism Spectrum Disorders from families with multiple affected members. *J. Dev. Behav. Pediatr.* **2011**, *32*, 351–360. [CrossRef] [PubMed]

83. Mazurek, M.O.; Vasa, R.A.; Kalb, L.G.; Kanne, S.M.; Rosenberg, D.; Keefer, A.; Murray, D.S.; Freedman, B.; Lowery, L.A. Anxiety, sensory over-responsivity, and gastrointestinal problems in children with Autism Spectrum Disorders. *J. Abnorm. Child Psychol.* **2013**, *41*, 165–176. [CrossRef] [PubMed]

84. Chaidez, V.; Hansen, R.L.; Hertz-Picciotto, I. Gastrointestinal problems in children with autism, developmental delays or typical development. *J. Autism Dev. Disord.* **2014**, *44*, 1117–1127. [CrossRef] [PubMed]

85. Agid, O.; Siu, C.O.; Potkin, S.G.; Kapur, S.; Watsky, E.; Vanderburg, D.; Zipursky, R.B.; Remington, G. Meta-regression analysis of placebo response in antipsychotic trials, 1970–2010. *Am. J. Psychiatry* **2013**, *170*, 1335–1344. [CrossRef] [PubMed]

86. Masi, A.; Lampit, A.; Glozier, N.; Hickie, I.B.; Guastella, A.J. Predictors of placebo response in pharmacological and dietary supplement treatment trials in pediatric Autism Spectrum Disorder: A meta-analysis. *Transl. Psychiatry* **2015**, *5*, e640. [CrossRef] [PubMed]

87. King, B.H.; Dukes, K.; Donnelly, C.L.; Sikich, L.; McCracken, J.T.; Scahill, L.; Hollander, E.; Bregman, J.D.; Anagnostou, E.; Robinson, F.; et al. Baseline factors predicting placebo response to treatment in children and adolescents with Autism Spectrum Disorders: A multisite randomized clinical trial. *JAMA Pediatr.* **2013**, *167*, 1045–1052. [CrossRef] [PubMed]

88. Das, U.N. Autism as a disorder of deficiency of brain-derived neurotrophic factor and altered metabolism of polyunsaturated fatty acids. *Nutrition* **2013**, *29*, 1175–1185. [CrossRef] [PubMed]

89. Das, U.N. Nutritional factors in the pathobiology of autism. *Nutrition* **2013**, *29*, 1066–1069. [CrossRef] [PubMed]

90. Singh, M. Essential fatty acids, DHA and human brain. *Indian J. Pediatr.* **2005**, *72*, 239–242. [CrossRef] [PubMed]

91. Petropoulos, H.; Friedman, S.D.; Shaw, D.W.; Artru, A.A.; Dawson, G.; Dager, S.R. Gray matter abnormalities in Autism Spectrum Disorder revealed by T2 relaxation. *Neurology* **2006**, *67*, 632–636. [CrossRef] [PubMed]

92. Rojas, D.C.; Peterson, E.; Winterrowd, E.; Reite, M.L.; Rogers, S.J.; Tregellas, J.R. Regional gray matter volumetric changes in autism associated with social and repetitive behavior symptoms. *BMC Psychiatry* **2006**, *6*, 56. [CrossRef] [PubMed]

93. Pryweller, J.R.; Schauder, K.B.; Anderson, A.W.; Heacock, J.L.; Foss-Feig, J.H.; Newsom, C.R.; Loring, W.A.; Cascio, C.J. White matter correlates of sensory processing in autism spectrum disorders. *NeuroImage Clin.* **2014**, *6*, 379–387. [CrossRef] [PubMed]

94. Conklin, S.M.; Gianaros, P.J.; Brown, S.M.; Yao, J.K.; Hariri, A.R.; Manuck, S.B.; Muldoon, M.F. Long-chain omega-3 fatty acid intake is associated positively with corticolimbic gray matter volume in healthy adults. *Neurosci. Lett.* **2007**, *421*, 209–212. [CrossRef] [PubMed]

95. Murphy, M.G. Dietary fatty acids and membrane protein function. *J. Nutr. Biochem.* **1990**, *1*, 68–79. [CrossRef]

96. Ibarguren, M.; López, D.J.; Escribá, P.V. The effect of natural and synthetic fatty acids on membrane structure, microdomain organization, cellular functions and human health. *Biochim. Biophys. Acta* **2014**, *1838*, 1518–1528. [CrossRef] [PubMed]

97. Donahue, R.J.; Venkataraman, A.; Carroll, F.I.; Meloni, E.G.; Carlezon, W.A., Jr. Pituitary adenylate cyclase activating polypeptide disrupts motivation, social interaction, and attention in male Sprague-Dawley rats. *Biol. Psychiatry* **2016**, *80*, 955–964. [CrossRef] [PubMed]

98. Abu Shmais, G.A.; Al-Ayadhi, L.Y.; Al-Dbass, A.M.; El-Ansary, A.K. Mechanism of nitrogen metabolism-related parameters and enzyme activities in the pathophysiology of autism. *J. Neurodev. Disord.* **2012**, *4*, 4. [CrossRef] [PubMed]

99. Cao, D.; Xue, R.; Xu, J.; Liu, Z. Effects of docosahexaenoic acid on the survival and neurite outgrowth of rat cortical neurons in primary cultures. *J. Nutr. Biochem.* **2005**, *16*, 538–546. [CrossRef] [PubMed]

100. Mita, T.; Mayanagi, T.; Ichijo, H.; Fukumoto, K.; Otsuka, K.; Sakai, A.; Sobue, K. Docosahexaenoic acid promotes axon outgrowth by translational regulation of tau and collapsin response mediator protein 2 expression. *J. Biol. Chem.* **2016**, *291*, 4955–4965. [CrossRef] [PubMed]

101. Liu, Z.-H.; Yip, P.K.; Adams, L.; Davies, M.; Lee, J.W.; Michael, G.J.; Priestley, J.V.; Michael-Titus, A.T. A single bolus of docosahexaenoic acid promotes neuroplastic changes in the innervation of spinal cord interneurons and motor neurons and improves functional recovery after spinal cord injury. *J. Neurosci.* **2015**, *35*, 12733–12752. [CrossRef]

102. Robson, L.G.; Dyall, S.; Sidloff, D.; Michael-Titus, A.T. Omega-3 polyunsaturated fatty acids increase the neurite outgrowth of rat sensory neurones throughout development and in aged animals. *Neurobiol. Aging* **2010**, *31*, 678–687. [CrossRef] [PubMed]

103. Calderon, F.; Kim, H.Y. Docosahexaenoic acid promotes neurite growth in hippocampal neurons. *J. Neurochem.* **2004**, *90*, 979–988. [CrossRef] [PubMed]

104. Nakato, M.; Matsuo, M.; Kono, N.; Arita, M.; Arai, H.; Ogawa, J.; Kioka, N.; Ueda, K. Neurite outgrowth stimulation by *n*-3 and *n*-6 PUFAs of phospholipids in apoE-containing lipoproteins secreted from glial cells. *J. Lipid Res.* **2015**, *56*, 1880–1890. [CrossRef] [PubMed]

105. Zikopoulos, B.; Barbas, H. Changes in prefrontal axons may disrupt the network in autism. *J. Neurosci.* **2010**, *30*, 14595–14609. [CrossRef] [PubMed]

106. Zikopoulos, B.; Barbas, H. Altered neural connectivity in excitatory and inhibitory cortical circuits in autism. *Front. Hum. Neurosci.* **2013**, *7*, 609. [CrossRef] [PubMed]

107. Kasarpalkar, N.J.; Kothari, S.T.; Dave, U.P. Brain-derived neurotrophic factor in children with autism spectrum disorder. *Ann. Neurosci.* **2014**, *21*, 129–133. [CrossRef] [PubMed]

108. Bryn, V.; Halvorsen, B.; Ueland, T.; Isaksen, J.; Kolkova, K.; Ravn, K.; Skjeldal, O.H. Brain derived neurotrophic factor (BDNF) and Autism Spectrum Disorders (ASD) in childhood. *Eur. J. Paediatr. Neurol.* **2015**, *19*, 411–414. [CrossRef] [PubMed]

109. Wu, A.; Ying, Z.; Gomez-Pinilla, F. Dietary omega-3 fatty acids normalize BDNF levels, reduce oxidative damage, and counteract learning disability after traumatic brain injury in rats. *J. Neurotrauma* **2004**, *21*, 1457–1467. [CrossRef] [PubMed]

110. Martineau, J.; Barthelemy, C.; Jouve, J.; Muh, J.P.; Lelord, G. Monoamines (serotonin and catecholamines) and their derivatives in infantile autism: Age-related changes and drug effects. *Dev. Med. Child Neurol.* **1992**, *34*, 593–603. [CrossRef] [PubMed]

111. Nakamura, K.; Sekine, Y.; Ouchi, Y.; Tsujii, M.; Yoshikawa, E.; Futatsubashi, M.; Tsuchiya, K.J.; Sugihara, G.; Iwata, Y.; Suzuki, K.; et al. Brain serotonin and dopamine transporter bindings in adults with high-functioning autism. *Arch. Gen. Psychiatry* **2010**, *67*, 59–68. [CrossRef] [PubMed]

112. Chugani, D.C.; Muzik, O.; Behen, M.; Rothermel, R.; Janisse, J.J.; Lee, J.; Chugani, H.T. Developmental changes in brain serotonin synthesis capacity in autistic and nonautistic children. *Ann. Neurol.* **1999**, *45*, 287–295. [CrossRef]

113. Mulder, E.J.; Anderson, G.M.; Kema, I.P.; de Bildt, A.; van Lang, N.D.; den Boer, J.A.; Minderaa, R.B. Platelet serotonin levels in pervasive developmental disorders and mental retardation: Diagnostic group differences, within-group distribution, and behavioral correlates. *J. Am. Acad. Child Adolesc. Psychiatry* **2004**, *43*, 491–499. [CrossRef] [PubMed]

114. Husarova, V.M.; Lakatosova, S.; Pivovarciova, A.; Babinska, K.; Bakos, J.; Durdiakova, J.; Kubranska, A.; Ondrejka, I.; Ostatnikova, D. Plasma oxytocin in children with autism and its correlations with behavioral parameters in children and parents. *Psychiatry Investig.* **2016**, *13*, 174–183. [CrossRef] [PubMed]

115. Modahl, C.; Green, L.; Fein, D.; Morris, M.; Waterhouse, L.; Feinstein, C.; Levin, H. Plasma oxytocin levels in autistic children. *Biol. Psychiatry* **1998**, *43*, 270–277. [CrossRef]

116. Horder, J.; Lavender, T.; Mendez, M.A.; O'Gorman, R.; Daly, E.; Craig, M.C.; Lythgoe, D.J.; Barker, G.J.; Murphy, D.G. Reduced subcortical glutamate/glutamine in adults with Autism Spectrum Disorders: A [lsqb]1H[rsqb]MRS study. *Transl. Psychiatry* **2013**, *3*, e279. [CrossRef] [PubMed]

117. Delion, S.; Chalon, S.; Herault, J.; Guilloteau, D.; Besnard, J.C.; Durand, G. Chronic dietary alpha-linolenic acid deficiency alters dopaminergic and serotoninergic neurotransmission in rats. *J. Nutr.* **1994**, *124*, 2466–2476. [PubMed]

118. Zimmer, L.; Hembert, S.; Durand, G.; Breton, P.; Guilloteau, D.; Besnard, J.C.; Chalon, S. Chronic *n*-3 polyunsaturated fatty acid diet-deficiency acts on dopamine metabolism in the rat frontal cortex: A microdialysis study. *Neurosci. Lett.* **1998**, *240*, 177–181. [CrossRef]

119. Kodas, E.; Galineau, L.; Bodard, S.; Vancassel, S.; Guilloteau, D.; Besnard, J.C.; Chalon, S. Serotoninergic neurotransmission is affected by *n*-3 polyunsaturated fatty acids in the rat. *J. Neurochem.* **2004**, *89*, 695–702. [CrossRef] [PubMed]

120. Moreira, J.D.; Knorr, L.; Ganzella, M.; Thomazi, A.P.; de Souza, C.G.; de Souza, D.G.; Pitta, C.F.; Mello e Souza, T.; Wofchuk, S.; Elisabetsky, E.; et al. Omega-3 fatty acids deprivation affects ontogeny of glutamatergic synapses in rats: Relevance for behavior alterations. *Neurochem. Int.* **2010**, *56*, 753–759. [CrossRef] [PubMed]

121. Kim, H.-Y.; Spector, A.A.; Xiong, Z.-M. A synaptogenic amide N-docosahexaenoylethanolamide promotes hippocampal development. *Prostaglandins Other Lipid Mediat.* **2011**, *96*, 114–120. [CrossRef] [PubMed]

122. Naik, U.S.; Gangadharan, C.; Abbagani, K.; Nagalla, B.; Dasari, N.; Manna, S.K. A Study of nuclear transcription factor-kappa b in childhood autism. *PLoS ONE* **2011**, *6*, e19488. [CrossRef] [PubMed]

123. Inga Jácome, M.; Morales ChacÈn, L.M.; Vera Cuesta, H.; Maragoto Rizo, C.; Whilby Santiesteban, M.; Ramos Hernandez, L.; Noris García, E.; González Fraguela, M.E.; Fernandez Verdecia, C.I.; Vegas Hurtado, Y.; et al. Peripheral Inflammatory Markers Contributing to Comorbidities in Autism. *Behav. Sci.* **2016**, *6*, 29. [CrossRef] [PubMed]

124. El-Ansary, A.; Hassan, W.M.; Qasem, H.; Das, U.N. Identification of biomarkers of impaired sensory profiles among autistic patients. *PLoS ONE* **2016**, *11*, e0164153. [CrossRef] [PubMed]

125. El-Ansary, A.; Al-Ayadhi, L. Lipid mediators in plasma of autism spectrum disorders. *Lipids Health Dis.* **2012**, *11*, 1–9. [CrossRef] [PubMed]

126. Adams, J.B.; Baral, M.; Geis, E.; Mitchell, J.; Ingram, J.; Hensley, A.; Zappia, I.; Newmark, S.; Gehn, E.; Rubin, R.A.; et al. The severity of autism is associated with toxic metal body burden and red blood cell glutathione levels. *J. Toxicol.* **2009**, *2009*, 532640. [CrossRef] [PubMed]

127. SalLam, M.M.; Motaleb, F.I.A.; Ahmed, M.B.; Mahmoud, A.A. Anti-inflammatory effect of omega-3 polyunsaturated fatty acids in children with bronchial asthma; relation to nuclear factor-kappa B (NF-κB) and inflammatory cytokines IL-12 and IL-13. Egypt. *J. Biochem. Mol. Biol.* **2010**, *28*, 51–66.

128. Zhang, R.; He, G.-Z.; Wang, Y.-K.; Zhou, K.-G.; Ma, E.-L. Omega-3 polyunsaturated fatty acids inhibit the increase in cytokines and chemotactic factors induced in vitro by lymph fluid from an intestinal ischemia-reperfusion injury model. *Nutrition* **2015**, *31*, 508–514. [CrossRef] [PubMed]

129. Zhao, Y.; Joshi-Barve, S.; Barve, S.; Chen, L.H. Eicosapentaenoic acid prevents LPS-induced TNF-α expression by preventing NF-κB activation. *J. Am. Coll. Nutr.* **2004**, *23*, 71–78. [CrossRef] [PubMed]

130. Allam-Ndoul, B.; Guénard, F.; Barbier, O.; Vohl, M.-C. Effect of *n*-3 fatty acids on the expression of inflammatory genes in THP-1 macrophages. *Lipids Health Dis.* **2016**, *15*, 69. [CrossRef] [PubMed]

131. Mathias, R.A.; Sergeant, S.; Ruczinski, I.; Torgerson, D.G.; Hugenschmidt, C.E.; Kubala, M.; Vaidya, D.; Suktitipat, B.; Ziegler, J.T.; Ivester, P.; et al. The impact of FADS genetic variants on ω6 polyunsaturated fatty acid metabolism in African Americans. *BMC Genet.* **2011**, *12*, 50. [CrossRef] [PubMed]

132. Abdelmagid, S.A.; Clarke, S.E.; Roke, K.; Nielsen, D.E.; Badawi, A.; El-Sohemy, A.; Mutch, D.M.; Ma, D.W.L. Ethnicity, sex, FADS genetic variation, and hormonal contraceptive use influence delta-5- and delta-6-desaturase indices and plasma docosahexaenoic acid concentration in young Canadian adults: A cross-sectional study. *Nutr. Metab. (Lond.)* **2015**, *12*, 14. [CrossRef] [PubMed]

133. Chouinard-Watkins, R.; Plourde, M. Fatty acid metabolism in carriers of apolipoprotein e epsilon 4 allele: Is it contributing to higher risk of cognitive decline and coronary heart disease? *Nutrients* **2014**, *6*, 4452–4471. [CrossRef] [PubMed]

134. Shimamoto, C.; Ohnishi, T.; Maekawa, M.; Watanabe, A.; Ohba, H.; Arai, R.; Iwayama, Y.; Hisano, Y.; Toyota, T.; Toyoshima, M.; et al. Functional characterization of FABP3, 5 and 7 gene variants identified in schizophrenia and autism spectrum disorder and mouse behavioral studies. *Hum. Mol. Genet.* **2014**, *23*, 6495–6511. [CrossRef] [PubMed]

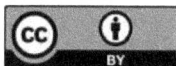

nutrients

MDPI

Article

Micronutrient-Fortified Milk and Academic Performance among Chinese Middle School Students: A Cluster-Randomized Controlled Trial

Xiaoqin Wang [1,*], Zhaozhao Hui [1], Xiaoling Dai [2], Paul D. Terry [3], Yue Zhang [1], Mei Ma [1], Mingxu Wang [1], Fu Deng [4], Wei Gu [1], Shuangyan Lei [1], Ling Li [1], Mingyue Ma [1] and Bin Zhang [1]

[1] Department of Public Health, Xi'an Jiaotong University Health Science Center, Xi'an 710061, China; huizhaozhao93@163.com (Z.H.); zymoon95@126.com (Y.Z.); wysun201314195@163.com (M.M.); wangmx601@mail.xjtu.edu.cn (M.W.); 232guwei@mail.xjtu.edu.cn (W.G.); shuangyan724@163.com (S.L.); liling-ch@163.com (L.L.); mamingyue66@163.com (M.M.); zhbin@mail.xjtu.edu.cn (B.Z.)

[2] Department of Nursing, Shaanxi Provincial Tumor Hospital, Xi'an 710061, China; Daixling113@126.com

[3] Department of Medicine, University of Tennessee Medical Center, Knoxville, TN 37996, USA; pdterry@utk.edu

[4] Xi'an Tie Yi High School, Xi'an 710000, China; dengfu01@126.com

* Correspondence: wangxiaoqin@mail.xjtu.edu.cn; Tel.: +86-29-8265-7015

Received: 13 January 2017; Accepted: 28 February 2017; Published: 2 March 2017

Abstract: Many children suffer from nutritional deficiencies that may negatively affect their academic performance. This cluster-randomized controlled trial aimed to test the effects of micronutrient-fortified milk in Chinese students. Participants received either micronutrient-fortified (n = 177) or unfortified (n = 183) milk for six months. Academic performance, motivation, and learning strategies were estimated by end-of-term tests and the Motivated Strategies for Learning Questionnaire. Blood samples were analyzed for micronutrients. In total, 296 students (82.2%) completed this study. Compared with the control group, students in the intervention group reported higher scores in several academic subjects (p < 0.05), including languages, mathematics, ethics, and physical performance at the end of follow-up. Students in the intervention group showed greater self-efficacy and use of cognitive strategies in learning, and reported less test anxiety (p < 0.001). Moreover, vitamin B_2 deficiency (odds ratio (OR) = 0.18, 95% confidence interval (CI): 0.11~0.30) and iron deficiency (OR = 0.34, 95% CI: 0.14~0.81) were less likely in the students of the intervention group, whereas vitamin D, vitamin B_{12}, and selenium deficiencies were not significantly different. "Cognitive strategy" had a partial mediating effect on the test scores of English (95% CI: 1.26~3.79) and Chinese (95% CI: 0.53~2.21). Our findings suggest that micronutrient-fortified milk may improve students' academic performance, motivation, and learning strategies.

Keywords: fortified milk; micronutrient; middle school students; academic performance; motivated strategies for learning

---

1. Introduction

More than 2 billion people suffer from micronutrient deficiencies worldwide, including many school-aged children and adolescents in developing countries [1]. A recent systematic review reported that China has a high prevalence of micronutrient deficiencies, and that 55.7%, 45.2%, and 84.7% of children have insufficient iron, vitamin D, and selenium, respectively [2]. For instance, iron deficiency can have a detrimental effect on physical performance in children and adolescents [3]. Vitamin D deficiency in early life may negatively affect neuronal differentiation, axonal connectivity, dopamine ontogeny, and brain structure and function [4]. Retinoic acid, the active metabolite of vitamin A, is tied to processes of neural plasticity, and may influence memory [5,6]. Micronutrient deficiencies have been linked to damaging physical performance [3], impaired cognitive functioning [7], suboptimal learning [8], and poor academic performance [9]. These endpoints, in turn, may lead to an increased risk of adulthood obesity [10,11], living in poverty [12], depression [13], and other psychiatric disorders [14]. Hence, there is a need to identify and evaluate safe, tolerable, and cost-effective nutritional interventions in school children and adolescents.

Food fortification has been an effective public health strategy to decrease micronutrient deficiencies [15,16], but the effect of micronutrient-fortified food on academic performance remains unclear [17,18]. A 2012 literature review [17] identified four studies, none of which showed a positive effect of micronutrient supplementations on school examination grades. On the other hand, a systematic review of randomized controlled trials (RCTs) in 2016 [18] reported a lack of consistency in school performance among students receiving micronutrient interventions. In the latter review, 8 of 19 trials incorporated assessment of academic performance, and one reported significant improvements in mathematics, while no improvement was observed in other academic subjects. Several factors might influence the effect of fortified food on academic performance, such as motivation and learning strategies, which also play important roles in the process of learning and have significant influences on academic performance [19]. In a cross-sectional study, milk intake showed significant positive correlations with testing technique and learning strategy in Korean male high school students [20]. However, there have been few studies investigating the effect of fortified food on both motivated strategies for learning and academic performance.

China has a considerable number of school-aged children and adolescents who would benefit from an integrated nutrition improvement policy approach. In 2011, the General Office of the State Council launched the Nutrition Improvement Program for Rural Compulsory Education Students (NIPRCES), which allots children undergoing compulsory education a daily container of milk and a chicken egg [21]. Although NIPRCES has been implemented for several years, it has not yet been utilized fully in many urban areas, and has yet to be studied for potential effects on school performance. Given this dearth of knowledge, we hypothesized that milk fortified with micronutrients would go further than regular milk in improving micronutrient status, and would positively influence academic performance, motivation, and use of effective studying strategies.

2. Materials and Methods

2.1. Study Design and Participants

We conducted a cluster-randomized controlled trial among healthy Chinese middle school students, aged 12 to 14 years between June 2015 and January 2016. This study was carried out according to the guidelines laid down in the Declaration of Helsinki and all procedures involving human subjects were approved by the Biomedical Ethics Committee of Xi'an Jiaotong University Health Science Center (Project identification code: 2015-356). Prior to the data collection, written informed consent was obtained from a parent or guardian of all participating students along with verbal assent from each student. The exclusion criteria for children included moderately/severely undernourished children (Body Mass Index (BMI) for age z-score < -2 SD) [22], severe anemia (Hemoglobin (Hb) < 8 g/dL), infection (White Blood Cell (WBC) $> 10.0 * 10^9$/L), history of food allergies, children consuming nutritional supplements, and those participating in another nutritional program.

A total of 681 students were recruited from Xi'an Middle School. After excluding 321 students (47.1%) who missed the screening examination, declined to participate, or were deemed ineligible, 360 students were enrolled in the present study. Participating children were allocated to either an intervention group ($n = 177$) or a control group ($n = 183$) with random number table by the research staff, considering each class as a cluster, such that each student in the class, if eligible, would be included. The schematic flow of the participants in the present study is shown in Figure 1. Subjects of the intervention group were given 250 mL micronutrient-fortified milk (Future Star, Mengniu Dairy Company Limited, Hohhot, China) per day for six months; students of the control group were provided pure milk with approximately the same caloric value of the fortified milk (Milk Deluxe, China Mengniu Dairy Company Limited, Hohhot, China) (Table 1). The milk was given to each student by the research assistants, and its consumption was supervised by the students' teachers. Academic performance, motivation, and learning strategies, and micronutrient status were all assessed at baseline and at the end of follow-up. Children, study investigators, and the data analyst were not blinded to treatment allocation.

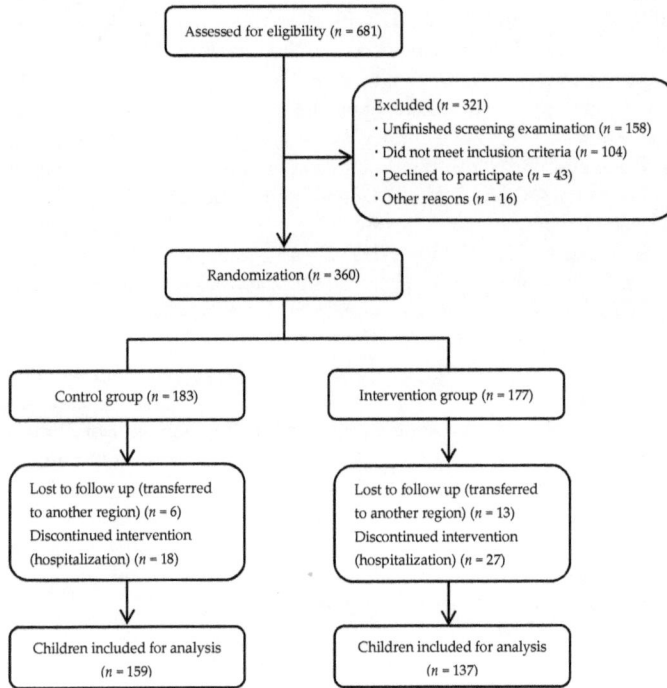

Figure 1. Schematic flow of the participants.

Table 1. Nutrient composition of the micronutrient fortified milk and pure milk in the present study.

Nutrients	Units	Fortified Milk per 100 mL	Pure Milk per 100 mL	FAO/WHO RNI for 10–18 Years [a]	Chinese DRIs EER/RNI/AI/EAR for 11–14 Years [b]
Energy	KJ	332	309	—	7530/8580 [c]
Protein	g	3.1	3.6	—	55/60
Fat	g	3.6	4.4	—	<60
Carbohydrate	g	8.6	5.0	—	150
Sodium	mg	58	65	—	1400
Vitamin A	µg RE	78	0	600	630/670 [c]
Vitamin D	µg	1.5	0	5	10
Vitamin E	mg α-TE	2.0	0	7.5/10.0 [c]	13
Vitamin B$_2$	mg	0.09	0	1.0/1.3 [c]	1.1/1.3 [c]
Pantothenic acid	mg	0.2	0	5.0	4.5
Phosphorus	mg	70	0	—	640
Calcium	mg	100	120	1300	1200
Zinc	mg	0.34	0	7.2/8.6 [c]	9.0/10.0 [c]

RNI: Recommended Nutrient Intake; DRIs: Dietary Reference Intakes; EER: Estimated Energy Requirement; AI: Adequate Intake; EAR: Estimated Average Requirement; RE: Retinol Equivalent; α-TE: α-Tocopherol Equivalent; [a] Food and Agriculture Organization of the United Nations (FAO) and World Health Organization (WHO), 2004. Vitamins and Mineral Requirements in Human Nutrition. Second Edition; [b] Chinese Nutrition Society, 2013. Chinese Dietary Reference Intakes; [c] Female/Male.

2.2. Screening Examination

The screening examination included anthropometric measurements and routine blood tests. Body height and weight were measured by trained personnel using standard anthropometric techniques. Subjects removed their shoes, emptied their pockets, and wore indoor clothing. Weight was recorded to the nearest 0.1 kg using a digital weighing scale. Height was measured to the nearest 0.1 cm using a stadiometer from head to foot. The weight and height of each participant were measured twice by study personnel. A third height and/or weight measurement was taken in the rare event that the first two measurements were not in agreement. BMI was derived from weight and height (kg/m^2), and thereafter BMI z-scores were calculated based on growth reference algorithms developed by the World Health Organization (WHO) for children and youth [23].

Hb and WBC counts were also assessed before the intervention to exclude children with severe anemia and infection. Non-fasting venous blood samples were collected in tubes containing anticoagulant (EDTA–K2). Blood samples were stored at 4 °C and analyzed within 4 hours. Hb and WBC counts were measured with an automatic hematology analyzer (XFA6100, PERLONG, Nanjing, China).

2.3. Academic Performance

Academic performance was measured using age- and gender-standardized end-of-term test scores retrieved from the school administration system. Academic tests were designed and administered by the Education Bureau of Xi'an, and scores obtained before the intervention were compared with those obtained at the end of follow-up. Test scores were analyzed using a percentage grading system, with 100 as the maximum grade and 60 percent as the minimum passing grade. The subjects of Chinese, mathematics, English, physics, social science, ethics, and physical performance were evaluated in the present study. Physical performance was assessed by a Physical Fitness Test, which includes a 1000-metre race for boys/800-metre race for girls, a 50-metre race, a standing long jump, sit-and-reach exercises, and pull-ups for boys/sit-ups for girls. Performance on the Physical Fitness Test was converted to a percentile score based on the national standard.

2.4. Motivation and Learning Strategies

Motivation and learning strategies were assessed by the Motivated Strategies for Learning Questionnaire (MSLQ) [24]. The MSLQ is a 44-item self-reported instrument consisting of three motivational belief subscales (Self-Efficacy, Intrinsic Value, and Test Anxiety), the Cognitive Strategy subscale and the Self-regulation subscale. The Self-Efficacy subscale is constructed by adding the scores of the students' responses to nine items regarding perceived competence and confidence in performance of class work. The Intrinsic Value subscale consists of nine items concerning intrinsic interest, perceived importance of course work, as well as preference for "challenge" and mastery of goals. Four items concerning worry about, and cognitive interference on, academic tests were used in the Test Anxiety subscale. The Cognitive Strategy Use subscale consists of 13 items pertaining to the use of rehearsal strategies, elaboration strategies, and organizational strategies. A Self-Regulation subscale was constructed from nine metacognitive and effort management items. Scores for each subscale were computed by summing the scores of specific items. Several items within the MSLQ are negatively worded and must be reversed before the respective score is calculated. Prior to the present study, the psychometric properties of the MSLQ were examined by a questionnaire survey with 30 subjects who did not participate in the present study, indicating a sound reliability (Cronbach's alpha = 0.79).

2.5. Micronutrient Status

Non-fasting venous blood specimens were collected by professional phlebotomist. Serum and plasma samples were separated within 4 hours of collection and stored at -80 °C until analysis. Micronutrient status was measured at baseline and at the end of follow-up for serum ferritin (SF), soluble transferrin receptor (sTfR), vitamin D, vitamin B_2, vitamin B_{12}, and selenium. SF, vitamin D, and vitamin B_{12} were measured with electrochemiluminescence technique (Elecsys 2010, Roche Diagnostics, Mannheim, Germany). sTfR was measured using immunoturbidimetry (IMMAGE 800, Beckman Coulter, Carlsbad, America). Vitamin B_2 was measured by the Erythrocyte Glutathione Reductase Activity Coefficient method using UV-VIS 1800 spectrophotometer by the modified ascorbic acid methodology [25]. The serum selenium levels were determined by atomic fluorescence spectrometry (RGF-8780, Bohui, Beijing, China). All biochemical analyses were carried out at the Micronutrient Laboratory, Division of Nutrition, Xi'an Jiaotong University Health Science Center. SF less than 15 mg/L or sTfR greater than 8.5 mg/L was considered to be a sign of iron deficiency. Deficiencies of vitamin D, vitamin B_2, vitamin B_{12}, and selenium were defined as vitamin D less than 11 ng/mL, the activity coefficient of vitamin B_2 greater than 1.2 AC, vitamin B_{12} less than 203 pg/mL, and body selenium less than 84.9 mg/mL, respectively. Body iron was calculated as Body Iron (mg/kg) = $-$[log (R/F ratio) $-$ 2.8229]/0.1207 where R/F ratio = sTfR/SF [26].

2.6. Statistical Analysis

Data management and data analysis were performed using Epidata (The Epidata Association, Odense, Denmark) and SPSS (Statistical Package for the Social Sciences for Windows, IBM, Armonk, NY, USA) version 23.0. The nominal variables are presented as frequency and proportion. The distribution normality of the quantitative variables was tested by One-Sample Kolmogorov-Smirnov test. The normally distributed variables are presented as mean $\pm$ standard deviation (SD). Student's *t*-tests were performed to analyze the differences in anthropometric parameters such as age, height, weight, and BMI, whereas gender difference and the prevalence of micronutrient deficiencies at baseline between the two groups were tested using Chi-square tests. For categories with small numbers (theoretical frequency < 5), the Fisher's exact test was used. After the intervention, the prevalence of micronutrient deficiencies was analyzed with logistic regression models. Analysis of covariance (ANCOVA) was used to test differences in academic performance, motivation and learning strategies while adjusting for baseline measures of independent variance. The mediating effects of motivation and learning strategies on academic performance in micronutrients were analyzed with nonparametric Bootstrap methods [27]. Statistical significance was set at $p < 0.05$; all tests were two-sided.

3. Results

3.1. Demographic and Anthropometric Characteristics of Subjects

The demographic and anthropometric characteristics of the subjects in this study are shown in Table 2. Overall, 137 students in the intervention group (77.4%) and 159 students in the control group (86.9%) completed this study. The mean age of the students at the time of enrollment was 13.2 ± 1.0 years and 13.4 ± 0.9 years in the intervention group and the control group, respectively. The study sample included more girls than boys, although the proportions did not differ significantly by intervention group ($p = 0.894$). There were also no significant differences in age ($p = 0.071$), height ($p = 0.283$), weight ($p = 0.100$), BMI ($p = 0.252$), or BMI z-scores ($p = 0.509$) between the two groups.

Table 2. Demographic and anthropometric characteristics of subjects in the intervention and control groups.

Variables	Intervention (*n* = 137)	Control (*n* = 159)	t/X^2	*p*
Age (years)	13.2 ± 1.0	13.4 ± 0.9	1.811	0.071
Gender			0.018	0.894
Male (*n* (%))	38 (27.7)	43 (27.0)		
Female (*n* (%))	99 (72.3)	116 (73.0)		
Height (cm)	163.9 ± 1.7	163.7 ± 1.5	1.075	0.283
Weight (kg)	58.8 ± 4.1	58.1 ± 3.2	1.648	0.100
BMI (kg/m^2)	21.2 ± 0.8	21.1 ± 0.7	1.147	0.252
BMI z-scores	0.1 ± 1.3	0.2 ± 1.3	0.660	0.509

BMI: Body Mass Index.

3.2. Micronutrient Deficiencies

Micronutrient deficiencies in students were comparable between the intervention group and the control group at baseline (Table 3). The effects of micronutrient-fortified milk consumption on iron, vitamin D, vitamin B$_2$, vitamin B$_{12}$, and selenium deficiencies analyzed with logistic regression models are shown in Table 4. After six months, students in the intervention group were less likely to be iron deficient (odds ratio (OR) = 0.34, 95% confidence interval (CI): 0.14~0.81) and vitamin B$_2$ deficient (OR = 0.18, 95% CI: 0.11~0.30) when compared with the control group. However, there was no statistically significant difference in the prevalence of vitamin D, vitamin B$_{12}$, and selenium deficiencies between the two groups.

Table 3. Prevalence of iron, vitamin D, vitamin B$_2$, vitamin B$_{12}$, and selenium deficiencies in subjects at baseline between the intervention and control group.

Micronutrients	Intervention (*n* = 137)	Control (*n* = 159)	X^2	*p*
Iron deficiency	10 (7.3)	13 (8.3)	0.079	0.779
Vitamin D deficiency	5 (3.6)	5 (3.1)		0.999 *
Vitamin B$_2$ deficiency	127 (92.7)	145 (91.2)	0.224	0.636
Vitamin B$_{12}$ deficiency	12 (8.8)	15 (9.4)	0.040	0.841
Selenium deficiency	68 (49.6)	77 (48.4)	0.043	0.836

* *p* value was compared using Fisher's exact test.

Table 4. The effects of micronutrient-fortified milk on the prevalence of iron, vitamin D, vitamin B$_2$, vitamin B$_{12}$, and selenium deficiencies.

Micronutrients	Intervention (*n* = 137)	Control (*n* = 159)	Adjusted OR	95% CI	*p*
Iron deficiency	7 (5.1)	22 (13.8)	0.34 [a]	0.14~0.81	0.012
Vitamin D deficiency	6 (4.4)	8 (5.0)	0.87 [b]	0.29~2.56	0.792
Vitamin B$_2$ deficiency	31 (22.6)	99 (62.3)	0.18 [c]	0.11~0.30	0.000
Vitamin B$_{12}$ deficiency	4 (2.9)	3 (1.9)	1.56 [d]	0.34~7.11	0.708
Selenium deficiency	53 (38.7)	59 (37.1)	1.07 [e]	0.67~1.71	0.780

OR: Odds Ratio; CI: Confidence Interval; [a] Adjusted by gender, age, BMI, vitamin D, vitamin B$_2$, vitamin B$_{12}$, selenium; [b] Adjusted by gender, age, BMI, iron, vitamin B$_2$, vitamin B$_{12}$, selenium; [c] Adjusted by gender, age, BMI, iron, vitamin D, vitamin B$_{12}$, selenium; [d] Adjusted by gender, age, BMI, iron, vitamin D, vitamin B$_2$, selenium; [e] Adjusted by gender, age, BMI, iron, vitamin D, vitamin B$_2$, vitamin B$_{12}$.

3.3. Academic Performance

The academic scores of trial participants are shown in Table 5. The academic performance of the subjects was comparable between the intervention group and the control group at baseline (*p* > 0.05). Compared with students receiving unfortified milk, students receiving micronutrient-fortified milk showed significantly higher scores in the subjects of Chinese, mathematics, English, ethics, and physical performance ($p < 0.05$), whereas the scores for physics were higher but not statistically significant ($p = 0.224$). No significant difference was observed in social science scores ($p = 0.428$). When modeled as independent variables, both iron and vitamin B_2 were associated with improved performance in the subjects of Chinese, mathematics, English, ethics, and physical performance ($p < 0.05$).

Table 5. Academic scores of the end-of-term tests between the control and intervention group in middle school students.

Subjects	Intervention (n = 137)		Control (n = 159)		F	p	F'	p'
	Baseline	Post-Trial	Baseline	Post-Trial				
Chinese	72.1 ± 2.0	81.2 ± 2.2	72.3 ± 2.1	78.5 ± 2.0	127.852	0.000	127.395	0.000
Mathematics	82.8 ± 2.0	86.1 ± 2.1	82.4 ± 2.0	85.6 ± 2.0	9.416	0.002	8.013	0.005
English	73.0 ± 2.0	84.1 ± 1.9	72.6 ± 2.0	79.3 ± 2.0	497.398	0.000	483.216	0.000
Physics	62.6 ± 2.1	70.0 ± 2.0	62.2 ± 2.2	69.5 ± 2.4	1.766	0.185	1.484	0.224
Social science	81.3 ± 2.1	84.9 ± 2.0	80.9 ± 1.8	85.2 ± 2.2	0.591	0.443	0.629	0.428
Ethics	72.6 ± 1.9	77.8 ± 2.1	72.4 ± 2.1	74.9 ± 2.0	127.497	0.000	127.637	0.000
Physical performance	68.7 ± 3.7	83.3 ± 4.7	69.3 ± 3.4	78.5 ± 4.4	79.162	0.000	59.090	0.000

F': Adjusted by gender, age, BMI, iron, vitamin D, vitamin B_2, vitamin B_{12}, selenium, self-efficacy, intrinsic value, test anxiety, cognitive strategy, and self-regulation. The effect sizes (Eta Square) are 0.303, 0.027, 0.623, 0.005, 0.002, 0.004, and 0.168 for Chinese, mathematics, English, physics, social science, ethics, and physical performance, respectively.

3.4. Motivation and Learning Strategies

Baseline motivation and learning strategy scores were comparable between the intervention groups for self-efficacy, intrinsic value, test anxiety, cognitive strategy, and self-regulation (Table 6). After the intervention, students in the fortified milk group showed higher scores for self-efficacy ($p < 0.001$), and lower scores for test anxiety ($p < 0.001$), than those in the control group. There was no significant difference in scores for "intrinsic value". Regarding use of learning strategies, students who consumed fortified milk were more likely to incorporate cognitive strategies into their study routines ($p < 0.001$). However, no significant difference was observed in "self-regulation" between the two groups. In addition, the use of cognitive strategies had a partial mediating effect on academic scores in relation to iron and vitamin B_2, accounting for 29.3% (95% CI: 1.26~3.79) of the improved performance in English and 14.7% (95% CI: 0.53~2.21) for Chinese.

Table 6. Motivation and learning strategy scores between the control and intervention group in middle school students.

Dimensions	Score				F	p	F'	p'
	Intervention (n = 137)		Control (n = 159)					
	Baseline	Post-Trial	Baseline	Post-Trial				
Self-efficacy	50.3 ± 2.7	52.5 ± 0.9	49.9 ± 2.0	51.9 ± 0.7	19.497	0.000	17.621	0.000
Intrinsic value	50.8 ± 3.3	53.0 ± 2.9	51.3 ± 2.5	52.6 ± 2.7	0.375	0.541	0.285	0.594
Test anxiety	22.0 ± 5.5	20.1 ± 4.3	21.4 ± 4.3	22.8 ± 3.7	41.278	0.000	40.905	0.000
Cognitive strategy	58.2 ± 2.8	61.1 ± 3.1	57.7 ± 2.6	60.1 ± 2.7	15.885	0.000	15.730	0.000
Self-regulation	47.6 ± 3.2	47.5 ± 1.7	48.0 ± 2.5	47.6 ± 2.1	0.987	0.321	1.174	0.279

F': Adjusted by gender, age, BMI, iron, vitamin D, vitamin B_2, vitamin B_{12}, and selenium. The effect sizes (Eta Square) are 0.057, 0.001, 0.123, 0.051, and 0.004 for self-efficacy, intrinsic value, test anxiety, cognitive strategy, and self-regulation, respectively.

4. Discussion

We conducted a cluster-randomized, controlled feeding intervention study to determine the effect of micronutrient-fortified milk versus unfortified milk on academic performance among Chinese middle school students aged 12 to 14 years. The micronutrient-fortified milk intervention raised blood vitamin B_2 and iron levels, and appeared to increase academic performance, physical performance, learning motivation, and the successful use of study strategies.

Children in our study who consumed micronutrient-fortified milk had significantly higher academic performance than those who consumed unfortified milk, not entirely consistent with findings in previous studies [9,17,28,29]. A recent literature review found that there was a correlation between micronutrients and the academic performance in school children [9]. However, another systematic review concluded no positive effect of multiple micronutrient supplementations on school examination grades [17]. For specific micronutrients, one cross-sectional study showed that iron insufficiency was related to disadvantages in learning, and insufficient serum iron concentration was correlated with significantly lower mathematic scores in female students ($r = 0.628$) [27]. Another interventional study suggested that improving iron status through fortified rice can enhance school performance ($p = 0.022$) [29]. In addition, a systematic review concluded that serum vitamin B_{12} levels were associated with cognitive function [30], which may further influence academic performance in school children [31]. Moreover, Babur demonstrated the negative effect of selenium deficiency on learning and memory in adult rats [32].

The beneficial effect on academic performance in the present study can be attributed to improved vitamin B_2 and iron status. Students who consumed fortified milk showed less iron deficiency, although iron was not added to the milk. The reason for this finding is unclear, although vitamin B_2 may influence iron status, possibly at the level of iron absorption [33]. Micronutrient levels have been linked in Indian school children to improved cognitive and physical performance [34]. Iron may alter the intracellular signaling pathways and electrophysiology of the developing hippocampus, the brain region responsible for recognition, learning, and memory [35]. In addition, we found that students in the intervention group had significantly higher physical performance than what was observed in controls. This may be attributed to improved iron status and oxygen carrying capacity in hemoglobin [36].

Another possible mechanism contributing to the improved academic performance might be the mediating role of learning strategies [37]. The present study found that students in the intervention group were more self-efficacious and had less test anxiety, and were also more likely to use cognitive strategies in the process of learning. Students' perception of self-efficacy and the evaluation of their own competence were significantly and positively related to academic achievement [38,39]. In a study of Finnish upper secondary school students [40], a statistically significant correlation was found between test anxiety levels and academic performance. Abdollahpour [41] also revealed that using cognitive strategies were positively correlated particularly with math achievement among male high school freshmen. Similarly, Zahrou [42] found that the consumption of fortified milk has a favorable effect on cognitive ability. Our data suggest that use of cognitive strategies may mediate the association between nutrient status and academic performance. Taken together with the results of these previous studies, our findings suggest a potentially long-term benefit to school-aged children from a relatively inexpensive intervention.

There are two strengths in the present study. Firstly, we not only examined the effect of fortified milk on students' nutritional status, but also on their academic performance, motivation, and use of learning strategies. Secondly, the cluster-randomized controlled trial design allows control of both measured and unmeasured confounding factors. Furthermore, the cluster-randomized design minimizes the possibility of contamination between the intervention and control group [43], because there is less opportunity to exchange the milk product for the participating students.

Several limitations of our study must be considered. Information on dietary factors other than nutritional supplements during the intervention period was not collected. Therefore, we cannot be certain that our results were not influenced by unmeasured dietary factors. Similarly, we did not account for factors such as "self-concept" [44], physical fitness [45], and cell phone use [46], which have been found to affect academic achievement. Lastly, the six-month follow-up period precluded the examination of longer-term effects of micronutrient-fortified milk on academic outcomes.

5. Conclusions

In conclusion, the results of the present study suggest that the consumption of micronutrient-fortified milk may improve academic performance, motivation, and learning strategies in Chinese school children. If our results are confirmed in future studies, additional studies will be needed to elucidate the underlying mechanisms and to identify subgroups of undernourished student populations that are most likely to benefit from this intervention.

Acknowledgments: We especially thank the teachers and administrators of Xi'an High School and gratefully acknowledge the students and their parents for their participation in the present study. This work was financially supported by a grant (Grant No. 81101333) from the National Natural Science Foundation of China and a grant (Grant No. 13-168-201608) from China Medical Board. The funders had no role in the design, analysis, or writing of this article.

Author Contributions: Xiaoqin Wang and Paul D. Terry conceived and designed the experiments; Xiaoling Dai, Mingxu Wang, Shuangyan Lei, Mingyue Ma, Ling Li, Fu Deng, Wei Gu, and Bin Zhang performed the experiments; Yue Zhang and Mei Ma analyzed the data; Zhaozhao Hui wrote the paper. Xiaoqin Wang and Paul D. Terry had primary responsibility for final content. All authors read and approved the final manuscript.

Conflicts of Interest: The authors declare no conflict of interest. The founding sponsors had no role in the design of the study; in the collection, analyses, or interpretation of data; in the writing of the manuscript, and in the decision to publish the results.

Abbreviations

The following abbreviations are used in this manuscript:

MSLQ	Motivated Strategies for Learning Questionnaire
EAR	Estimated Average Requirement
NIPRCES	Nutrition Improvement Program for Rural Compulsory Education Students
BMI	Body Mass Index
Hb	Hemoglobin
WBC	White Blood Cell
RNI	Recommended Nutrient Intake
DRIs	Chinese Dietary Reference Intakes
EER	Estimated Energy Requirement
AI	Adequate Intake
SF	Serum Ferritin
STfR	Soluble Transferrin Receptor
SPSS	Statistical Package for the Social Sciences
SD	Standard Deviation

References

1. Allen, L.; Benoist, B.D.; Dary, O.; Hurrell, R. *Guidelines on Food Fortification with Micronutrients*; World Health Organization and Food and Agriculture Organization: Geneva, Switzerland, 2006.
2. Wong, A.Y.; Chan, E.W.; Chui, C.S.; Sutcliffe, A.G.; Wong, I.C. The phenomenon of micronutrient deficiency among children in China: A systematic review of the literature. *Public Health Nutr.* **2014**, *17*, 2605–2618. [CrossRef] [PubMed]
3. Gera, T.; Sachdev, H.P.; Nestel, P. Effect of iron supplementation on physical performance in children and adolescents: Systematic review of randomized controlled trials. *Indian Pediatr.* **2007**, *44*, 15–24. [PubMed]
4. Eyles, D.W.; Burne, T.H.; McGrath, J.J. Vitamin D, effects on brain development, adult brain function and the links between low levels of vitamin D and neuropsychiatric disease. *Front. Neuroendocrinol.* **2013**, *34*, 47–64. [CrossRef] [PubMed]
5. Shearer, K.D.; Stoney, P.N.; Morgan, P.J.; McCaffery, P.J. A vitamin for the brain. *Trends Neurosci.* **2012**, *35*, 733–741. [CrossRef] [PubMed]
6. Ormerod, A.D.; Thind, C.K.; Rice, S.A.; Reid, I.C.; Williams, J.H.; McCaffery, P.J. Influence of isotretinoin on hippocampal based learning in human subjects. *Psychopharmacology* **2012**, *221*, 667–674. [CrossRef] [PubMed]
7. Black, M.M. Micronutrient deficiencies and cognitive functioning. *J. Nutr.* **2003**, *133*, 3927S–3931S. [PubMed]

8.   Osendarp, S.J.; Baghurst, K.I.; Bryan, J.; Calvaresi, E.; Hughes, D.; Hussaini, M.; Karyadi, S.J.; van Klinken, B.J.; van der Knaap, H.C.; Lukito, W.; et al. Effect of a 12-mo micronutrient intervention on learning and memory in well-nourished and marginally nourished school-aged children: 2 parallel, randomized, placebo-controlled studies in Australia and Indonesia. *Am. J. Clin. Nutr.* **2007**, *86*, 1082–1093. [PubMed]

9.   Syam, A.; Palutturi, S.; Djafar, N.; Astuti, N.; Thaha, A.R. Micronutrients, Academic Performance and Concentration of Study: A Literature Review. 2016. Available online: http://repository.unhas.ac.id/bitstream/handle/123456789/20833/IJABER?sequence = 1 (accessed on 13 January 2016).

10. Alatupa, S.; Pulkki-Råback, L.; Hintsanen, M.; Ravaja, N.; Raitakari, O.T.; Telama, R.; Viikari, J.S.; Keltikangas-Järvinen, L. School performance as a predictor of adulthood obesity: A 21-year follow-up study. *Eur. J. Epidemiol.* **2010**, *25*, 267–274. [CrossRef] [PubMed]

11. Sobol-Goldberg, S.; Rabinowitz, J. Association of childhood and teen school performance and obesity in young adulthood in the US National Longitudinal Survey of Youth. *Prev. Med.* **2016**, *89*, 57–63. [CrossRef] [PubMed]

12. Hoddinott, J.; Behrman, J.R.; Maluccio, J.A.; Melgar, P.; Quisumbing, A.R.; Ramirezzea, M.; Stein, A.D.; Yount, K.M.; Martorell, R. Adult consequences of growth failure in early childhood. *Am. J. Clin. Nutr.* **2013**, *98*, 1170–1178. [CrossRef] [PubMed]

13. Lehtinen, H.; Raikkonen, K.; Heinonen, K.; Raitakari, O.T.; Keltikangas-Jarvinen, L. School performance in childhood and adolescence as a predictor of depressive symptoms in adulthood. *Sch. Psychol. Int.* **2006**, *27*, 281–295. [CrossRef]

14. Bjorkenstam, E.; Dalman, C.; Vinnerljung, B.; Weitoft, G.R.; Walder, D.J.; Burstrom, B. Childhood household dysfunction, school performance and psychiatric care utilisation in young adults: A register study of 96 399 individuals in stockholm county. *J. Epidemiol. Community Health* **2016**, *70*, 473–480. [CrossRef] [PubMed]

15. Nga, T.T.; Winichagoon, P.; Dijkhuizen, M.A.; Khan, N.C.; Wasantwisut, E.; Furr, H.; Wieringa, F.T. Multi-micronutrient-fortified biscuits decreased prevalence of anemia and improved micronutrient status and effectiveness of deworming in rural Vietnamese school children. *J. Nutr.* **2009**, *139*, 1013–1021. [CrossRef] [PubMed]

16. Goyle, A.; Prakash, S. Effect of supplementation of micronutrient fortified biscuits on haemoglobin and serum iron levels of adolescent girls from Jaipur city, India. *Nutr. Food Sci.* **2010**, *40*, 477–484. [CrossRef]

17. Eilander, A.; Gera, T.; Sachdev, H.S.; Transler, C.; van der Knaap, H.C.; Kok, F.J.; Osendarp, S.J. Multiple micronutrient supplementation for improving cognitive performance in children: Systematic review of randomized controlled trials. *Am. J. Clin. Nutr.* **2010**, *91*, 115–130. [CrossRef] [PubMed]

18. Long, F.L.; Lawlis, T.R. Feeding the brain-The effects of micronutrient interventions on cognitive performance among school-aged children: A systematic review of randomized controlled trials. *Clin. Nutr.* **2016**, *2016*, 1–8. [CrossRef]

19. Pintrich, P.R.; De Groot, E.V. Motivation and self regulated learning components of academic performance. In Proceedings of the 39th EUCEN Conference, Rovaniemi, Finland, 27–29 May 2010.

20. Kim, S.H.; Kim, W.K.; Kang, M.H. Relationships between milk consumption and academic performance, learning motivation and strategy, and personality in Korean adolescents. *Nutr. Res. Pract.* **2016**, *10*, 198–205. [CrossRef] [PubMed]

21. Zhang, F.; Hu, X.; Tian, Z.; Ma, G. Literature research of the Nutrition Improvement Programme for Rural Compulsory Education Students in China. *Public Health Nutr.* **2014**, *18*, 1–8. [CrossRef] [PubMed]

22. WHO Multicentre Growth Reference Study Group. WHO Child Growth Standards based on length/height, weight and age. *Acta Paediatr. Suppl.* **2006**, *450*, 76–85.

23. de Onis, M.; Onyango, A.W.; Borghi, E.; Siyam, A.; Nishida, C.; Siekmann, J. Development of a WHO growth reference for school-aged children and adolescents. *Bull. World Health Organ.* **2007**, *85*, 660–667. [CrossRef] [PubMed]

24. Pintrich, P.R.; de Groot, E.V. Motivational and self-regulated learning components of classroom academic performance. *J. Educ. Psychol.* **1990**, *82*, 33–40. [CrossRef]

25. Dror, Y.; Stern, F.; Komarnitsky, M. Optimal and stable conditions for the determination of erythrocyte glutathione reductase activation coefficient to evaluate riboflavin status. *Int. J. Vitam. Nutr. Res.* **1994**, *64*, 257–262. [PubMed]

26. Cook, J.D.; Flowers, C.H.; Skikne, B.S. The quantitative assessment of body iron. *Blood* **2003**, *101*, 3359–3364. [CrossRef] [PubMed]

27. Hayes, A.F. Introduction to mediation, moderation, and conditional process analysis: A regression-based approach. *J. Educ. Meas.* **2013**, *51*, 335–337.

28. Soleimani, N.; Abbaszadeh, N. Relationship between anaemia, caused from the iron deficiency, and academic achievement among third grade high school female students. *Procedia-Soc. Behav. Sci.* **2011**, *29*, 1877–1884. [CrossRef]

29. Fiorentino, M.; Perignon, M.; Kuong, K.; Burja, K.; Kong, K.; Parker, M.; Berger, J.; Wieringa, F.T. Rice fortified with iron in school meals improves cognitive performance in Cambodian school children. In Proceedings of the Micronutrient Forum Global Conference, Addis Ababa, Ethiopia, 2–6 July 2014.

30. Vogel, T.; Dali-Youcef, N.; Kaltenbach, G.; Andres, E. Homocysteine, vitamin B12, folate and cognitive functions: A systematic and critical review of the literature. *Int. J. Clin. Pract.* **2009**, *63*, 1061–1067. [CrossRef] [PubMed]

31. Haile, D.; Nigatu, D.; Gashaw, K.; Demelash, H. Height for age z score and cognitive function are associated with academic performance among school children aged 8–11 years old. *Arch. Public Health* **2016**, *74*, 17. [CrossRef] [PubMed]

32. Babur, E.; Bakkaloglu, U.; Erol, E.; Dursun, N.; Suer, C. The effect of selenium deficiency on learning and memory in adult rats. *Acta Physiol.* **2015**, *215*, 42.

33. Powers, H.J. Riboflavin (vitamin B-2) and health. *Am. J. Clin. Nutr.* **2003**, *77*, 1352–1360. [PubMed]

34. Swaminathan, S.; Edward, B.S.; Kurpad, A.V. Micronutrient deficiency and cognitive and physical performance in Indian children. *Eur. J. Clin. Nutr.* **2013**, *67*, 467–474. [CrossRef] [PubMed]

35. Fretham, S.J.; Carlson, E.S.; Georgieff, M.K. The role of iron in learning and memory. *Adv. Nutr.* **2011**, *2*, 112–121. [CrossRef] [PubMed]

36. Waldvogel-Abramowski, S.; Waeber, G.; Gassner, C.; Buser, A.; Frey, B.M.; Favrat, B.; Tissot, J.D. Physiology of iron metabolism. *Transfus. Med. Hemother.* **2014**, *41*, 213–221. [CrossRef] [PubMed]

37. Ning, H.K.; Downing, K. Influence of student learning experience on academic performance: The mediator and moderator effects of self-regulation and motivation. *Br. Educ. Res. J.* **2012**, *38*, 219–237. [CrossRef]

38. Mothabeng, D.J. The relationship between the self-efficacy, academic performance and clinical performance. In Proceedings of the World Confederation for Physical Therapy Congress, Singapore, 1–4 May 2015.

39. Tenaw, Y.A. Relationship between self-efficacy, academic achievement and gender in analytical chemistry at Debre Markos College of teacher education. *Afr. J. Chem. Educ.* **2013**, *3*, 3–28.

40. Green, E. Test Anxiety, Coping, Gender and Academic Performance in English Exams: A Study of Finnish upper Secondary School Students. 2016. Available online: http://www.doria.fi/handle/10024/124720 (accessed on 15 August 2016).

41. Abdollahpour, M.A.; Kadivar, P.; Abdollahi, M.H. Relationships between cognitive styles, cognitive and meta-cognitive strategies with academic achievement. *Psychol. Res.* **2006**, *8*, 30–44.

42. Zahrou, F.E.; Azlaf, M.; El Menchawy, I.; El Mzibri, M.; El Kari, K.; El Hamdouchi, A.; Mouzouni, F.Z.; Barkat, A.; Aguenaou, H. Fortified iodine milk improves iodine status and cognitive abilities in schoolchildren aged 7–9 years living in a rural mountainous area of Morocco. *J. Nutr. Metab.* **2016**, *2016*, 8468594. [CrossRef] [PubMed]

43. Chenot, J.F. Cluster randomised trials: An important method in primary care research. *Z. Evidenz Fortbild. Qual. Gesundhwes.* **2009**, *103*, 475–480. [CrossRef]

44. Pottebaum, S.M.; Keith, T.Z.; Ehly, S.W. Is there a causal relation between self-concept and academic achievement? *J. Educ. Res.* **2015**, *79*, 140–144. [CrossRef]

45. Torrijos-Niño, C.; Martínez-Vizcaíno, V.; Pardo-Guijarro, M.J.; García-Prieto, J.C.; Arias-Palencia, N.M.; Sánchez-López, M. Physical fitness, obesity, and academic achievement in schoolchildren. *J. Pediatr.* **2014**, *165*, 104–109. [CrossRef] [PubMed]

46. Lepp, A.; Barkley, J.E.; Karpinski, A.C. The relationship between cell phone use, academic performance, anxiety, and satisfaction with life in college students. *Comput. Hum. Behav.* **2014**, *31*, 343–350. [CrossRef]

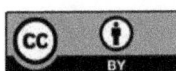

Article

Prevalence and Correlates of Preschool Overweight and Obesity Amidst the Nutrition Transition: Findings from a National Cross-Sectional Study in Lebanon

Lara Nasreddine [1,2], Nahla Hwalla [1,2], Angie Saliba [1], Christelle Akl [1] and Farah Naja [1,2,*]

[1] Department of Nutrition and Food Science, Faculty of Agricultural and Food Sciences,
American University of Beirut, P.O. Box 11-0236, Riad El Solh, Beirut, Lebanon;
ln10@aub.edu.lb (L.N.); nahla@aub.edu.lb (N.H.); aes10@mail.aub.edu (A.S.); cristell@gmail.com (C.A.)

[2] Nutrition, Obesity and Related Diseases (NORD), Office of Strategic Health Initiatives,
American University of Beirut, P.O. Box 11-0236, Riad El Solh, Beirut, Lebanon

* Correspondence: fn14@aub.edu.lb; Tel.: +961-1-35-0000 (ext. 4504)

Received: 17 January 2017; Accepted: 13 February 2017; Published: 11 March 2017

Abstract: There is increasing evidence linking early life adiposity to disease risk later in life. This study aims at determining the prevalence and correlates of overweight and obesity among preschoolers in Lebanon. A national cross-sectional survey was conducted amongst 2–5 years old children (n = 525). Socio-demographic, lifestyle, dietary, and anthropometric data were obtained. The prevalence of overweight and obesity was estimated at 6.5% and 2.7%, respectively. Based on stepwise logistic regression for the prediction of overweight and obesity (combined), the variance accounted for by the first block (socioeconomic, parental characteristics) was 11.9%, with higher father's education (OR = 5.31, 95% CI: 1.04–27.26) and the presence of household helper (OR = 2.19, 95% CI: 1.05–4.56) being significant predictors. The second block of variables (eating habits) significantly improved the prediction of overweight/obesity to reach 21%, with eating in front of the television (OR = 1.07, 95% CI: 1.02–1.13) and satiety responsiveness (OR = 0.83, 95% CI: 0.70–0.99) being significantly associated with overweight/obesity. In the third block, fat intake remained a significant predictor of overweight/obesity (OR = 2.31, 95% CI: 1.13–4.75). This study identified specific risk factors for preschool overweight/obesity in Lebanon and characterized children from high socioeconomic backgrounds as important target groups for preventive interventions. These findings may be of significance to other middle-income countries in similar stages of nutrition transition.

Keywords: obesity; preschoolers; prevalence; correlates; diet; socioeconomic status; Lebanon

1. Introduction

Childhood obesity is increasingly recognized as a serious public health concern, with available evidence suggesting a dramatic increase in its worldwide prevalence over the past few decades [1,2]. This increase is documented as early as the preschool years. De Onis et al. [2] showed that the global prevalence of preschool overweight and obesity has escalated from 4.2% in 1990 to 6.7% in 2010, with a projected increase to 9.1% in 2020 [2]. The highest prevalence rates of preschool overweight and obesity in 2010 were reported for the regions of Northern Africa and Western Asia, with an estimate of 17% and 14.7%, respectively [2]. The prevalence of preschool overweight and obesity in these regions, which largely represent the Middle East and North Africa (MENA) region, is projected to rise to over 25% by 2020 [2].

Excess body weight usually results from a complex interaction of genetic, environmental, behavioral and social factors, which may, in concert, modulate the child's propensity for becoming overweight [3]. Increased food intake, frequent consumption of high-calorie sweetened beverages and television viewing have been frequently reported as key determinants of the risk of pediatric overweight and obesity [3,4]. Socioeconomic status (SES) has also been identified as an important modulator of the risk of childhood obesity, although discrepancies have been reported in the direction of the relationship between SES and pediatric obesity [5]. In high-income countries, the risk of childhood obesity has been shown to be the highest in lower socioeconomic groups [5], while the opposite was reported for low-income countries [5,6]. Less is known about the relationship between SES and childhood obesity in middle-income countries, particularly those undergoing the nutrition transition [5,6].

Pediatric obesity is associated with adverse physical and psychological effects that may appear in childhood and track into the adult years [7–9]. Short-term health consequences of pediatric obesity include metabolic abnormalities such as high blood pressure, dyslipidemia, impaired glucose homeostasis, and metabolic syndrome [7]. In the long term, pediatric obesity tends to persist into adulthood, increasing the risk for obesity-associated morbidities such as cardiovascular disease, type 2 diabetes and some types of cancer [8,9]. Psychologically, obese children commonly suffer from negative body image and low self-esteem [7], that often progress into anxiety and depression in adulthood [8]. Consequently, the early prevention of overweight and obesity is increasingly recognized as a vital strategy to decrease the burden of associated short- and long-term morbidity [10]. The preschool years are identified as an important stage for preventive interventions, as eating patterns established in young childhood tend to track into later life [11].

The development of effective intervention programs aiming at the prevention of pediatric obesity should be based on rigorous investigations of its determinants and associated factors [10]. Most of the studies investigating obesity correlates in preschoolers have been conducted in high-income countries [12] and, as such, findings may not be applicable to low and middle-income countries, where the highest increases in preschool obesity are projected to take place. Among the latter, the Middle East and North Africa (MENA) region has been largely under-represented [12]. In Lebanon, an upper-middle income country of the Eastern Mediterranean basin that is currently undergoing the nutrition transition [13], available evidence documents an increase in obesity prevalence amongst 6–18 years old children and adolescents [14]. However, data on the prevalence and correlates of preschool obesity are lacking. Based on a nationally representative survey, the present study aims at (1) determining the prevalence of overweight and obesity among 2–5 years old preschool children in Lebanon and (2) investigating the association of preschool overweight and obesity with socioeconomic factors, parental characteristics, dietary intakes and eating behavior. Gaining greater insight into factors that are associated with preschool overweight and obesity should orient further studies investigating early life obesity and assist policy makers in setting forth successful culture-specific obesity prevention strategies in the region. The present study undertaken in Lebanon, and particularly the identification of factors that modulate the risk of under-five overweight, may be viewed as a case-study for other middle-income countries in similar stages of the nutrition transition. The study responds to the United Nation's call for a worldwide commitment to address preschool overweight and reverse its rising trends, as included in the General Assembly's resolution proclaiming the UN Decade of Action on Nutrition (2016–2025) [15].

2. Materials and Methods

2.1. Study Population

The data for this study was drawn from the national survey, "Early Life Nutrition and Health in Lebanon", conducted on a representative sample of Lebanese children (0–5 years) and their mothers. The survey was undertaken between September 2011 and August 2012. A stratified cluster sampling strategy was followed, whereby the strata were the six Lebanese governorates and the clusters were selected further at the level of districts. Within each district, households were selected following a probability proportional to size approach, whereby a higher number of participating households were drawn from more populous districts. The selection of the households was carried out using systematic sampling. Housing units constituted the primary sampling units in the different districts of Lebanon. To participate in the study, the household ought to include a mother and a child below five years of age. The child had to be Lebanese, born at term (of gestational age at birth ≥37 weeks), not suffering from any chronic illness, inborn errors of metabolism or physical malformations that may interfere with his/her feeding patterns and body composition, and not reported as being ill during the past 24 h (i.e., on the day that would be recalled for food intake). Of the 1194 eligible households that were contacted, 1029 participated in the survey (response rate 86%). The main reasons for refusal were time constraint, child being sick, lack of husband's consent or disinterest in the study. In face to face interviews with participating mothers, trained nutritionists collected data, using age-specific multi-component questionnaires covering information on demographic, socioeconomic, eating habits and dietary intakes. Anthropometric measurements were obtained from both mother and child. Dietary intake was assessed using the United States Department of Agriculture (USDA) multiple pass 24-h recall (24-HR) [16]. Interviews were held in the household setting and lasted for approximately one hour. Quality control measures including pre-testing of the study instruments, equipment and data collection procedure in addition to training and field monitoring, were applied. All questionnaires were designed by a panel of experts including scientists in the fields of epidemiology and nutrition and were tested on a convenience sample of 100 households to check for clarity and cultural sensitivity.

2.2. Ethical Considerations

The design and conduct of the survey were performed according to the guidelines laid down in the Declaration of Helsinki, and all procedures involving human subjects were approved by the Institutional Review Board of the American University of Beirut. A written informed consent was obtained from all mothers prior to participation.

2.3. Data Collection

For the purpose of this study, data of children aged between 2 and 5 years were used (n = 531). The availability of this sample size allowed the estimation of a 10% prevalence of overweight and obesity at a 95% confidence interval and a precision of ±2.5% [17]. Survey data used in this study included demographic, socioeconomic, and parental characteristics, eating habits, anthropometric measurements, as well as dietary intakes. Demographic characteristics consisted of the following: sex of the child, age of the child and the mother (in years), mother's marital status (married, not married) and number of children in the family; socioeconomic indicators included father's and mother's education levels (primary or less, intermediate, high school, and above) and household's monthly income, which are the most commonly utilized indicators of socioeconomic status [18], in addition to mother's employment (working, not working), presence of paid household helper, and household crowding index. Moreover, given that the formal age at which children enroll in the preprimary level of schools is three years in Lebanon [19], information on the type of school the child attends (private vs. public) was also obtained as one of the socioeconomic indicators. In fact, in Lebanon, there exist strong social inequalities among those attending private and public schools, with the private schools enrolling the highest proportion of students from a high SES, and the public schools enrolling those from a low SES [19,20]. The assessment of the child's eating habits included weekly frequency of breakfast consumption, eating in front of the television (TV), eating out, and eating the same meal with the family. In addition, early life feeding practices were assessed by the mother's retrospective recall of breastfeeding duration, age of introduction of formula and of solid food. The child satiety responsiveness and food responsiveness were evaluated using questions derived from the Child Eating Behaviour Questionnaire (CEBQ) [21].

2.4. Anthropometric Assessment

Information on birth weight of the child was obtained from the mother. Anthropometric measurements were performed, including weight and height of both mothers and children. Participants were weighed to the nearest 0.1 kg in light indoor clothing and with bare feet or stockings, using a standard clinical balance (Seca, model 770, Hamburg, Germany). Measurements of the weight were taken twice and repeated a third time if the first two measurements differed by more than 0.3 kg. Using a portable stadiometer (Seca, model 213, Hamburg, Germany) height was measured without shoes. Measurements of the height were taken twice and repeated a third time if the first two measurements differ by more than 0.5 cm. The average values of weight and height were used for the calculation of BMI, which is computed as the ratio of weight (kilograms) to the square of height (meters). Weight and height were not collected from women who were pregnant at the time of the interview ($n = 42$), due to the limitations of BMI use during pregnancy.

Overweight and obesity among mothers were assessed using the World Health Organization (WHO) criteria for body mass index (BMI) [22]. For children, the prevalence of overweight and obesity was assessed using the WHO-2006 criteria based on sex and age specific BMI z-scores, which were calculated using the WHO AnthroPlus software (WHO 2009, Department of Nutrition for Health and Development, Switzerland, Geneva) [23,24]. Accordingly, the following cutoffs were adopted: $+1 <$ BMI-for-age z-score $\leq +2$ (at risk of overweight), $+2 <$ BMI-for-age z-score $\leq +3$ (overweight), and BMI-for-age z-score $> +3$ (obesity). In addition, and in order to allow for comparability with other studies, the prevalence of overweight and obesity was assessed using two other definitions, including the Center for Disease Control and Prevention-2000 (CDC-2000) and International Obesity Task Force (IOTF):

1. According to the CDC 2000 reference [25,26] cut-off values were defined based on sex and age specific BMI percentiles: 85th to <95th percentile (overweight) and ≥95th percentile (obesity).
2. According to the IOTF standard [27], overweight and obesity were based on centiles passing at age 18 years through BMI 25 kg/m^2 and 30 kg/m^2, respectively.

2.5. Dietary Intake of Children

Dietary intake of children was assessed by a single multiple pass 24 HR. Even though various methods have been developed for the assessment of dietary consumption, including dietary recalls, food frequency questionnaires (FFQs) and food records [28], the choice of the 24 HR approach in this study may be explained by (1) the lack of validated culture-specific FFQs targeting under-five children in Lebanon and the MENA region; and (2) the practical difficulties of using food records in the context of national surveys, given the burden that this method may impose on participants and given its literacy requirements [28]. In addition, acknowledging the practical challenges of administering repeated multiple 24 HRs in the context of a national survey and the impact that this approach may have on response rate [29], we have opted to use a single 24 HR, with mothers serving as the main proxy. In case another caretaker shared the responsibility of feeding the child, the mother directly consulted with him/her for additional information pertinent to the dietary interview. The 24-HRs were carried using the multiple pass food recall five-step approach, developed by the USDA [16]. This approach has consistently showed attenuation in the 24-HRs' limitations [30]. The steps followed included (1) quick food list recall; (2) forgotten food list probe; (3) time and occasion at which foods were consumed; (4) detailed overall cycle; and (5) a final probe review of the foods consumed. While collecting the dietary data, specific reference was made to solicit information about food that were consumed at daycare or school. The Nutritionist Pro software (version 5.1.0, 2014, First Data Bank, Nutritionist Pro, Axxya Systems, San Bruno, CA, USA) was used for the analysis of the dietary intake data and to estimate energy and macronutrients' intakes. For composite and mixed dishes, standardized recipes were added to the Nutritionist Pro software using single food items. Within the Nutritionist Pro, the USDA database was selected for analysis (SR 24, published September 2011). Food composition of specific Lebanese foods (not included in the Nutritionist Pro software database) was obtained from food composition tables for use in the Middle East [31].

2.6. Data Analysis

Frequencies and percentages, as well as means and standard deviations (SD), were used to describe categorical and continuous variables, respectively. Crowding index was calculated as the total number of co-residents per household divided by the total number of rooms, excluding the kitchen and bathrooms. Bivariate logistic regression was used to examine the sociodemographic, eating habits and dietary intake correlates of overweight and obesity in the study population. In this regression, the dependent variable was 'overweight/obesity', as defined by the WHO-2006 (BMI-for-age z-score > +2) [23]. In order to examine the independent effect of each group of variables (sociodemographic and parental characteristics, eating habits and dietary intake) in predicting overweight and obesity, a stepwise logistic regression was conducted. Block 1 consisted of sociodemographic and parental characteristics, block 2 included eating habits variables and block 3 was comprised of dietary intake data. Variables chosen to be included in the multivariate modeling were either significant in the bi-variate analysis and/or were important according to the literature. Data analysis was carried out using Statistical Package for Social Sciences 22.0 (SPSS for Windows, 2013, SPSS Inc., Chicago, IL, USA). A *p*-value less than 0.05 was considered statistically significant.

3. Results

Out of the 531 survey participants, six children had incomplete sociodemographic and dietary data and, hence, were excluded from the remaining analyses and results. Among children participating in this study (*n* = 525), prevalence rates of overweight and obesity using the four definitions are presented in Table 1. According to the WHO-2006 criteria, prevalence estimates of overweight and obesity were 6.5% and 2.7%, respectively. Higher estimates were obtained using IOTF and CDC-2000 reference cutoffs, with the latter presenting the highest estimates (overweight 16.1% and obesity 10.6%). Although the WHO-2006 presented lowest estimates of overweight and obesity compared to other references, it also had the lowest prevalence of normal weight (64.6%) since, according to this reference, a proportion of normal weight are grouped under a distinct category called 'at risk of overweight', with a prevalence of 26.3%. This particular category does not exist within the other references. No significant difference in overweight or obesity rates were observed between boys and girls (Table 1).

Table 1. Overweight/obesity prevalence among 2–5 years old Lebanese preschoolers, according to WHO-2006, IOTF and CDC-2000 criteria.

Weight Status	Total (*n* = 525)	Boys (*n* = 281)	Girls (*n* = 244)
	n (%)		
WHO-2006 reference [a]			
Normal weight [b]	339 (64.6)	177 (63.0)	162 (66.4)
At risk of overweight	138 (26.3)	78 (27.8)	60 (24.6)
Overweight [c]	34 (6.5)	18 (6.4)	16 (6.6)
Obese	14 (2.7)	8 (2.8)	6 (2.5)
Overweight and obese	48 (9.1)	26 (9.3)	22 (9.0)
IOTF reference [d]			
Normal weight [b]	433 (82.8)	235 (84.2)	198 (81.1)
Overweight [c]	70 (13.4)	36 (12.9)	34 (13.9)
Obese	20 (3.8)	8 (2.9)	12 (4.9)
Overweight and obese	90 (17.2)	44 (15.8)	46 (18.8)
CDC-2000 reference [e]			
Normal weight [b]	383 (73.1)	207 (74.2)	176 (72.1)
Overweight [c]	84 (16.1)	41 (14.7)	43 (17.6)
Obese	56 (10.6)	31 (11.1)	25 (10.2)
Overweight and obese	140 (26.8)	72 (25.8)	68 (27.9)

No significant differences between genders were observed. [a] World Health Organization-2006 reference [23]; [b] The normal weight category included thinness, with only one child identified as thin based on the WHO 2006 criteria [23], 18 based on IOTF criteria [32], and 16 based on CDC [25,26]; [c] "Overweight" category does not include "Obese"; [d] International Obesity Task Force reference [27]; [e] Center for Disease Control and Prevention-2000 reference [25,26].

Table 2 presents descriptive statistics for the sociodemographic, socioeconomic, and parental characteristics, eating habits, and dietary intake of study participants, in addition to the univariate associations of these correlates with overweight (including obesity) (BMI-for-age z-score > +2). The mean age of preschoolers was of 3.3 ± 0.87 years, with 53.5% boys and 46.5% girls. Most parents had intermediate level education (62.8% of fathers and 61.5% of mothers). The majority of mothers did not work (85.1%) and most of the households did not have a household helper (84.1%). Average maternal BMI was estimated at 26.71 ± 5.18 kg/m^2 (Table 2), with the prevalence of overweight and obesity being estimated at 58.4% among mothers (34.3% overweight and 24.1% obese) (data not shown). When looking at early life feeding practices, almost half of the participating preschoolers were breastfed for less than six months (47.8%), 16.8% for 6–11 months (data not shown) and 35.4% for more than 12 months. The average breastfeeding duration was estimated at 8.9 ± 8.7 months, while the average age of formula milk introduction and of solid food introduction were estimated at 1.3 ± 1.7 and 5.8 ± 2.49 months, respectively. In the study sample, the average weekly frequency of eating breakfast was of 6.7 ± 1.6, while the mean frequencies of "eating in front of the TV" and of "eating the same meal as the family" were estimated at 4.8 ± 6 and 10.7 ± 6.2, respectively. As for dietary intake variables, energy and macronutrient consumption were categorized as above or below the respective median values. These median values corresponded to 1509 kcal/day for energy, 39.3% for "energy consumption from fat", 48.6% for "energy consumption from CHO", and 13.15% for energy consumption from protein. As shown in Table 2, lower odds of overweight/obesity were found in families with number of children ≥3, attending a public school, a crowding index ≥1, longer duration of breastfeeding (≥12 months), eating the same meal with the family at home and a higher satiety responsiveness. The odds of overweight/obesity increased significantly with father's education level, mother's education level, presence of paid helper at home, income higher than 1,500,000 Lebanese lira (LL), mother's BMI, higher frequency of eating while watching TV, eating out, and a greater food responsiveness. Among dietary intake variables, energy consumption from fat was associated with a higher odd of overweight/obesity (Table 2).

Table 2. Association of demographic, socioeconomic, eating habits and dietary intakes with preschoolers' weight status, Lebanon (*n* = 525) [a].

Variables	Children Adiposity Status [c]				
	Total [b] (*n* = 525)	Normal Weight (Including at Risk of Overweight) (*n* = 477)	Overweight (Not Including Obese) (*n* = 34)	Obese (*n* = 14)	Univariate Analysis [d]
	Demographic, socioeconomic and parental characteristics *n* (%)				OR [95% CI]
Gender					
Boys	281 (53.5)	255 (53.5)	18 (52.9)	8 (57.1)	1 [ref]
Girls	244 (46.5)	222 (46.5)	16 (47.1)	6 (42.9)	0.97 [0.53–1.76]
Child's Age (years)					
mean ± SD	3.32 + 0.87	3.32 + 0.88	3.33 + 0.78	3.53 + 0.57	1.08 [0.77–1.53]
Mother's Age (years)					
mean ± SD	32.78 + 5.97	32.68 + 5.92	33.11 + 6.49	35.21 + 6.27	1.02 [0.98–1.08]
Mother's marital status					
Married	514 (97.9)	468 (98.1)	33 (97.1)	13 (92.9)	1 [ref]
Unmarried (divorced or widowed)	11 (2.1)	9 (1.9)	1 (2.9)	1 (7.1)	2.26 [0.47–10.77]
Number of children in the family					
≤2 children	272 (51.8)	236 (49.5)	26 (76.5)	10 (71.4)	1 [ref]
≥3 children	253 (48.2)	241 (50.5)	8 (23.5)	4 (28.6)	**0.32 [0.16–0.64]**
Type of school attended [e]					
Private	310 (74.5)	274 (72.9)	25 (89.3)	11 (91.7)	1 [ref]
Public	106 (25.5)	102 (27.1)	3 (10.7)	1 (8.3)	**0.29 [0.10–0.86]**

Table 2. *Cont.*

Variables	Total [b] (*n* = 525)	Normal Weight (Including at Risk of Overweight) (*n* = 477)	Overweight (Not Including Obese) (*n* = 34)	Obese (*n* = 14)	Univariate Analysis [d]
			Children Adiposity Status [c]		
	Demographic, socioeconomic and parental characteristics *n* (%)				OR [95% CI]
Father's education					
Primary or less	116 (22.1)	114 (24.3)	2 (6.1)	0 (0.0)	1 [ref]
Intermediate	324 (62.8)	290 (61.8)	26 (78.8)	8 (57.1)	**6.68** [1.57–28.27]
High school and above	76 (14.7)	65 (13.9)	5 (15.2)	6 (42.9)	**9.64** [2.07–44.86]
Mother's education					
Primary or less	101 (19.2)	98 (20.5)	2 (5.9)	1 (7.1)	1 [ref]
Intermediate	323 (61.5)	292 (61.2)	23 (67.6)	8 (57.1)	**3.46** [1.03–11.59]
High school and above	101 (19.2)	87 (18.2)	9 (26.5)	5 (35.7)	**5.25** [1.46–18.90]
Mother's employment					
Working	78 (14.9)	68 (14.3)	5 (14.7)	5 (35.7)	1 [ref]
Not Working	447 (85.1)	409 (85.7)	29 (85.3)	9 (64.3)	0.63 [0.30–1.32]
Presence of paid helper					
No	439 (84.1)	406 (85.7)	25 (73.5)	8 (57.1)	1 [ref]
Yes	83 (15.9)	68 (14.3)	9 (26.5)	6 (42.9)	**2.71** [1.40–5.26]
Crowding index					
<1 person/room	60 (11.5)	50 (10.5)	6 (17.6)	4 (28.6)	1 [ref]
≥1 person/room	464 (88.5)	426 (89.5)	28 (82.4)	10 (71.4)	**0.45** [0.21–0.96]
Monthly income					
Low (<1,000,000 LL)	172 (39.3)	161 (40.6)	10 (33.3)	1 (9.1)	1 [ref]
Medium (1,000,000–1,500,000 LL)	108 (24.7)	100 (25.2)	8 (26.7)	0 (0.0)	1.17 [0.45–3.01]
High (>1,500,000 LL)	158 (36.1)	136 (34.3)	12 (40.0)	10 (90.9)	**2.36** [1.10–5.05]
Mother's BMI (Kg/m^2) *	26.71 ± 5.18	26.59 ± 5.17	27.99 ± 5.63	27.51 ± 4.40	**1.05** [1.00–1.10]
	Breastfeeding history and eating habits				OR [95% CI]
Breastfeeding duration					
<12 months	339 (64.6)	300 (62.9)	26 (76.5)	13 (92.9)	1 [ref]
≥12 months	186 (35.4)	177 (37.1)	8 (23.5)	1 (7.1)	**0.39** [0.18–0.82]
Breastfeeding duration (in months)	8.94 ± 8.73	9.11 ± 8.92	8.10 ± 6.84	4.92 ± 3.85	1 [ref] 0.97 [0.94–1.01]
Age of formula/cow's milk's introduction (months)	1.34 ± 1.71	1.34 ± 1.70	1.66 ± 2.07	0.70 ± 0.89	1 [ref] 0.99 [0.78–1.27]
Age of solid food's introduction (months)	5.80 ± 2.49	5.75 ± 2.51	6.48 ± 2.57	5.89 ± 1.47	1 [ref] 1.07 [0.98–1.18]
Child's birth weight (kg)	3.19 ± 0.55	3.18 ± 0.56	3.30 ± 0.52	3.32 ± 0.49	1.00 [1.00–1.01]
Eating breakfast (weekly frequency)	6.74 ± 1.64	6.75 ± 1.68	6.88 ± 0.53	6.21 ± 2.00	0.97 [0.81–1.16]
Eating in front of the TV (weekly frequency)	4.81 ± 6.00	4.61 ± 5.59	6.67 ± 9.87	7.14 ± 6.58	**1.04** [1.01–1.09]
Eating out (weekly frequency)	0.40 ± 0.87	0.38 ± 0.78	0.70 ± 1.65	0.57 ± 0.82	**1.27** [1.01–1.62]
Eating the same meal as the family at home (weekly frequency)	10.74 ± 6.24	10.92 ± 6.29	9.55 ± 5.55	7.60 ± 5.54	**0.94** [0.89–0.99]
Satiety responsiveness	8.56 ± 2.15	8.63 ± 2.15	7.94 ± 2.02	7.71 ± 2.05	**0.84** [0.73–0.97]
Food responsiveness	3.87 ± 1.39	3.82 ± 1.37	3.97 ± 1.50	5.14 ± 1.46	**1.28** [1.03–1.58]

Table 2. *Cont.*

Variables	Total [b] (*n* = 525)	Normal Weight (Including at Risk of Overweight) (*n* = 477)	Overweight (Not Including Obese) (*n* = 34)	Obese (*n* = 14)	Univariate Analysis [d]
	Children Adiposity Status [c]				
	Dietary intake (per day) [f] *n* (%)				OR [95% CI]
Total energy (Kcal)					
Below the median [f]	258 (50.1)	234 (50.1)	18 (52.9)	61 (42.9)	1 [ref]
Above the median [f]	257 (49.9)	233 (49.9)	16 (47.1)	8 (57.1)	1.00 [0.55–1.81]
Energy consumption from fat (%)					
Below the median [f]	259 (50.3)	243 (52.0)	11 (32.4)	5 (35.7)	1 [ref]
Above the median [f]	256 (49.7)	224 (48.0)	23 (67.6)	9 (64.3)	**2.17 [1.15–4.06]**
Energy consumption from CHO (%)					
Below the median [f]	257 (49.9)	227 (48.6)	22 (64.7)	8 (57.1)	1 [ref]
Above the median [f]	258 (50.1)	240 (51.4)	12 (35.3)	6 (42.9)	0.56 [0.30–1.04]
Energy consumption from protein (%)					
Below the median [f]	260 (50.5)	240 (51.4)	11 (32.4)	9 (64.3)	1 [ref]
Above the median [f]	255 (49.5)	227 (48.6)	23 (67.6)	5 (35.7)	1.48 [0.81–2.70]

OR: odds ratio for overweight/obesity vs. normal weight; CI: confidence interval; TV: television; CHO: carbohydrates. [a] In this table, continuous and categorical variables are presented as mean ± SD and *n* (%), respectively; [b] Lack of corresponding sum of frequencies with total sample size is due to missing data; [c] Children adiposity status based on the WHO 2006 BMI-for-age *z*-score cut-offs [23]; Normal weight (including at risk of overweight): −2 ≤ *z*-score ≤ +2; Overweight (not including obese): +2 < *z*-score ≤ +3; Obese: *z*-score > +3; [d] Crude logistic regression was conducted with the outcome variable being "overweight" and "obese"combined; [e] The sum of frequencies does not correspond to the total sample size given that preschoolers below the age of three years do not go to school. [f] Median for "total energy" corresponds to 1509 kcal; median for "energy consumption from fat" corresponds to 39.3%; median for "energy consumption from CHO" corresponds to 48.6%; median for "energy consumption from protein" corresponds to 13.15%; * The number of mothers included in this variable is 483, after exclusion of pregnant women (*n* = 42). Bolded numbers are significant at *p* < 0.05.

The results of the stepwise logistic regression examining the independent effects of socioeconomic and parental characteristics, eating habits, as well as dietary intakes on the odds of overweight/obesity are presented in Table 3. The variance accounted for by the first block (socioeconomic and parental characteristics) was 11.9%. Within this block, father's education, mother's BMI, presence of a paid helper, and crowding index made significant contributions (*p* < 0.05) to the prediction of overweight/obesity among study participants. The second block of variables was related to early life feeding and eating habits, including breastfeeding duration, eating while watching TV, eating out, eating the same meal with the family at home, satiety responsiveness, and food responsiveness. After controlling for the socioeconomic and parental characteristics, these variables significantly improved the prediction of overweight/obesity to reach 21% (*p* < 0.01). Eating in front of the TV was associated with an 8% increase in the odds of overweight/obesity (OR: 1.08, 95% CI: 1.02–1.1), while a higher score of satiety responsiveness was associated with lower odds of overweight/obesity in the study population (OR: 0.8, 95% CI: 0.68–0.99). As for the third block (dietary intakes), energy consumption from fat remained a significant predictor of preschool overweight/obesity, after adjusting for other variables (OR: 2.31, 95% CI: 1.13–4.75). (Table 3).

Given the association between preschool overweight/obesity and fat intake, additional analyses were conducted to assess the major food contributors to fat and energy intakes in the study sample. The results showed that, besides milk and dairy products which appeared as the largest contributor to fat intake (24.4%), the main sources of fat were fast food and salty snacks (21.6%), followed by beef, poultry, and eggs (12.3%), rice and rice-based dishes (8.7%), and sweet deserts (8.2%). Similarly, the main contributor to daily energy intake was milk and dairy products (17.6%), followed by fast food and salty snacks (16.2%), breads (12.5%), sweets (9.6%), meat, poultry, and eggs (9.04%), rice and rice-based dishes (7.8%), and sweetened beverages (6.1%) (data not shown).

Table 3. Associations of overweight [a] with selected demographic, socioeconomic, parental, and dietary variables among preschoolers (n = 525).

Variables	Model 1 [b]	Model 2 [b]	Model 3 [b]
	OR [95% CI]		
Demographic, socioeconomic and parental variables			
Gender			
Boys	1 [ref]	1 [ref]	1 [ref]
Girls	0.97 [0.52–1.83]	1.07 [0.56–2.07]	0.96 [0.49–1.88]
Child's age (years)			
mean ± SD	0.99 [0.68–1.44]	0.91 [0.63–1.33]	0.92 [0.63–1.35]
Father's education [c]			
Primary or less	1 [ref]	1 [ref]	1 [ref]
Intermediate	**5.16 [1.19–22.41]**	**5.81 [1.27–26.51]**	**5.77 [1.24–26.96]**
High school and above	**5.31 [1.04–27.26]**	5.22 [0.96–28.39]	**5.02 [1.03–27.91]**
Mother's BMI (Kg/m^2)			
mean ± SD	**1.06 [1.01–1.13]**	**1.09 [1.03–1.16]**	**1.08 [1.02–1.15]**
Presence of paid helper			
No	1 [ref]	1 [ref]	1 [ref]
Yes	**2.19 [1.05–4.56]**	**2.34 [1.05–5.21]**	**2.30 [1.02–5.17]**
Crowding index			
<1 person/room	1 [ref]	1 [ref]	1 [ref]
≥1 person/room	**0.42 [0.19–0.97]**	0.47 [0.19–1.15]	0.41 [0.17–1.02]
Breastfeeding history and eating habits			
Breastfeeding duration			
<12 months	------------	1 [ref]	1 [ref]
≥12 months		0.62 [0.27–1.42]	0.62 [0.27–1.44]
Eating in front of the TV	------------	**1.07 [1.02–1.13]**	**1.08 [1.02–1.14]**
Eating out	------------	1.23 [0.93–1.63]	1.22 [0.92–1.62]
Eating the same meal as the family at home	------------	0.95 [0.89–1.01]	0.95 [0.89–1.01]
Satiety responsiveness	------------	**0.83 [0.70–0.99]**	**0.8 [0.68–0.99]**
Food responsiveness	------------	1.14 [0.87–1.49]	1.16 [0.88–1.52]
Dietary variables			
Total daily energy (Kcal) [d]			
Low	------------	------------	1 [ref]
High			0.72 [0.35–1.50]
Energy consumption from Fat (%) [d,e]			
Low	------------	------------	1 [ref]
High			**2.31 [1.13–4.75]**
−2 Log Likelihood	274.89	252.82	247.2
Nagelkerke R^2	0.12	0.21	0.23
Nagelkerke R^2 difference	0.12	0.09	0.02

OR: odds ratio; CI: confidence interval. [a] Overweight (including obesity) defined based on the WHO 2006 sex and age specific + 2 BMI z-scores [23]; [b] Model 1: adjusted for gender, age, father's education, presence of paid helper, crowding index and mother's BMI; Model 2 = Model 1 + adjustment for eating behavior variables; Model 3 = Model 2 + adjustment for dietary variables; [c] Low, medium and high education levels refer to primary or less, intermediate or high school and above, respectively; [d] Low and high total energy and energy from fat refer to first and second median, respectively; [e] Fat intake based on percent contribution to daily energy intake. Bolded numbers are significant at $p < 0.05$.

4. Discussion

This paper reports on the national prevalence of overweight and obesity in Lebanese 2–5 years old preschoolers and provides evidence linking specific socioeconomic, dietary, and lifestyle factors to increased risk of overweight and obesity in this age group. In view of the scarcity of data on the determinants of childhood obesity in the MENA, the present study's findings may be viewed as a case-study for other middle-income countries of the region, in similar stages of the nutrition transition.

Using the WHO-2006 BMI criteria, findings of this study show that the prevalence of overweight/obesity combined (BMI-for-age z-score > +2) (9.1%) amongst Lebanese preschoolers exceeds the global prevalence estimate of preschool overweight/obesity for 2010 (6.7%), as well as the estimate reported for developing countries (6.1%) [2]. The prevalence rates of overweight (6.4% in boys and 6.6% in girls) and obesity (2.8% in boys and 2.5% in girls) amongst Lebanese preschoolers are similar to those reported from several European countries, while being lower than those reported from some other MENA countries such as Bahrain and Qatar [33–44]. (Table 4). To allow for a comparison with findings reported from other countries, data were re-analyzed according to the IOTF and CDC criteria. Based on the IOTF criteria, current prevalence estimates of overweight (12.9% in boys and 13.9% in girls) and obesity (2.9% in boys and 4.9% in girls) amongst Lebanese preschoolers are within the range reported from developed countries such as Australia and Canada [33,44–46]. When using the CDC criteria, the prevalence estimates of preschool overweight (14.7% in boys and 17.6% in girls) and obesity (11.1% in boys and 10.2% in girls) in Lebanon are found to be higher than those reported from Iran (overweight: 9.8 and 10.3% respectively; obesity: 4.8 and 4.5% respectively) [47], with the prevalence of obesity being also higher than that reported from the United States of America [48].

Table 4. Prevalence of overweight and obesity among Lebanese preschool children compared to those in selected countries.

Country	Date of Surveys	Criteria Used	Age (Years)	Overweight [b] (%) Boys	Overweight [b] (%) Girls	Obesity (%) Boys	Obesity (%) Girls
		WHO-2006 [c]					
Lebanon [a]	2010		2–5	6.4	6.6	2.8	2.5
China (Beijing) [41]	2004		2–5	4.6	2.7	2.9	1.7
Bahrain [39]	2003		2–5	9.8	10.1	7.1	5.9
Jordan [42]	2010		1–5	6.7	7.3	2.5	1.1
Qatar (Doha) [40]	2009–2010		2–5	10.6	15.2	15.5	12.5
The Netherlands [34]	2002–2006		2–5	6	4.1	5	2.9
Romania [35]	2004		2–5	5.7	4.2	2.1	2.2
Spain [43]	2006		2–5	9.6	12.2	8.8	4.4
Italy [36]	2005		2–5	5.9	5.7	4.1	2.6
Cyprus [37,38]	2004		2–5	3.3	4.7	1.8	1.3
England [44]	2002		2–5	9.8	7.5	2.5	2.2
		IOTF [d]					
Lebanon [a]	2010		2–5	12.9	13.9	2.9	4.9
Canada [46]	2004		2–5	13	19	6	6
Australia [45]	2007		2–3	17	14	4	4
		CDC [e]					
Lebanon [a]	2010		2–5	14.7	17.6	11.1	10.2
Iran (Tehran) [47]	2009–2010		3–6	9.8	10.3	4.8	4.5
United States of America [48]	2011–2012		2–5	23.9	21.7	9.5	7.2
Saudi Arabia (Khobar) [49]	2006		2–4	19.6	16.3	20	18.1

[a] Current study; [b] Overweight (not including obesity); [c] WHO-2006: World Health organization 2006 reference [23]; [d] IOTF: International Obesity Task Force [27]; [e] CDC: Center for Disease Control and Prevention-2000 [25,26].

Pediatric obesity and excess body weight often result from a complex interaction between genetic and lifestyle factors [10]. Our finding of a positive significant association between preschool overweight/obesity and maternal BMI corroborates those reported from other studies and underscores the importance of genetic factors in the etiology of body fatness [10,50]. Our study's findings also underscore the importance of socioeconomic and lifestyle factors in modulating the risk of pediatric overweight. To our knowledge, this study is the first from the MENA region to investigate and document a positive association between preschool overweight/obesity and SES as assessed by several indicators, including type of school attended, father's educational level, mother's educational level, presence of a paid helper, crowding index, and monthly income. Socioeconomic and parental characteristics made the highest contributions to the prediction of overweight/obesity among study participants, accounting for 12% of the model variance. Previous studies conducted in other parts of the world suggest that SES affects the risk of developing obesity in children, but available evidence highlights disparities in the relationship between SES and pediatric obesity in industrialized vs. developing countries [51]. While children from low SES groups are at higher risk of obesity in industrialized countries, pediatric obesity appears to be predominantly a problem of the rich in low-income countries [18,51]. Less is, however, known about the relationship between SES and childhood obesity in middle-income countries, particularly those undergoing the nutrition transition [5,6]. The present study showed that, in Lebanon, a middle-income country undergoing the nutrition transition, the odds of preschool overweight/obesity were positively associated with SES. In fact, higher paternal education, which is one of the most commonly adopted SES indicators [18], was associated with a five-fold increase in the odds of preschool overweight/obesity, and a higher crowding index, which reflects a lower SES, was associated with lower odds of overweight/obesity in this age group. These findings are in agreement with those reported from several developing countries [52,53] and highlight the role of upward mobility and SES in modulating the family's economic and cultural resources, all of which may bear ramifications on lifestyle and, therefore, obesity risk in childhood. The observed positive association between SES and preschool overweight/obesity in Lebanon may be explained by the fact that children from affluent families may have higher access to energy-rich diets and electronic games as well as more opportunities for eating out, putting them at a higher risk for positive energy balance and weight gain [5]. Additional analyses conducted in this study have in fact shown significant associations between "eating out", "eating the same meal with the family", and main drivers of SES, such as paternal education (data not shown).

Of interest, the study findings showed that the presence of a paid helper in the household was associated with a two-fold increase in the odds of overweight/obesity in Lebanese preschoolers, even after adjustment for other SES indicators including father's education and crowding index. It is important to note that in the Lebanese context, the responsibility of feeding the child is often shared with the household helper, and this type of child care is becoming increasingly common in the country. Available estimates suggest that, in 2010, Lebanon hosted 117,941 paid sleep-in domestic workers who come from foreign countries, including the Philippines, Sri Lanka, Ethiopia, and Bangladesh, and who live in their employer's house for the duration of their contract [54]. Our findings of a positive association between preschool overweight/obesity and the presence of a household helper echo those reported by a population-based birth cohort of Chinese children, where "informal" non-parental child care at each of 3, 5, or 11 years of age was independently associated with higher BMI-for-age z-scores and with the presence of childhood overweight levels [55]. Our results are also in agreement with findings stemming from Western societies, where several studies [56–58] have reported an association between pediatric obesity and "informal" rather than parental child care [55]. Needless to say that caregivers, including household helpers, may play an important role in influencing the child's dietary practices and eating habits [59]. While parents may play a more active role in supervising the child's eating behavior, household helpers, who are usually hired for housework as well as child care, may not be able to spend much time and effort on enforcing dietary recommendations, limiting the child's consumption of energy-dense favorite foods or restraining TV viewing [55]. In our study, the time spent on TV viewing was not directly assessed, but a positive association was found between preschool overweight/obesity and eating while watching TV. Several studies have shown that eating in front of the TV is positively associated with higher BMI among children, an association that is independent of the overall time spent watching TV or the sedentary behavior that accompanies it [60,61]. Dubois et al. showed that four- to five-year-old children who frequently ate in front of the TV had higher BMI relative to their peers, while no significant associations were found between the child's BMI and the overall time spent watching TV [3]. There are several mechanisms that could link preschool obesity to the act of eating while watching TV. First, children who eat in front of the TV may miss out on the nutritional and psychosocial benefits of family meals [3,61]. In addition, eating in front of the TV is associated with increased exposure to the advertisements of unhealthy foods at meal time hours and with mindless eating that often results in the consumption of larger food portions [62]. Available evidence suggests that children who are given the opportunity to eat while watching TV may become less sensitive to internal cues of satiety [63]. In this study, higher satiety responsiveness was associated with significantly lower odds of overweight/obesity in preschoolers. These findings are in agreement with previously reported inverse association between satiety response and preschoolers' BMI [64,65].

The results of the present study showed that higher dietary fat intake was associated with a two-fold increase in the prevalence of preschool overweight/obesity. Even though the evidence in the literature is inconsistent, several studies have shown that percentage energy intake from fat was greater in obese children compared with their non-obese counterparts, although total energy intake was not different, a finding that is in agreement with the results of the present study [66–68]. Other studies using BMI and or skinfold measures to estimate adiposity have documented a positive association between the percentage of energy intake from fat and body fatness in children before and after controlling for maternal BMI, a finding that is also in agreement with the results of the present study [69,70]. There are a number of mechanisms through which dietary fat may play a role in the development of overweight and obesity. Compared to protein and carbohydrate, fat is more palatable and energy dense, has less ability to regulate hunger and satiety and, hence, is more likely to lead to passive over-consumption [69,71,72]. In addition, and in contrast to protein and carbohydrate, which have comparatively limited storage capacity and are therefore preferentially oxidized when energy intake exceeds expenditure, there is no regulation of fat balance or limit on storage of excess energy from fat, making it more efficiently (about 96%) stored than excess carbohydrate energy (60% $\pm$ 80%) [66,73]. Thus, given the poor regulation of fat at both the levels of consumption and oxidation, a chronically high fat diet may compromise the regulation of energy balance and lead to weight gain [71,72]. The study findings may thus call for dietary intervention strategies aiming at reducing fat intake amongst preschoolers in Lebanon [74]. These interventions should, at least partly, focus on the observed main sources of fat in this age group, which included fast food, salty snacks, and sweets.

The strengths of the study include the national design of the survey, the use of a culture and population specific questionnaire in data collection and the measurements of anthropometric characteristics instead of self-reporting. In addition, several indicators were used in this study for the assessment of SES, all of which have converged in documenting a positive association with preschool overweight/obesity in Lebanon. The results of this study should, however, be considered in light of the following limitations. Though every effort was exerted in order to ensure the representativeness of the sample, a comparison of the study sample distribution across governorates with that of the Lebanese population for the same age group showed a few discrepancies. For instance, while South Lebanon constitutes 21.1% of the population, this percentage was only 16.8% in the study population. This difference was compensated by a higher representation of Mount Lebanon (32% in the study sample vs. 28.8% in the population), and Beirut (10.5% in the study sample vs. 7.7% in the population). Such discrepancies resulted from the fact that the research team faced security clearance challenges in South Lebanon, whereby access to this governorate is controlled by tight security measures. In our study, dietary information was based on the collection of one 24-HR, which may not be representative of dietary intakes at the individual level. However, despite its well-known limitations, such as reliance on memory and day-to-day variation, the 24-HR may provide accurate estimates of energy intake at the population level [75]. In the present study, dietary information was collected by the multiple pass 24-HR approach, which was shown to provide accurate estimates of dietary intake in children [76]. In addition, the recalls were taken by research nutritionists who went through extensive training prior to data collection in order to minimize interviewer errors. Similarly, inter-observer measurement error in anthropometric assessment was minimized by extensive training and follow up to maintain quality of measurement among all research nutritionists. It is important to note that physical activity was not assessed in the present study, and as such its association with preschool overweight/obesity was not investigated. However, variability in physical activity tends to be rather limited in this age group and engagement in structured exercise is quite uncommon [77,78]. It is important to note that no information was available regarding whether the participating mothers have recently delivered and/or are currently breastfeeding at the time of the interview. For these two groups of mothers, given that BMI may not be reflective of their usual weight status, their inclusion in the analysis may have attenuated the results found in this study. Similarly, data on access to non-traditional food markets, body image of children, means of transportation and the built environment, which may play an important role in influencing the risk of childhood obesity [79,80] were not collected in this study. Finally, the cross-sectional design of the study allows us to test associations rather than to assess any causal relationships.

5. Conclusions

This study showed that the rates of overweight and obesity amongst Lebanese preschoolers exceed the global prevalence estimate of preschool overweight/obesity, as well as the estimate reported for developing countries [2]. This study has also provided the first evidence from the MENA region on the link between preschool overweight/obesity and higher SES, thus, potentially serving as a case-study for other middle-income countries in similar stages of the nutrition transition. In addition, specific dietary behaviors, including eating while watching TV and consuming a high fat diet, were shown to be associated with increased risk of overweight and obesity in Lebanese preschoolers, which corroborate findings stemming from previous studies on this age group. Taken together, the study's findings highlight the importance of the home environment in modulating the young child's lifestyle and dietary habits and hence obesity risk early in life. In this context, the results of the study call for education interventions aiming at raising parental awareness on preschool overweight in Lebanon, a country where early life "chubbiness" may not be perceived as a health threat but is rather culturally believed to be a sign of good health and an inherent component of the child's "cuteness".

Recognizing that the development of early life obesity prevention strategies should rely on evidence-based public health approaches, the results of this paper could represent a stepping stone for the formulation of effective interventions and policies aiming at curbing the epidemic of pediatric obesity in Lebanon. Family-focused interventions and behavioral strategies, coupled with school-based interventions and policies, are needed to instill healthy lifestyle and dietary habits early in life [6].

Acknowledgments: Funding for this study was provided by the Lebanese National Council for Scientific Research (Beirut, Lebanon) through its support of the Associated Research Unit (ARU) on 'Nutrition and Non-communicable Diseases in Lebanon' and by the University Research Board (American University of Beirut, Lebanon). The authors are indebted to every subject who took the time to participate in the study. The authors would also like to acknowledge the services of Nada Adra for her help in statistical analyses, Joana Abou-Rizk for her help in dietary analyses and Jennifer Ayoub for editing the manuscript.

Author Contributions: L.N., as the principal investigator, was responsible for the conceptualization of the study objectives and methodology and contributed to the write-up of the manuscript. N.H. critically reviewed the manuscript and provided valuable input for data interpretation. A.S. was involved in data collection and analysis in partial fulfilment of her MSc Degree. C.A. was responsible for the statistical evaluation of the data; F.N. contributed to data analysis and write-up of the manuscript and played a central role in integrating the dietary and anthropometric results. All authors participated in the drafting of the manuscript and have approved the final version of the manuscript.

Conflicts of Interest: The authors declare no conflict of interest.

References

1. Wang, Y.; Lobstein, T. Worldwide trends in childhood overweight and obesity. *Int. J. Pediatr. Obes.* **2006**, *1*, 11–25. [CrossRef] [PubMed]
2. De Onis, M.; Blössner, M.; Borghi, E. Global prevalence and trends of overweight and obesity among preschool children. *Am. J. Clin. Nutr.* **2010**, *92*, 1257–1264. [CrossRef] [PubMed]
3. Dubois, L.; Farmer, A.; Girard, M.; Peterson, K. Social factors and television use during meals and snacks is associated with higher BMI among pre-school children. *Public Health Nutr.* **2008**, *11*, 1267–1279. [CrossRef] [PubMed]
4. Gupta, N.; Goel, K.; Shah, P.; Misra, A. Childhood obesity in developing countries: Epidemiology, determinants, and prevention. *Endocr. Rev.* **2012**, *33*, 48–70. [CrossRef] [PubMed]
5. Mirmiran, P.; Sherafat Kazemzadeh, R.; Jalali Farahani, S.; Azizi, F. Childhood obesity in the Middle East: A review. *East. Mediterr. Health J.* **2010**, *16*, 1009–1017. [PubMed]
6. World Health Organization. Report of the Commission on Ending Childhood Obesity. 2016. Available online: http://www.who.int/end-childhood-obesity/final-report/en/ (accessed on 10 July 2016).
7. Mirza, N.M.; Yanovski, J.A. Prevalence and consequences of pediatric obesity. In *Handbook of Obesity: Epidemiology, Etiology, and Physiopathology*; Taylor & Francis Ltd.: Boca Raton, FL, USA, 2014; pp. 55–74.
8. Kelsey, M.M.; Zaepfel, A.; Bjornstad, P.; Nadeau, K.J. Age-related consequences of childhood obesity. *Gerontology* **2014**, *60*, 222–228. [CrossRef] [PubMed]
9. Park, M.H.; Falconer, C.; Viner, R.M.; Kinra, S. The impact of childhood obesity on morbidity and mortality in adulthood: A systematic review. *Obes. Rev.* **2012**, *13*, 985–1000. [CrossRef] [PubMed]
10. Jouret, B.; Ahluwalia, N.; Cristini, C.; Dupuy, M.; Nègre-Pages, L.; Grandjean, H.; Tauber, M. Factors associated with overweight in preschool-age children in southwestern France. *Am. J. Clin. Nutr.* **2007**, *85*, 1643–1649. [PubMed]
11. World Health Organization. Global Strategy on Diet, Physical Activity and Health. 2004, Resolution WHA55.23. WHO, Geneva. A57/59. 17 April 2004. Available online: http://www.who.int/dietphysicalactivity/strategy/eb11344/en/ (accessed on 10 July 2016).
12. Monasta, L.; Batty, G.; Cattaneo, A.; Lutje, V.; Ronfani, L.; Van Lenthe, F.; Brug, J. Early-life determinants of overweight and obesity: A review of systematic reviews. *Obes. Rev.* **2010**, *11*, 695–708. [CrossRef] [PubMed]
13. World Health Organization. Technical Paper. Regional Strategy on Nutrition 2010–2019. 2010. Fifty-Seventh Session. Agenda Item 4 (b). Available online: http://applications.emro.who.int/docs/EM_RC57_54_en.pdf (accessed on 10 July 2016).
14. Nasreddine, L.; Naja, F.; Chamieh, M.C.; Adra, N.; Sibai, A.-M.; Hwalla, N. Trends in overweight and obesity in Lebanon: Evidence from two national cross-sectional surveys (1997 and 2009). *BMC Public Health* **2012**, *12*, 798. [CrossRef] [PubMed]
15. World Health Organization. Nutrition—General Assembly Proclaims the Decade of Action on Nutrition. Available online: http://www.who.int/nutrition/GA_decade_action/en/ (accessed on 10 July 2016).
16. Moshfegh, A.J.; Borrud, L.; Perloff, B.; LaComb, R. Improved method for the 24-hour dietary recall for use in national surveys. *FASEB J.* **1999**, *13*, A603.
17. Naing, L.; Than, W.; Rusli, B. Practical issues in calculating the sample size for prevalence studies. *Arch. Orofac. Sci.* **2006**, *1*, 9–14.
18. Dinsa, G.; Goryakin, Y.; Fumagalli, E.; Suhrcke, M. Obesity and socioeconomic status in developing countries: A systematic review. *Obes. Rev.* **2012**, *13*, 1067–1079. [CrossRef] [PubMed]
19. Banque Bemo. *Education in Lebanon Growth Drivers, Structure, Primary and Secondary Cycles, Tertiary Cycle, Challenges and Recommendations*; BEMO Industry Report; Banque Bemo: Beirut, Lebanon, 2014.
20. Yaacoub, N.; Badre, L. *Education in Lebanon*; Statistics in Focus (SIF), Central Administration of Statistics: Beirut, Lebanon, 2012.
21. Wardle, J.; Guthrie, C.A.; Sanderson, S.; Rapoport, L. Development of the children's eating behaviour questionnaire. *J. Child Psychol. Psychiatry* **2001**, *42*, 963–970. [CrossRef] [PubMed]
22. National Institutes of Health. Clinical guidelines on the identification, evaluation, and treatment of overweight and obesity in adults: The evidence report. *Obes. Res.* **1998**, *6*, 51–209.

23. WHO Multicentre Growth Reference Study Group. *Who Child Growth Standards: Length/Height-for-Age, Weight-for-Age, Weight-for-Length, Weight-for-Height and Body Mass Index-for-Age: Methods and Development*; World Health Organization: Geneva, Switzerland, 2006; Available online: http://www.who.int/childgrowth/standards/Growth_standard.pdf (accessed on 8 July 2016).

24. World Health Organization. *Who Anthro Plus for Personal Computers Manual: Software for Assessing Growth of the World's Children and Adolescents*; World Health Organization: Geneva, Switzerland, 2009; Available online: http://www.who.int/growthref/tools/who_anthroplus_manual.pdf (accessed on 8 July 2016).

25. Kuczmarski, R.J.; Ogden, C.L.; Grummer-Strawn, L.M.; Flegal, K.M.; Guo, S.S.; Wei, R.; Mei, Z.; Curtin, L.R.; Roche, A.F.; Johnson, C.L. CDC growth charts: United states. *Adv. Data* **2000**, *314*, 1–27.

26. Kuczmarski, R.J.; Ogden, C.L.; Guo, S.S.; Grummer-Strawn, L.M.; Flegal, K.M.; Mei, Z.; Wei, R.; Curtin, L.R.; Roche, A.F.; Johnson, C.L. 2000 CDC growth charts for the united states: Methods and development. *Vital Health Stat.* **2002**, *11*, 1–190.

27. Cole, T.J.; Bellizzi, M.C.; Flegal, K.M.; Dietz, W.H. Establishing a standard definition for child overweight and obesity worldwide: International survey. *BMJ* **2000**, *320*, 1240. [CrossRef] [PubMed]

28. Willett, W. *Nutritional Epidemiology*, 2nd ed.; Oxford University Press: New York, NY, USA, 1998.

29. Shim, J.-S.; Oh, K.; Kim, H.C. Dietary assessment methods in epidemiologic studies. *Epidemiol. Health* **2014**, *36*, e2014009. [CrossRef] [PubMed]

30. Moshfegh, A.; Rhodes, D.; Baer, D.; Murayi, T.; Clemens, J.; Rumpler, W. The U.S. Department of agriculture automated multiple-pass method reduces bias in the collection of energy intakes. *Am. J. Clin. Nutr.* **2008**, *88*, 324–332. [PubMed]

31. Pellet, P.; Shadarevian, S. *Food Composition Tables for Use in the Middle East*; American University of Beirut: Beirut, Lebanon, 2013.

32. Cole, T.J.; Flegal, K.M.; Nicholls, D.; Jackson, A.A. Body mass index cut offs to define thinness in children and adolescents: International survey. *BMJ* **2007**, *335*, 194. [CrossRef] [PubMed]

33. Cattaneo, A.; Monasta, L.; Stamatakis, E.; Lioret, S.; Castetbon, K.; Frenken, F.; Manios, Y.; Moschonis, G.; Savva, S.; Zaborskis, A. Overweight and obesity in infants and pre-school children in the European Union: A review of existing data. *Obes. Rev.* **2010**, *11*, 389–398. [CrossRef] [PubMed]

34. Frenken, F. *Health Interview Survey 1981–2006*; Statistics Netherlands: Herleen, The Netherlands, 2007.

35. Nanu, M. *Nutritional Status of Children under 5 Years Old. National Nutritional Surveillance Programme 1993–2002*; Alfred Rusescu Institute for Mother and Child Care: Bucharest, Romania, 2003.

36. Onyango, A.W.; de Onis, M.; Caroli, M.; Shah, U.; Sguassero, Y.; Redondo, N.; Carroli, B. Field-testing the who child growth standards in four countries. *J. Nutr.* **2007**, *137*, 149–152. [PubMed]

37. Savva, S.; Tornaritis, M.; Chadjigeorgiou, C.; Kourides, Y.; Savva, M.; Panagi, A.; Chrictodoulou, E.; Kafatos, A. Prevalence and socio-demographic associations of undernutrition and obesity among preschool children in Cyprus. *Eur. J. Clin. Nutr.* **2005**, *59*, 1259–1265. [CrossRef] [PubMed]

38. Savva, S.; Tornaritis, M.; Chadjigeorgiou, C.; Kourides, Y.; Epiphaniou-Savva, M.; Panagi, A.; Chrictodoulou, E.; Kafatos, A. *Research and Education Institute of Child Health (REICH) Crosssectional Study, May–June 2004*; Research and Education Institute of Child Health (REICH): Nicosia, Cyprus, 2005.

39. Al-Raees, G.Y.; Al-Amer, M.A.; Musaiger, A.O.; D'Souza, R. Prevalence of overweight and obesity among children aged 2–5 years in Bahrain: A comparison between two reference standards. *Int. J. Pediatr. Obes.* **2009**, *4*, 414–416. [CrossRef] [PubMed]

40. Rady, M.; Al-Muslemani, M.; Salama, R. Determinants of overweight and obesity among Qatari children (2–5 years) in Doha, Qatar-2010. *Can. J. Clin. Nutr.* **2013**, *1*, 16–26. [CrossRef]

41. Shan, X.-Y.; Xi, B.; Cheng, H.; Hou, D.-Q.; Wang, Y.; Mi, J. Prevalence and behavioral risk factors of overweight and obesity among children aged 2–18 in Beijing, china. *Int. J. Pediatr. Obes.* **2010**, *5*, 383–389. [CrossRef] [PubMed]

42. Jordan Ministry of Health. National Micronutrient Survey Jordan 2010. 2011. Available online: http://www.gainhealth.org/wp-content/uploads/2014/05/56.-Jordan-Micronutrient-Survey-Report.pdf (accessed on 15 July 2016).

43. Instituto Nacional de Estadística; Ministerio de Sanidad y Consumo. *Encuesta Nacional de Salud 2006—Estilos de Vida y Prácticas Preventivas*; INE: Madrid, Spain, 2008.

44. Stamatakis, E. Anthropometric measurements, overweight, and obesity. In *Health Survey for England 2002—The Health for Children and Young People*; Sproston, K., Primatesta, P., Eds.; Highline Medical Services Organization: London, UK, 2003; Volume 1.

45. Commonwealth Scientific Industrial Research Organisation (CSIRO); Preventative Health National Research Flagship; The University of South Australia. 2007 Australian National Children's Nutrition and Physical Activity Survey—Main Findings. 2008. Available online: https://www.health.gov.au/internet/main/publishing.nsf/Content/8F4516D5FAC0700ACA257BF0001E0109/\protect\T1\textdollarFile/childrens-nut-phys-survey.pdf (accessed on 16 July 2016).

46. Shields, M. Measured Obesity: Overweight Canadian Children and Adolescents. Statistics Canada, 2005. Nutrition: Findings from the Canadian Community Health Survey; Issue No. 1 2005. Available online: http://www.statcan.gc.ca/pub/82-620-m/2005001/pdf/4193660-eng.pd (accessed on 16 July 2016).

47. Gaeini, A.; Kashef, M.; Samadi, A.; Fallahi, A. Prevalence of underweight, overweight and obesity in preschool children of Tehran, Iran. *J. Res. Med. Sci.* **2011**, *16*, 821–827. [PubMed]

48. Ogden, C.L.; Carroll, M.D.; Kit, B.K.; Flegal, K.M. Prevalence of childhood and adult obesity in the United States, 2011–2012. *J. Am. Med. Assoc.* **2014**, *311*, 806–814. [CrossRef] [PubMed]

49. Al Dossary, S.; Sarkis, P.; Hassan, A.; Ezz El Regal, M.; Fouda, A. Obesity in Saudi children: A dangerous reality. *East. Mediterr. Health J.* **2010**, *16*, 1003–1008. [PubMed]

50. Hui, L.; Nelson, E.; Yu, L.; Li, A.; Fok, T. Risk factors for childhood overweight in 6-to 7-y-old Hong Kong children. *Int. J. Obes.* **2003**, *27*, 1411–1418. [CrossRef] [PubMed]

51. Wang, Y.; Lim, H. The global childhood obesity epidemic and the association between socio-economic status and childhood obesity. *Int. Rev. Psychiatry* **2012**, *24*, 176–188. [CrossRef] [PubMed]

52. Nasreddine, L.; Mehio-Sibai, A.; Mrayati, M.; Adra, N.; Hwalla, N. Adolescent obesity in Syria: Prevalence and associated factors. *Child Care Health Dev.* **2010**, *36*, 404–413. [CrossRef] [PubMed]

53. Mushtaq, M.U.; Gull, S.; Shahid, U.; Shafique, M.M.; Abdullah, H.M.; Shad, M.A.; Siddiqui, A.M. Family-based factors associated with overweight and obesity among Pakistani primary school children. *BMC Pediatr.* **2011**, *11*, 114. [CrossRef] [PubMed]

54. Fakih, A.; Marrouch, W. Determinants of Domestic Workers' Employment: Evidence from Lebanese Household Survey Data. 2012. Available online: http://ftp.iza.org/dp6822.pdf (accessed on 18 July 2016).

55. Lin, S.L.; Leung, G.M.; Hui, L.L.; Lam, T.H.; Schooling, C.M. Is informal child care associated with childhood obesity? Evidence from Hong Kong's "children of 1997" birth cohort. *Int. J. Epidemiol.* **2011**, *40*, 1238–1246. [CrossRef] [PubMed]

56. Benjamin, S.E.; Rifas-Shiman, S.L.; Taveras, E.M.; Haines, J.; Finkelstein, J.; Kleinman, K.; Gillman, M.W. Early child care and adiposity at ages 1 and 3 years. *Pediatrics* **2009**, *124*, 555–562. [CrossRef] [PubMed]

57. Pearce, A.; Li, L.; Abbas, J.; Ferguson, B.; Graham, H.; Law, C. Is childcare associated with the risk of overweight and obesity in the early years? Findings from the UK millennium cohort study. *Int. J. Obes.* **2010**, *34*, 1160–1168. [CrossRef] [PubMed]

58. Schooling, C.M.; Yau, C.; Cowling, B.J.; Lam, T.H.; Leung, G.M. Socio-economic disparities of childhood body mass index in a newly developed population: Evidence from Hong Kong's 'children of 1997' birth cohort. *Arch. Disease Child.* **2010**, *95*, 437–443. [CrossRef] [PubMed]

59. Story, M.; Kaphingst, K.M.; French, S. The role of child care settings in obesity prevention. *Future Child.* **2006**, *16*, 143–168. [CrossRef] [PubMed]

60. Utter, J.; Neumark-Sztainer, D.; Jeffery, R.; Story, M. Couch potatoes or French fries: Are sedentary behaviors associated with body mass index, physical activity, and dietary behaviors among adolescents? *J. Am. Diet. Assoc.* **2003**, *103*, 1298–1305. [CrossRef]

61. Vik, F.N.; Bjørnarå, H.B.; Øverby, N.C.; Lien, N.; Androutsos, O.; Maes, L.; Jan, N.; Kovacs, E.; Moreno, L.A.; Dössegger, A. Associations between eating meals, watching TV while eating meals and weight status among children, ages 10–12 years in eight European countries: The energy cross-sectional study. *Int. J. Behav. Nutr. Phys. Act.* **2013**, *10*, 58. [CrossRef] [PubMed]

62. Chandon, P.; Wansink, B. Does food marketing need to make us fat? A review and solutions. *Nutr. Rev.* **2012**, *70*, 571–593. [CrossRef] [PubMed]

63. Francis, L.A.; Birch, L.L. Does eating during television viewing affect preschool children's intake? *J. Am. Diet. Assoc.* **2006**, *106*, 598–600. [CrossRef] [PubMed]

64. Jansen, P.W.; Roza, S.J.; Jaddoe, V.; Mackenbach, J.D.; Raat, H.; Hofman, A.; Verhulst, F.C.; Tiemeier, H. Children's eating behavior, feeding practices of parents and weight problems in early childhood: Results from the population-based Generation R Study. *Int. J. Behav. Nutr. Phys. Act.* **2012**, *9*, 130. [CrossRef] [PubMed]

65. Santos, J.L.; Ho-Urriola, J.A.; González, A.; Smalley, S.V.; Domínguez-Vásquez, P.; Cataldo, R.; Obregón, A.M.; Amador, P.; Weisstaub, G.; Hodgson, M.I. Association between eating behavior scores and obesity in Chilean children. *Nutr. J.* **2011**, *10*, 108. [CrossRef] [PubMed]

66. Gazzaniga, J.M.; Burns, T.L. Relationship between diet composition and body fatness, with adjustment for resting energy expenditure and physical activity, in preadolescent children. *Am. J. Clin. Nutr.* **1993**, *58*, 21–28. [PubMed]

67. Maffeis, C.; Talamini, G.; Tato, L. Influence of diet, physical activity and parents' obesity on children's adiposity: A four-year longitudinal study. *Int. J. Obes. Relat. Metab. Disord.* **1998**, *22*, 758–764. [CrossRef] [PubMed]

68. United States Department of Agriculture (USDA). Is Intake of Dietary Fat Associated with Adiposity in Children? Available online: http://www.nel.gov/evidence.cfm?evidence_summary_id=250348 (accessed on 20 July 2016).

69. Magarey, A.; Daniels, L.; Boulton, T.; Cockington, R. Does fat intake predict adiposity in healthy children and adolescents aged 2–15 years? A longitudinal analysis. *Eur. J. Clin. Nutr.* **2001**, *55*, 471–481. [CrossRef] [PubMed]

70. Skinner, J.; Bounds, W.; Carruth, B.; Morris, M.; Ziegler, P. Predictors of children's body mass index: A longitudinal study of diet and growth in children aged 2–8 years. *Int. J. Obes. Relat. Metab. Disord.* **2004**, *28*, 476–482. [CrossRef] [PubMed]

71. World Health Organization. *Obesity. Preventing and Managing the Global Epidemic*; Report of a WHO Consultation on Obesity; World Health Organisation: Geneva, Switzerland, 1998; Available online: http://www.who.int/nutrition/publications/obesity/WHO_TRS_894/en/ (accessed on 20 July 2016).

72. Little, T.J.; Horowitz, M.; Feinle-Bisset, C. Modulation by high-fat diets of gastrointestinal function and hormones associated with the regulation of energy intake: Implications for the pathophysiology of obesity. *Am. J. Clin. Nutr.* **2007**, *86*, 531–541. [PubMed]

73. Horton, T.J.; Drougas, H.; Brachey, A.; Reed, G.W.; Peters, J.C.; Hill, J. Fat and carbohydrate overfeeding in humans: Different effects on energy storage. *Am. J. Clin. Nutr.* **1995**, *62*, 19–29. [PubMed]

74. Campbell, K.; Hesketh, K. Strategies which aim to positively impact on weight, physical activity, diet and sedentary behaviours in children from zero to five years. A systematic review of the literature. *Obes. Rev.* **2007**, *8*, 327–338. [CrossRef] [PubMed]

75. Livingstone, M.; Robson, P. Measurement of dietary intake in children. *Proc. Nutr. Soc.* **2000**, *59*, 279–293. [CrossRef] [PubMed]

76. Burrows, T.L.; Martin, R.J.; Collins, C.E. A systematic review of the validity of dietary assessment methods in children when compared with the method of doubly labeled water. *J. Am. Diet. Assoc.* **2010**, *110*, 1501–1510. [CrossRef] [PubMed]

77. Penpraze, V.; Reilly, J.J.; MacLean, C.M.; Montgomery, C.; Kelly, L.A.; Paton, J.Y.; Aitchison, T.; Grant, S. Monitoring of physical activity in young children: How much is enough? *Pediatr. Exerc. Sci.* **2006**, *18*, 483. [CrossRef]

78. Corder, K.; Ekelund, U.; Steele, R.M.; Wareham, N.J.; Brage, S. Assessment of physical activity in youth. *J. Appl. Physiol.* **2008**, *105*, 977–987. [CrossRef] [PubMed]

79. Griffiths, L.J.; Parsons, T.J.; Hill, A.J. Self-esteem and quality of life in obese children and adolescents: A systematic review. *Int. J. Pediatr. Obes.* **2010**, *5*, 282–304. [CrossRef] [PubMed]

80. Booth, K.M.; Pinkston, M.M.; Poston, W.S.C. Obesity and the built environment. *J. Am. Diet. Assoc.* **2005**, *105*, 110–117. [CrossRef] [PubMed]

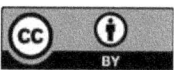

nutrients

MDPI

Article

Intake Levels of Fish in the UK Paediatric Population

Sibylle Kranz [1,*,†]**, Nicholas R. V. Jones** [2] **and Pablo Monsivais** [2,‡]

1   Centre for Exercise, Nutrition and Health Sciences, University of Bristol, Bristol BS8 1TH, UK
2   UKCRC Centre for Diet and Activity Research (CEDAR), Cambridge CB2 0QQ, UK;
     nrvj2@cantab.net (N.R.V.J.); pm491@medschl.cam.ac.uk (P.M.)
*   Correspondence: Sibylle.kranz@virginia.edu; Tel.: +1-434-924-7904
†   Current address: Department of Kinesiology, University of Virginia, Charlottesville 22904, USA.
‡   Current address: Department of Nutrition and Exercise Physiology, Washington State University,
     Spokane, WA 99210, USA.

Received: 6 February 2017; Accepted: 1 April 2017; Published: 16 April 2017

Abstract: The United Kingdom (UK) is an island and its culture, including diet, is heavily influenced by the maritime resources. Dietary guidance in the UK recommends intake of fish, which provides important nutrients, such as long-chain omega-3 polyunsaturated fatty acids (*n*-3 PUFA). This study was designed to describe the fish intake habits of UK children using a nationally representative sample. Dietary and socio-demographic data of children 2–18 (N = 2096) in the National Diet and Nutrition Survey Rolling Program (NDNS) Years 1–4 (2008–2012) were extracted. Average nutrient and food intakes were estimated. Logistic regression models were used to predict the meeting of fish intake recommendations, controlling for age, sex, income, total energy intake, and survey year. All analyses were conducted using survey routines and dietary survey weights. In this nationally representative study, 4.7% of children met the fish and 4.5% the oily fish intake recommendations; only 1.3% of the population met both recommendations. Fish intake levels did not significantly change with children's increasing age. Higher vegetable but lower meat consumption predicted meeting the fish intake recommendations, indicating that children eating fish have better diet quality than non-consumers. Further research is needed to explore how intake behaviours can be changed to improve children's diet quality.

Keywords: fish intake; diet quality; nutrition monitoring; NDNS-RP; child nutrition

1. Introduction

Fish contains very specific nutrients, including eicosapentanoic acid (EPA) and docosahexaenoic acid (DHA), which considered critical, as these long-chain n(omega)-3 polyunsaturated fatty acids (PUFA) have important roles in health [1], such as heart health [2], brain [3], and eye development [4–6]. Since EPA and DHA are not easily synthesized in the human body and the conversion rate from medium-chain *n*-3 fatty acids, such as alpha linoleic acid (ALA), is only approximately 1% [7], dietary intake of fish is considered part of a healthy diet [8–10].

Public health guidance recommends the consumption of fish, especially oily fish (i.e., salmon, herring, anchovy, smelt, and mackerel). The *Dietary Guidelines for Americans* [11] and United Kingdom (UK) Scientific Advisory Committee on Nutrition (SACN) [12] both suggest the consumption of two servings of fish (140 g each) per week, one serving of which should be from oily fish. This is equivalent to a calculated daily average minimum of 40 g of fish, of which 20 g should be from oily fish. Meeting these intake recommendations would contribute approximately 450 mg of EPA/DHA, which is considered as the adequate intake level by the two agencies. The Joint Food and Agriculture Organization (FAO) and World Health Organization (WHO) Expert Consultation on Fats and Fatty Acids in Human Nutrition provide a similar recommendation, namely 300 mg/day EPA and DHA, of which at least 200 mg/day should be DHA [13].

Studies of children's diets in Germany indicated that children consuming even small amounts of fish had significantly improved long-chain n-3 PUFA consumption levels compared to non-consumers [14]. A study of national fish consumption trends in American children reported overall low intake of fish; moreover, only one of the three most frequently consumed fish species was an oily variety [15]. Likewise, another analysis of the diets of one through five year old American children found very low intake of fish and long-chain n-3 PUFA [16].

The countries of the UK (England, Wales, Scotland, and Northern Ireland) are geographically maritime—islands surrounded by waters that are traditionally harvested for fish and seafood. Although slightly varied between these four countries, the historic diet culture in the UK includes many fish- and seafood-based dishes, such as baked or pickled fish, seafood salads or pies, and smoked/dried fish. The most recognized dishes internationally include "fish and chips" (battered and deep fried cod, haddock or plaice served with large-cut potato fries), "kippers" (salted and smoked herring), or smoked mackerel. These dishes are found on the menu of most eateries in the UK. They are offered as low-cost street-food but also in higher-end restaurants as "traditional fare".

The national dietary intake guidance for the UK is issued by the Food Standards Agency in form of the "The Eatwell Plate" and reflects the SACN recommendations for fish and oily fish [17]. Survey data shows that fish intake is recognized as a healthy choice by young people, although opinions somewhat vary [18]. Despite the relatively high availability of fish and seafood and consistent public health guidance to consume more fish, just like American children, UK children may not meet the intake recommendation.

The primary goal of this study was to use nationally representative data to examine the fish and seafood consumption of children in the UK, and to compare reported consumption levels with the intake recommendations for total fish and oily fish. A secondary goal was to examine the association of fish intake to other indicators of diet quality, in this case vegetable and meat intake.

2. Materials and Methods

2.1. Population Sample

Data from 2–18 year-old children ($N = 2096$) of the survey years 1–4 of the National Diet and Nutrition Survey rolling programme (NDNS-RP, 2008–2012) were included in this study. Children's age was used to stratify the population in three distinct age groups: 2–5 year olds, 6–11 year olds, and 12–18 year olds. All analyses were conducted for the total sample, as well as separately for those who reported consuming any fish. NDNS is publicly available and de-identified data, thus this study does not fall under the scope of research in human subjects.

Dietary, demographic, and socioeconomic data were obtained from the dataset. Demographic and socio-economic data (sex, race/ethnicity, and income) were used to describe the sample. Income was not available for 21 (1%) children in the sample, leaving $N = 2075$ children for whom the household income was categorized and equalised using a method previously used [16]. Income was coded as missing when household income was not provided.

2.2. Nutritional Variables

To estimate dietary intake, four consecutive 24-h estimated diet diaries (records) were collected from participants. Participants kept dietary intake records for four consecutive days. Dietary intake data collection was conducted year-round. No information as to the season of the data collected here is available. Weekend days were over-sampled in year one of the survey and under-sampled in the remaining years of the dataset used here, thus providing a fair estimate of usual daily intake of the participants. Each participant aged 12 and older was instructed on how to complete his or her own diary using household measures (i.e., measuring cups and spoons) and information from product packages to estimate the amounts of food and drink consumed. Children 16 and older were asked to estimate the portions of food and drink consumed by referring to a photo booklet of commonly-consumed items. For children younger than 12, parents or care-givers were asked to complete the diary, with information from the child. By the second or third diary day, survey staff met with the participant to review the diary days completed so far and provide feedback for improving the quality of diet data collection for the remaining diary days. Daily average food group and nutrient consumptions are reported in the dataset. Completed diaries were coded and entered by trained survey staff. Data were entered into the MRC-Human Nutrition Research dietary assessment system DINO (Diet IN Nutrients Out), an analysis system written in Microsoft Access. Nutrient intake assessed by DINO is based on a food composition database derived from UK food tables and supplemented with additional information from the food industry. Details of the use of DINO to estimate nutrient intakes in NDNS has been reported [19].

For the purpose of this study, total energy (kilocalories per day (kcal)), food group (in percent of total energy consumed for protein, fat, carbohydrates, and total sugars) and individual food items (in grams per 1000 kcal consumed or fruits and vegetables, total meat, red meat, white meat, eggs, nuts and seeds, total fish, white fish, oily fish, canned tuna, and shellfish) were calculated. This approach allows for comparison across age groups, which consume different levels of total energy and therefore increasing amounts of each food group with increasing age. Based on the reported diet, children were classified as "fish consumers" if they consumed any amount of fish or seafood (NDNS Variable 33 "White fish coated or fried", Variable 34 "Other white fish, shellfish and fish dishes", and Variable 35 "Oily fish") or as non-consumers otherwise. All data were reported for all children and disaggregated by age group for the total sample and the fish consumers and non-consumers separately. In the NDNS dataset, the n-3 PUFA are estimated as one variable, thus, no differentiation between the intake of long-chain n-3 PUFA, such as EPA and DHA, and short- or medium-chain PUFA can be made.

2.3. Statistical Analysis

All analyses were conducted using survey routines and the dietary survey weights to maintain the nationally representative character of the data. Analyses were conducted in STATA Version 13 (STATA Corporation, College Station, TX, USA). Mean consumption of food groups and nutrients was calculated for the total population and for each age group separately and reported as mean ± standard error. Intakes of macronutrients were expressed as percent energy and food groups were expressed on a gram (g) per-1000 kcal basis in order to facilitate comparisons across age groups. Since fish and seafood consumption was highly skewed, so median and interquartile range were estimated to describe the consumption in the population. Non-parametric test for trend across ordered groups was used to determine if consumption increased or decreased with increasing age across three age groups (2–5, 6–11, 12–18 years old). Significant differences in mean consumption between the group of children who consume fish and non-consumers was determined using the *lincom* command, the survey routine equivalent to the Student's *T*-test to compare means. Logistic regression modelling was employed to determine the contributors to children's odds of (a) meeting the dietary intake recommendation for total fish (40 g/day); (b) for oily fish (20 g/day); and (c) for any consumption of fish. All models controlled for age, sex, household income, total energy intake, and NDNS survey year. Statistical significance was assumed using a 95% level of significance.

3. Results

Based on the nature of this study, the demographic profile of the population included in the sample is representative of all children in the UK (data not shown). More than half of the population (55%, $N = 1142$) consumed any fish/seafood during the four days of dietary intake measurement (Table 1). Of those, 4.7% met the total fish intake recommendation, 4.5% the oily fish intake recommendation, and only 1.3% ($N = 28$ children) of 2–18 year olds met both (the total fish and the oily fish intake recommendations).

Table 1. Proportion of children meeting the recommended fish and seafood intake of the "Eatwell Plate" UK national intake recommendations in the National Diet and Nutrition Survey 2008–2012 in the total sample (*N* = 2075).

Characteristic	Total Sample (*N* = 2096)	2–5 Year Olds (*N* = 634)	6–11 Year Olds (*N* = 664)	12–18 Year Olds (*N* = 798)
Fish consumers [1]	54.9	62.9	58.3	45.5
Meet fish recommendation (≥40 g of fish/day)	4.2	2.5	4.6	5.3
Meet oily fish recommendation (≥20 g of fish/day)	4.0	2.4	4.8	4.7
Meet fish and oily fish recommendations	1.3	0.6	1.4	1.0

[1] Includes NDNS food groups "White fish coated or fried", "Other white fish, shellfish and fish dishes", and "Oily fish".

Fish and seafood intake was highly skewed, hence, both mean and standard error (SE) as well as median and interquartile range (IQR), the 25th and 75th percentile of intake, were calculated. Total fish and seafood consumption was low (mean ± SE = 10.41 ± 0.42; median and IQR: 3.78 g/day and 0; 16.5 g/day); oily fish consumption was even lower (mean ± SE = 1.78 ± 0.17; median and IQR: 0 g/day and 0; 0 g/day); the 90th percentile of oily fish intake was only 2.55 g/day.

Analysis of the average dietary intake of foods and food groups in the total sample and the subsamples of fish consumers, and those children meeting the intake recommendations, showed that children who consumed fish had better diet quality (Table 2). Those children consumed more vegetables and less meat. Most nutrient and food group intake vary with age in the total population, in that total energy, meat density (red and white meat density) and shellfish increased while percent of energy from added sugar, fruit and vegetable density, total- and white fish density decreased. Comparison of intake between fish consumers and non-consumers showed that children who consume fish have higher fruit and vegetable density in their diet and lower meat density.

Logistic regression models showed that neither household income nor ethnic group was associated with total fish or oily fish intake (data not shown) and subsequent modelling including age, sex, equalised household income, total energy consumed and NDNS survey year as covariates (Table 3).

Consuming any fish was strongly and positively associated with being in the medium or highest tertile of vegetable intake and negatively associated with eating the medium or highest tertile of meat (OR = 1.55, 95% CI 1.19–2.12; OR = 1.88, 95% CI 1.39–2.58; OR = 0.72, 95% CI 0.55–0.98; OR = 0.47, 95% CI 0.34–0.66, respectively). Consuming the recommended amount of two servings of fish was significantly and positively predicted by consuming the highest tertile of vegetables (OR = 2.51, 95% CI 1.30–4.84) and significantly but negatively associated with consuming the highest tertile of meat (OR = 0.32, 95% CI 0.16–0.64). The odds of meeting the intake recommendation for oily fish was increased with eating the highest tertile of vegetables (OR = 3.49, 95% CI 1.21–9.96) and the medium or highest tertile of meat consumption (OR = 2.84, 95% CI 1.20-6.75 and OR = 2.65, 95% CI 1.90–7.84, respectively).

Table 2. Estimated intakes of select food groups and foods † by children in the National Diet and Nutrition Survey 2008–2012 in the total sample and by age group (N = 2096).

	All Children	2–5 Year Olds	6–11 Year Olds	12–18 Year Olds	Test for Trend ‡ p-Value
		Total sample (N = 2096)			
Total energy (kcal/day)	1554 ± 14	1205 ± 17	1608 ± 18	1801 ± 24	<0.001 ***
Protein (% energy/day)	14.8 ± 0.8	15.1 ± 0.1	14.4 ± 0.1	14.8 ± 0.1	0.172
Fat (% energy/day)	33.7 ± 0.1	33.8 ± 0.3	33.4 ± 0.2	33.8 ± 0.2	0.783
Carbohydrates (% energy/day)	51.2 ± 0.2	51.2 ± 0.3	52.2 ± 0.2	50.5 ± 0.3	0.011 *
	Energy-adjusted intakes of food groups (g/1000 kcal consumed)				
Fruits and vegetables	126.3 ± 2.4	158.9 ± 5.1	129.4 ± 3.7	96.8 ± 2.7	<0.001 ***
Total meat	47.2 ± 0.8	37.7 ± 4.1	46.4 ± 1.1	44.8 ± 1.4	<0.001 ***
Red meat	30.6 ± 0.7	25.7 ± 1.2	30.6 ± 1.1	34.8 ± 1.2	<0.001 ***
White meat	16.6 ± 0.5	12.1 ± 0.7	15.8 ± 0.7	21.0 ± 0.8	<0.001 ***
Eggs	6.9 ± 0.4	6.8 ± 0.6	6.1 ± 0.6	7.6 ± 0.7	0.345
Nuts and seeds	0.6 ± 0.1	0.7 ± 0.6	0.6 ± 0.1	0.6 ± 0.1	0.263
Total fish	7.1 ± 0.3	7.9 ± 0.5	7.2 ± 0.5	6.2 ± 0.4	<0.001 ***
White fish	4.0 ± 0.2	4.9 ± 0.4	4.2 ± 0.4	2.3 ± 0.2	<0.001 ***
Oily fish	1.2 ± 0.1	1.1 ± 0.2	1.3 ± 0.2	1.1 ± 0.2	0.164
Canned tuna	1.6 ± 0.1	1.6 ± 0.3	1.1 ± 0.1	1.9 ± 0.3	0.152
Shellfish	0.6 ± 0.1	0.2 ± 0.1	0.6 ± 0.1	0.8 ± 0.2	<0.001 ***
	Consumers of fish/seafood (N = 1142)				
Total energy (kcal/day)	1522 ± 18 ⊥	1211 ± 18	1621 ± 26	1776 ± 34	<0.001 ***
Protein (% energy/day)	15.1 ± 0.1 ⊥	15.3 ± 0.2 ⊥	14.7 ± 0.2 ⊥	15.2 ± 0.2 ⊥	0.812
Fat (% energy/day)	33.8 ± 0.2	33.7 ± 0.4	33.6 ± 0.3	34.2 ± 0.3	0.875
Carbohydrates (% energy/day)	50.9 ± 0.2 ⊥	51.0 ± 0.4	51.8 ± 0.3 ⊥	50.0 ± 0.4	0.055

Table 2. *Cont.*

	All Children	2–5 Year Olds	6–11 Year Olds	12–18 Year Olds	Test for Trend [‡] p-Value
Energy-adjusted intakes of food groups (g/1000 kcal consumed)					
Fruits and vegetables	135.3 ± 3.2 ⊥	162.9 ± 0.006.2	138.3 ± 4.1 ⊥	100.4 ± 3.7	<0.001 ***
Total meat	43.4 ± 1.1 ⊥	35.3 ± 1.8 ⊥	43.7 ± 1.5 ⊥	52.3 ± 2.0 ⊥	<0.001 ***
Red meat	27.6 ± 0.7 ⊥	23.6 ± 1.4 ⊥	28.4 ± 1.3 ⊥	31.2 ± 1.6 ⊥	<0.001 ***
White meat	15.8 ± 0.6	11.7 ± 1.0	15.3 ± 0.8	21.1 ± 1.3	<0.001 ***
Eggs	6.6 ± 0.5	7.0 ± 0.8	6.1 ± 0.9	6.9 ± 0.8	0.247
Nuts and seeds	0.7 ± 0.1 ⊥	0.7 ± 0.2	0.7 ± 0.2 ⊥	0.6 ± 0.2	0.153
Total fish	12.9 ± 0.4	12.6 ± 0.8	12.5 ± 0.6	13.7 ± 0.7	0.064
White fish	4.0 ± 0.2	7.8 ± 0.6	7.2 ± 0.5	5.0 ± 0.5	<0.001 ***
Oily fish	1.2 ± 0.1	1.8 ± 0.3	2.3 ± 0.3	2.5 ± 0.4	0.406
Canned tuna	1.6 ± 0.1	2.6 ± 0.5	1.9 ± 0.2	4.4 ± 0.5	<0.001 ***
Shellfish	0.6 ± 0.1	0.3 ± 0.1	1.1 ± 0.2	1.9 ± 0.4	<0.001 ***
Non-consumers of fish/seafood (N = 954)					
Total energy (kcal/day)	1594 ± 22 ⊥	1196 ± 30	1590 ± 25	1821 ± 34	<0.001 ***
Protein (% energy/day)	14.4 ± 0.12 ⊥	14.7 ± 0.2 ⊥	14.1 ± 0.2 ⊥	14.5 ± 0.2	0.314
Fat (% energy/day)	33.6 ± 0.2	34.0 ± 0.5	33.2 ± 0.4	33.6 ± 0.4	0.565
Carbohydrates (% energy/day)	51.5 ± 0.2 ⊥	51.4 ± 0.5	52.8 ± 0.4	50.9 ± 0.4	0.062
Energy-adjusted intakes of food groups (g/1000 kcal consumed)					
Fruits and vegetables	115.5 ± 3.7 ⊥	152.2 ± 8.7	116.9 ± 6.8 ⊥	93.8 ± 3.9	<0.001 ***
Total meat	51.9 ± 1.2 ⊥	41.8 ± 2.2 ⊥	50.1 ± 1.9 ⊥	58.8 ± 1.8 ⊥	<0.001 ***
Red meat	34.4 ± 1.1 ⊥	29.2 ± 1.9 ⊥	33.6 ± 1.8 ⊥	37.8 ± 1.7 ⊥	0.002 **
White meat	17.6 ± 0.7	12.6 ± 1.1	16.5 ± 1.1	21.0 ± 1.1	<0.001 ***
Eggs	7.1 ± 0.6	6.6 ± 1.0	6.0 ± 0.8	8.1 ± 1.0	0.945
Nuts and seeds	0.5 ± 0.1 ⊥	0.6 ± 0.2	0.3 ± 0.1 ⊥	0.6 ± 0.1	0.878

[†] Includes NDNS food groups "White fish coated or fried", "Other white fish, shellfish and fish dishes", and "Oily fish"; [‡] across ordered groups by age group; Asterisks indicate significant trend with increasing age * $p < 0.05$; ** $p < 0.01$; *** $p < 0.0001$; ⊥ significantly different between fish consumers and non-consumers.

Table 3. Association (odds ratios and 95% confidence intervals) of children's dietary characteristics for children, who (a) are fish consumers and (b) meet the fish intake recommendation of 280 g/week (or 40 g/day), and (c) meet the oily fish intake recommendation of 140 g/week (or 20 g/day) ($N = 2096$).

		Odds Ratio	95% Confidence Interval
(a) Consume any fish/seafood			
Tertile of vegetable	Lowest	1.00	
	Medium	1.55 **	1.19, 2.12
	Highest	1.88 ***	1.39, 2.58
Tertile of meat	Lowest	1.00	
	Medium	0.72 *	0.55, 0.98
	Highest	0.47 ***	0.34, 0.66
(b) Meet fish intake recommendation			
Tertile of vegetable	Lowest	1.00	
	Medium	0.99	0.45, 2.16
	Highest	2.51 **	1.30, 4.84
Tertile of meat	Lowest	1.00	
	Medium	0.55	0.27, 1.09
	Highest	0.32 **	0.16, 0.64
(c) Meet oily fish intake recommendation			
Total fish intake (g/day)		1.07 ***	1.05, 1.09
Tertile of vegetable	Lowest	1.00	
	Medium	1.89	0.67, 5.97
	Highest	3.47 **	1.21, 9.96
Tertile of meat	Lowest	1.00	
	Medium	2.84 **	1.20, 6.75
	Highest	2.65 *	1.90, 7.84

Values were significantly different at: * $p < 0.05$; ** $p < 0.01$; *** $p < 0.0001$, all models controlling for age, sex, total energy intake, equalized household income, and NDNS survey year.

4. Discussion

Recommendations for fish intake, especially those focussing on oily fish, are in part designed to promote adequate intakes of EPA and DHA in children and adults. Low intake of EPA/DHA is commonly observed in the Western diet [17] and might negatively affect children's brain development and function [18,19]. Data from observational studies indicated that low levels of EPA/DHA may be associated with rising prevalence of childhood developmental disorders, such as attention-deficit hyperactivity disorder and dyslexia [20]. Overall, EPA and DHA have a recognized role in health and disease prevention [1–6]. As our results show, the proportion of children in the UK meeting the intake recommendations for total fish and oily fish intake is extremely small. This is reason for concern.

Although small amounts of EPA and DHA can be found in foods other than fish, those foods (predominantly eggs and dark poultry meats) are also very high in saturated fatty acids [21]. Although we showed that a very large proportion of 2–18 year-old children in the UK fail to meet the intake recommendation for total fish and/or oily fish, we are not able to directly assess if children meet the targeted daily minimum consumption amounts for EPA and DHA because EPA and DHA are not reported separately from medium- and short-chain fatty acids in the NDNS data set. This particular problem with the UK national dietary data survey system has been noted previously [22]. It would be very beneficial for policy purposes if future releases of the NDNS nutrient data wold be modified to allow a direct measurement of the individual dietary fatty acids. However, it is noteworthy to point out that the measurement of EPA and DHA in free-living individuals is a challenge, due to tissue storage, conversion rate, and saturable plasma levels [20]. In the future, other approaches might be possible to better estimate fish intake, such as a metabolomic study of biomarkers of meat and fish intake [21].

Despite the lack of direct measurement of EPA and DHA intake levels in this sample, our analysis showed that the vast majority of 2–18 year old children in the UK fail to meet the intake recommendations for fish. Interestingly, the density of fish in the diet increased with increasing age for most categories of fish, but consumption of white fish dropped and oily fish remained almost the same in 12–18 year olds while intake of canned tuna and shellfish experienced a marked increase compared to the two younger age groups. While the similar findings in the US paediatric population [22] may be explained by the relatively low availability of affordable fish, especially oily fish, the same phenomenon in the UK must have different reasons and begs to be explored further. In the US, especially young children from low-income households may have limited access to fish, due to their mothers dietary intake practices, which have been shown to be low in fish and other healthy items [23]. However, as the authors for that research report explain, there is severe lack of evidence on the possible venues to rectify the problem of low diet quality in low-income women. Some possible contributing factors may be the lack of access (i.e., family ability to obtain seafood from local vendors) and availability (i.e., the quantity and quality of food provided), the relatively higher cost of some oily fish compared to (for example) cheaper processed meats [23]. Also, parents' and carers' knowledge and ability to prepare fish, as well as their role-modelling of eating fish and seafood [24] may contribute. Other changes in local culture, such as the lack of family meals and a preference to consume foods from other cuisines are potential contributing to the low intake of fish in children. These phenomena may also be the underlying cause of reduction of fish intake in Mediterranean countries, which used to be traditionally high in fish intake [24,25]. A published research report for an intervention study to increase dietary EPA and DHA consumption of preschool-age children showed that the substitution of meats usually used for the lunch meal in child care settings can be replaced with oily fish [25]. Since oily fish, such as salmon, herring, and sardines, are so high in EPA and DHA that even a small increase in intake results in significantly improved intakes, adding fish to mixed dishes, such as pasta and sauce, may significantly improve children's EPA and DHA consumption.

One possible limitation of this study was the use of four estimated dietary records to estimate intake. Although this method has been accepted for large nutrition surveys, intake of rarely consumed foods, such as seafood, may be misrepresented using this somewhat short-term data collection method. On the other hand, the level of detail provided by multiple-day records is superior to diet information obtained from long-term food frequency questionnaires. Compared to the intake estimates used in US national surveys (using two 24-hour recalls), the use of four days of food records doubled the odds of capturing those rarely consumed foods. Ideally, future research on fish intake would include a biomarker of intake levels, such as trimethylamine-N-oxide [21].

One major strength of this study was the use of a nationally-representative data set, which allows generalizability of the results. Some might expect that younger children have different intake patterns than teenagers. However, the consumption levels of all fish and seafood types available in the dataset show that intake increases with age, with the exception of white fish.

A key finding was that only approximately 2% of the population met the recommendations for both total fish and oily fish intake. Interestingly, our data show that children who consumed any fish or seafood also had healthier eating patterns, characterized by higher vegetable intake but lower meat intake. This relationship between higher vegetable but lower meat intake showed a significant trend, in that the odds for meeting the fish intake recommendations were even better in the children consuming in the highest tertile of vegetable compared to the medium tertile. Likewise, the odds for meeting the intake recommendations were lower for the children consuming in the highest tertile for meat intake compared to the medium tertile of meat consumption. This finding suggests for the first time that in the UK paediatric population, fish intake may be a useful proxy for overall healthy eating patterns.

Results of this study indicate that programmes and policies to promote the consumption of fish in the UK are not heeded. Although some might recommend more frequent and larger amounts of fish intake in the paediatric population, even a small intake of predatory fish raises the concern for the possible nutrition-toxicity issues [26]. Supplying sufficient amounts of safe fish to meet EPA and DHA intake recommendations may also be at odds with the sustainability of marine ecosystems [27]. At the same time, exploring other dietary sources of EPA and DHA that are low-cost, widely available, and acceptable to children might be beneficial for all children, not only in the UK.

5. Conclusions

Our study indicates that children in the UK do not consume sufficient amounts of fish. However, due to the lack of data on the EPA and DHA consumption, it is not clear whether or not the low fish intake is associated with inadequate levels of these two important nutrients for brain development and functioning. Further research is needed to pursue this question and to identify the barriers to fish intake in a population of traditionally high fish- and seafood diets.

Acknowledgments: N.R.V.J. and P.M. were supported by the Centre for Diet and Activity Research (CEDAR), a UKCRC Public Health Research Centre of Excellence. Funding from the British Heart Foundation, Cancer Research UK, Economic and Social Research Council, Medical Research Council, the National Institute for Health Research, and the Wellcome Trust, under the auspices of the UK Clinical Research Collaboration, is gratefully acknowledged. The funders had no role in the design or conduct of the study or the writing of the manuscript. This research received no specific grant from any funding agency, commercial or not-for-profit sectors.

Author Contributions: S.K. is the primary author and led the analysis and writing. N.R.V.J. and P.M. contributed to analysis and writing. All authors have read and approved the final manuscript.

Conflicts of Interest: No conflicts of interest are declared.

References

1. Yashodhara, B.M.; Umakanth, S.; Pappachan, J.M.; Bhat, S.K.; Kamath, R.; Choo, B.H. Omega-3 fatty acids: A comprehensive review of their role in health and disease. *Postgrad. Med. J.* **2009**, *85*, 84–90. [CrossRef] [PubMed]
2. Mozzaffarian, D.; Wu, J.H.Y. (*n*-3) fatty acids and cardiovascular health: Are effects of EPA and DHA shared or complementary? *J. Nutr.* **2012**, *142*, 614S–625S. [CrossRef] [PubMed]
3. Innis, S.M. Dietary omega 3 fatty acids and the developing brain. *Brain Res.* **2008**, *1237*, 35–43. [CrossRef] [PubMed]
4. Birch, E.E.; Garfield, S.; Castaneda, Y.; Hughbankswheaton, D.; Uauy, R.; Hoffman, D. Visual acuity and cognitive outcomes at 4 years of age in a double-blind, randomized trial of long-chain polyunsaturated fatty acid-supplemented infant formula. *Early Hum. Dev.* **2007**, *83*, 279–284. [CrossRef] [PubMed]
5. Jacques, C.; Levy, E.; Muckle, G.; Jacobson, S.W.; Bastien, C.; Dewailly, E.; Ayotte, P.; Jacobson, J.L.; Saint-Amour, D. Long-term effects of prenatal omega-3 fatty acid intake on visual function in school-age children. *J. Pediatr.* **2011**, *158*, 73. [CrossRef] [PubMed]
6. SanGiovanni, J.P.; Chew, E.Y. The role of omega-3 long-chain polyunsaturated fatty acids in health and disease of the retina. *Prog. Retin. Eye Res.* **2005**, *24*, 87–138. [CrossRef] [PubMed]
7. Gebauer, S.K.; Psota, T.L.; Harris, W.S.; Kris-Etherton, P.M. N-3 fatty acid dietary recommendations and food sources to achieve essentiality and cardiovascular benefits. *Am. J. Clin. Nutr.* **2006**, *83*, 1526S–1535S. [PubMed]
8. Institute of Medicine of the National Academy of Sciences. *Dietary Reference Intakes for Energy, Carbohydrate, Fiber, Fat, Fatty Acids, Cholesterol, Protein, and Amino Acids (Macronutrients)*; National Academy Press: Washington, DC, USA, 2002.
9. Flock, M.R.; Harris, W.S.; Kris-Etherton, P.M. Long-chain omega-3 fatty acids: Time to establish a dietary reference intake. *Nutr. Rev.* **2013**, *71*, 692–707. [CrossRef] [PubMed]
10. Scientific Advisory Committee for Nutrition (SCAN). *Advice on Fish Consumption: Benefits and Risks*; Food Standards Agency and the Department of Health: London, UK, 2004.
11. World Health Organization Study Group. Interim summary of conclusions and dietary recommendations on total fat and fatty acids. In Proceedings of the Joint FAO/WHO Expert Consultation on Fats and Fatty Acids in Human Nutrition, Geneva, Switzerland, 10–14 November 2008.

12. Kris-Etherton, P.M.; Taylor, D.S.; Yu-Poth, S.; Huth, P.; Moriarty, K.; Fishell, V.; Hargrove, R.L.; Zhao, G.; Etherton, T.D. Polyunsaturated fatty acids in the food chain in the United States. *Am. J. Clin. Nutr.* **2000**, *71*, 179S–188S. [PubMed]

13. Sichert-Hellert, W.; Wicher, M.; Kersting, M. Age and time trends in fish consumption pattern of children and adolescents, and consequences for the intake of long-chain *n*-3 polyunsaturated fatty acids. *Eur. J. Clin. Nutr.* **2009**, *63*, 1071–1075. [CrossRef] [PubMed]

14. Tran, N.L.; Barraj, L.M.; Bi, X.; Schuda, L.C.; Moya, J. Estimated long-term fish and shellfish intake—National health and nutrition examination survey. *J. Expo. Sci. Environ. Epidemiol.* **2013**, *23*, 128–136. [CrossRef] [PubMed]

15. Keim, S.A.; Branum, A.M. Dietary intake of polyunsaturated fatty acids and fish among US children 12–60 months of age. *Matern. Child. Nutr.* **2013**, *11*, 987–998. [CrossRef] [PubMed]

16. Maguire, E.R.; Monsivais, P. Socio-economic dietary inequalities in UK adults: An updated picture of key food groups and nutrients from national surveillance data. *Br. J. Nutr.* **2014**, *113*, 1–9. [CrossRef] [PubMed]

17. Van Elst, K.; Bruining, H.; Birtoli, B.; Terreaux, C.; Buitelaar, J.K. Food for thought: Dietary changes in essential fatty acid ratios and the increase in autism spectrum disorders. *Neurosci. Biobehav. Rev.* **2014**, *45C*, 369–378. [CrossRef] [PubMed]

18. Rosales, F.J.; Reznick, J.S.; Zeisel, S.H. Understanding the role of nutrition in the brain and behavioral development of toddlers and preschool children: Identifying and addressing methodological barriers. *Nutr. Neurosci.* **2009**, *12*, 190–202. [CrossRef] [PubMed]

19. Simopoulos, A.P. The importance of the ratio of omega-6/omega-3 essential fatty acids. *Biomed. Pharmacother.* **2002**, *56*, 365–379. [CrossRef]

20. Schuchardt, J.P.; Huss, M.; Stauss-Grabo, M.; Hahn, A. Significance of long-chain polyunsaturated fatty acids (PUFAs) for the development and behaviour of children. *Eur. J. Pediatr.* **2010**, *169*, 149–164. [CrossRef] [PubMed]

21. Butler, G. Manipulating dietary PUFA in animal feed: Implications for human health. *Proc. Nutr. Soc.* **2014**, *73*, 87–95. [CrossRef] [PubMed]

22. Pot, G.K.; Prynne, C.J.; Roberts, C.; Olson, A.; Nicholson, S.K.; Whitton, C.; Teucher, B.; Bates, B.; Henderson, H.; Pigott, S.; et al. National diet and nutrition survey: Fat and fatty acid intake from the first year of the rolling programme and comparison with previous surveys. *Br. J. Nutr.* **2012**, *107*, 405–415. [CrossRef] [PubMed]

23. Jones, N.R.; Conklin, A.I.; Suhrcke, M.; Monsivais, P. The growing price gap between more and less healthy foods: Analysis of a novel longitudinal UK dataset. *PLoS ONE* **2014**, *9*, e109343. [CrossRef] [PubMed]

24. Santiago-Torres, M.; Adams, A.K.; Carrel, A.L.; Larowe, T.L.; Schoeller, D.A. Home food availability, parental dietary intake, and familial eating habits influence the diet quality of urban Hispanic children. *Child. Obes.* **2014**, *10*, 408–415. [CrossRef] [PubMed]

25. Huss, L.R.; McCabe, S.D.; Dobbs-Oates, J.; Burgess, J.; Behnke, C.; Santerre, C.R.; Kranz, S. Development of child-friendly fish dishes to increase young children's acceptance and consumption of fish. *Food Nutr. Sci.* **2013**, *4*, 78–87. [CrossRef]

26. Mahaffey, K.R.; Clickner, R.P.; Jeffries, R.A. Methylmercury and omega-3 fatty acids: Co-occurrence of dietary sources with emphasis on fish and shellfish. *Environ. Res.* **2008**, *107*, 20–29. [CrossRef] [PubMed]

27. Brunner, E.J.; Jones, P.J.; Friel, S.; Bartley, M. Fish, human health and marine ecosystem health: Policies in collision. *Int. J. Epidemiol.* **2009**, *38*, 93–100. [CrossRef] [PubMed]

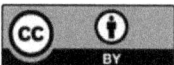

nutrients

Article

Snacking Quality Is Associated with Secondary School Academic Achievement and the Intention to Enroll in Higher Education: A Cross-Sectional Study in Adolescents from Santiago, Chile

Paulina Correa-Burrows [1,*], **Yanina Rodríguez** [1], **Estela Blanco** [2], **Sheila Gahagan** [2] **and Raquel Burrows** [1]

[1]   Institute of Nutrition and Food Technology, University of Chile, Santiago 7830490, Chile; yanirod77@hotmail.com (Y.R.); rburrows@inta.uchile.cl (R.B.)

[2]   Division of Child Development and Community Health, University of California, San Diego, CA 92093, USA; esblanco@ucsd.edu (E.B.); sgahagan@ucsd.edu (S.G.)

*   Correspondence: paulina.correa@inta.uchile.cl; Tel.: +56-229-78-1492

Received: 16 March 2017; Accepted: 24 April 2017; Published: 27 April 2017

Abstract: Although numerous studies have approached the effects of exposure to a Western diet (WD) on academic outcomes, very few have focused on foods consumed during snack times. We explored whether there is a link between nutritious snacking habits and academic achievement in high school (HS) students from Santiago, Chile. We conducted a cross-sectional study with 678 adolescents. The nutritional quality of snacks consumed by 16-year-old was assessed using a validated food frequency questionnaire. The academic outcomes measured were HS grade point average (GPA), the likelihood of HS completion, and the likelihood of taking college entrance exams. A multivariate analysis was performed to determine the independent associations of nutritious snacking with having completed HS and having taken college entrance exams. An analysis of covariance (ANCOVA) estimated the differences in GPA by the quality of snacks. Compared to students with healthy in-home snacking behaviors, adolescents having unhealthy in-home snacks had significantly lower GPAs (M difference: -40.1 points, 95% confidence interval (CI): -59.2, -16.9, $d = 0.41$), significantly lower odds of HS completion (adjusted odds ratio (aOR): 0.47; 95% CI: 0.25–0.88), and significantly lower odds of taking college entrance exams (aOR: 0.53; 95% CI: 0.31–0.88). Unhealthy at-school snacking showed similar associations with the outcome variables. Poor nutritional quality snacking at school and at home was associated with poor secondary school academic achievement and the intention to enroll in higher education.

Keywords: adolescents; unhealthy eating; snacks; academic performance; diet quality

1. Introduction

In spite of efforts by public agencies to monitor the types of food sold in school settings or regulate food advertising aimed at young people, their exposure to energy-dense foods (those with a high caloric concentration per bite) at and away from school remains high [1]. A recent study on the consumption of fast food in 36 developed and developing countries showed that more than 50% of adolescents consume fast food frequently or very frequently [2]. In Latin America, the Global School-based Health Survey (GSHS) showed that two-thirds of adolescents (13–17 years old) in Argentina, Chile and Uruguay reported daily intake of sugar-sweetened beverages [3]. In the early 2010s, among European 15-year-old, daily soft drink consumption was more than 40% in England, the Netherlands, Belgium, Slovakia and Slovenia [4].

Evidence is available on the role of Western-type diets (WD) in limiting cognitive abilities in critical brain maturation periods (i.e., infancy and childhood) [5,6]. Animal models show that exposure to a high-fat, high-sugar (HFS) diet in adolescence is related to impairment in hippocampal learning and memory processes, regardless of weight status [7,8]. One important mechanism that is proposed to underlie HFS-induced impaired hippocampal function is the reduced synthesis, secretion, and action of the brain-derived neurotrophic factor (BDNF). BDNF facilitates synaptic efficacy by converting changes in electrical activity to long-lasting changes in synaptic function, which is a suggested key process for memory formation [9]. Reduced levels of BDNF in association with impaired memory function has been well documented in the literature [10,11].

Impairment of memory consolidation and memory performance is a risk factor for learning difficulties and poor academic progress [12]. Thus, a diet of poor nutritional value may compromise students' ability to perform well in school. Longitudinal and cross-sectional studies, mostly conducted in developed countries, have examined the relationship between diet and school grades [13–15], as well as the relationship between diet and performance on standardized academic tests [16–18]. Results collectively suggest that better educational outcomes are associated with regular consumption of nutritious breakfasts, lower intake of energy-dense, nutrient-poor foods, and maintaining a healthy diet [19].

The effect of WDs on academic results can be used to strengthen health promotion strategies. While the connection between unhealthy diet and poor academic performance (as measured by school grades and standardized test scores) in elementary and middle schoolers has been well described, less is known about the relationship between dietary habits and postsecondary educational aspirations—that is, the intention to pursue higher education after secondary school. The increasing number of HS graduates seeking entrance to higher education institutions, including in non-industrialized nations, has made this a particularly important topic for students, families and policymakers.

Since the question of how WD foods may compromise students' intention to pursue higher education is also of interest to non-academic audiences, we used a translational-research approach to provide evidence that can be translated from research and applied to practice and policy. Thus, we examined the relationship of nutritional quality of snacks with academic outcomes using functional cognition measures like grade point average (GPA), high school (HS) completion, and college entrance examination participation rates. Our decision to concentrate on snacks rather than overall diet or meals such as breakfast, lunch or supper was based on wanting to focus on food choices made by adolescents rather than consumption of foods over which they may have little volition. We hypothesized that students habitually eating unhealthy snacks would have lower grades and be less likely to complete HS and take college admission exams.

2. Materials and Methods

2.1. Study Design and Population

We studied 16–17-year-old adolescents living in Santiago, Chile, from low-to-middle socioeconomic status (SES), who were part of an infancy cohort. Participants were recruited at 4 months from public healthcare facilities in the southeast area of Santiago (n = 1791). They were born at term of uncomplicated vaginal births, weighed >3.0 kg, and were free of acute or chronic health problems. At 6 months, infants free of iron deficiency anemia (n = 1657) were randomly assigned to receive iron supplementation or no added iron (ages 6–12 months). They were assessed for developmental outcomes in infancy, and at 5, 10 and 15 years [20]. At 16–17 years, those with complete data in each wave (n = 678) were also assessed for obesity risk and the presence of cardiovascular risk factors in a half-day evaluation that included assessment of dietary habits and nutritional content of food intake. Ethical approval was obtained by the institutional review boards of the University of Michigan, Institute of Nutrition and Food Technology (INTA), University of Chile, and the University of California, San Diego. Participants and their primary caregiver provided informed and written consent, according to the norms for Human Experimentation, Code of Ethics of the World Medical Association (Declaration of Helsinki, 1995).

2.2. Nutritional Quality of Snacking at Age 16

Nutritional quality of in-school and at-home snacking was measured considering the amount of saturated fat, fiber, sugar and salt in the food. Assessment was performed with a food frequency questionnaire, validated using three 24 h recalls to include weekends [21,22]. A section of this questionnaire was specially designed to assess the usual diet during the snack time at school and at home, by asking about the frequency of food consumption within the past three months. A list of 50 foods and beverages was used. The frequency of food consumption was assessed by a multiple response grid; respondents were asked to estimate how often a particular food or beverage was consumed. Categories ranged from "never" to "five or more times a week". The electronic version of the Chilean Food Composition Tables/Database was used to assess the quality of snacks composition [23]. Food items were classified as unhealthy (poor nutritional value items, high in fat, sugar, salt and calories), unhealthy-to-fair (highly processed items although low in fat) and healthy (nutrient rich foods). We assigned adjustment weights to each food item conditioned to its nutritional quality. A score ranging from 0–10 was computed by adjusting the frequency of food consumption to the nutritional quality of foods consumed during the snack time. For each snacking type (in-school or at-home), participants had a continuous score, with higher scores representing healthier snacking habits. We applied quartile cutoffs for the Chilean adolescent population (comprising students of high-, middle- and low-SES) to classify the nutritional quality of in-home and at-school snacking of participants into three groups: unhealthy ($\leq$4.3 or $\leq$25th percentile), unhealthy-to-fair (from 4.4 to 5.9 or >25th percentile and <75th percentile) and healthy ($\geq$6.0 or $\geq$75th percentile) [21].

2.3. Academic Outcomes

The academic outcomes measured were HS GPA, the likelihood of HS completion, and the likelihood of taking college entrance exams. Data on GPA and high school completion were obtained from publicly available records at the Academic Assessment Unit of the Ministry of Education of Chile. Following the Ministry of Education criteria, GPA (on a scale of 1–7) was transformed into standardized scores (ranging from 210–825), and adjusted by type of secondary education (academic, vocational or adult school). Data on college examination rates were derived from publicly available information from the Assessment and Measurement Department of the University of Chile, which administers the tests for college entrance on behalf of the Ministry of Education. Although the exams for college admission are non-mandatory for HS graduates (only for those aiming at enrolling in higher education), more than 85% of Chilean HS graduates take the tests and, thus, have plans for future schooling [24].

2.4. Weight Status at Age 16

A research physician used standardized procedures to measure the adolescent's height (cm) and weight (kg) in duplicate. Body mass index (BMI = kg/m^2) at age 16 was evaluated and z-scores were estimated according to the World Health Organization (WHO) 2007 references [25]. Weight status was defined as follows: underweight (BMI-z < -1 SD), normal weight (BMI-z from -1 SD to 1 SD), overweight (BMI-z from 1 SD to <2 SD) and obesity (BMI-z $\geq$ 2 SD).

2.5. Physical Activity at Age 16

Physical activity has been found to be associated with academic achievement in studies conducted in Chile [26,27]; therefore, it could be a relevant confounder for the association between diet and academic results. We approached physical activity habits with scheduled, repetitive and planned exercise, accounting for the number of weekly hours devoted to Physical Education (PE), and extracurricular sports. To measure this, we used a questionnaire that was validated in a previous study using accelerometry-based activity monitors in both elementary and high school children [28]. The questionnaire was administered by a researcher to all students at the time they attended the anthropometric examination. Participants were asked: (1) On average, over the past week, how often did you engage in PE? (2) On average, over the past week, how often did you engage in extracurricular sports, either school- or non-school-organized? (3) On those days, on average, how long did you engage in such activities? With this information, we estimated the average hours per week of scheduled physical activity. Participants having ≤90 min of weekly scheduled physical activity, which is the mandatory time for school-based PE, were considered to be physically inactive.

2.6. Other Covariates Collected in Previous Waves

Parental educational attainment is an important measure of human capital level among populations and, also, is an important predictor of children's educational outcomes [29]. In infancy, participant's mother and father were asked to report the highest schooling level they have been enrolled in, as well as the highest grade they completed at that level. In our analysis, five standard hierarchic levels were defined according to the 2011 International Standard Classification of Education: (1) no education completed; (2) first level (primary school or 1st–8th); (3) secondary level (first phase or 9th–10th); (4) secondary level (second phase or 11th–12th); and (5) post-secondary non-tertiary educations or short-cycle tertiary education [30]. Then, we merged these categories into two: incomplete secondary education (1 + 2 + 3), and complete secondary education or higher (4 + 5). In health research, parental education has been often used as proxy for socioeconomic background [31]. Also, because the literature describes correlations between children's educational outcomes and family structure [32], we include a variable denoting whether the participant was raised in a fatherless family. This information was reported by the participant's parents or guardian. Finally, to control potential design biases, we used a categorical variable denoting whether the participant had received iron supplementation or no added iron at 6–12 months.

2.7. Statistical Analysis

Data were processed using Stata SE for Windows 12.0 (Lakeway Drive College Station, TX, USA). All categorical data were expressed as absolute and relative frequencies, while continuous data were expressed as means and standard deviations. Statistical analysis included χ^2 for categorical variables, and analysis of variance (ANOVA) with Bonferroni correction for comparison of means. We tested for effect measure modification (interaction) by weight status and physical activity, in the association between quality of snacking and academic outcomes using two-way ANOVA. The interaction of quality of snacking with weight status and physical activity was non-significant at $p < 0.05$ and, therefore, we did not stratify the analysis. Unadjusted logistic models were used to explore cross-sectional patterns of variation in academic behavior across snack categories (unhealthy and unhealthy-to-fair vs. healthy). Next, the models were adjusted for sex, weight status, physical activity, familial background and a variable to control potential design biases. Odds ratios are presented in the tables with 95% CI to evaluate the strength and precision of the associations. Analysis of covariance (ANCOVA) was used to determine whether high school GPA differed by nutritional quality of snacking, accounting for the same potential confounders. Because GPA scores do not have an intrinsic meaning, the effect size for difference was estimated using Cohen's *d* coefficients. A $p < 0.05$ denoted statistical significance.

3. Results

As shown in Table 1, our sample was composed of 16.8-year-old (0.3 SD) adolescents (47% males). Eighty-four percent completed HS ($n = 571$) and were allowed to take the exams for college admission. Of them, 68% ($n = 388$) took the college entrance exam. High school GPA ranged from 269–795 points, and mean value was 481.1 (92.3 SD) points. Mean value of BMI-z was 0.65 (1.2 SD). Of the participants, 25% and 14% were overweight and obese, respectively. In the sample, 60% were physically inactive.

Table 1. Descriptive statistics of the sample: adolescent students from Santiago, Chile ($n = 678$).

Variables	Mean or n	SD or Percentage
Chronological age		
Age (years)	16.8	0.3
In-home snacking		
Healthy	180	26.55
Unhealthy-to-fair	337	49.71
Unhealthy	161	23.74
At-school snacking		
Healthy	183	26.99
Unhealthy-to-fair	302	44.54
Unhealthy	193	28.47
Academic outcomes		
Graduated high school	571	84.09
Took college admission exams * ($n = 571$)	387	67.76
High school GPA (score) ($n = 571$)	481.1	92.3
Sex		
Male	357	52.58
Anthropometrics		
BMI (z-score)	0.65	1.2
Weight status		
Normal	417	61.42
Overweight	167	24.59
Obesity	95	14.99
Physical activity		
Weekly scheduled PA $\leq$ 90 min	403	59.35
Parental education		
Maternal education: incomplete secondary	240	35.40
Paternal education: incomplete secondary	192	28.32
Family structure		
Fatherless family	274	40.4
Iron supplementation in infancy		
No added Fe (6–12 months)	286	42.18

* Only those students graduating from high school ($n = 571$) are allowed to take the exams for college admission. BMI: Body-Mass Index. Normal weight: BMI-z from −1 SD to +1 SD. Overweight: BMI-z from >1 SD to 2 SD. Obesity: BMI-z $\geq$ 2 SD. GPA: grade point average; SD: standard deviation; PA: physical activity.

The share of students completing the secondary education significantly increased with better nutritional quality of at-school ($\chi^2 = 6.73$, $p < 0.05$) and in-home ($\chi^2 = 7.19$, $p < 0.05$) snacking (Figure 1). Likewise, the proportion of students taking the exams for higher education was significantly higher among participants having healthy in-home ($\chi^2 = 12.40$, $p < 0.01$) and at-school ($\chi^2 = 11.66$, $p < 0.01$) snacking (Figure 2).

Table 2 shows the estimated cross-sectional association between graduating HS and the nutritional quality of in-home and at-school snacking. After adjusting for sex, weight status, physical activity, parental education, family structure and iron supplementation in infancy, unhealthy snacking significantly reduced the odds of completing the secondary education. For instance, students having unhealthy in-home snacks were 53% (odds ratio (OR): 0.47, 95% CI: 0.25–0.88) less likely to complete HS than students having healthy in-home snacks. Odds were lower but non-significant among students eating foods of unhealthy-to-fair nutritional quality at home compared to those eating healthy snacks at home. When school snacking was the exposure, we also found a positive significant association of nutritional quality of snacks with the likelihood of getting the HS diploma (aOR: 0.49, 95% CI: 0.27–0.89). In all these models, sex and physical activity were also related to the chances of HS graduation.

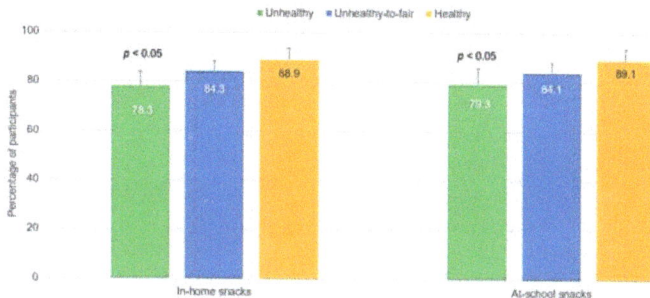

Figure 1. Proportion of students getting their high school diploma (outcome) by nutritional quality of in-home and at-school snacking (exposure) (*n* = 678). Error bars are 95% CI (upper limit). CI: confidence interval.

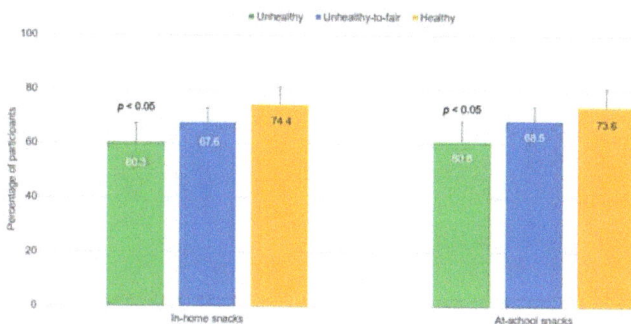

Figure 2. Proportion of participants taking the exams for college admission (outcome) by nutritional quality of in-home and at-school snacking (exposure) (*n* = 571). Only those students graduating from high school (*n* = 571) are allowed to take the exams for college admission. Error bars are 95% CI (upper limit).

Table 2. Estimated cross-sectional association between achieving the high school diploma (outcomes) and nutritional quality of in-home and at-school snacking (exposure) in students from Santiago, Chile, after adjusting other influences (*n* = 678).

	In-Home Snacking				At-School Snacking			
	OR	95% CI	aOR	95% CI	OR	95% CI	aOR	95% CI
Unhealthy	0.44 **	0.25–0.82	0.47 *	0.25–0.88	0.47 *	0.26–0.83	0.49 *	0.27–0.89
Unhealthy-to-fair	0.67	0.39–1.16	0.70	0.39–1.24	0.65	0.37–1.13	0.67	0.37–1.20
Male	(…)	–	0.42 ***	0.27–0.67	(…)	–	0.43 ***	0.27–0.68
Overweight	(…)	–	0.88	0.52–1.46	(…)	–	0.89	0.53–1.48
Obesity	(…)	–	0.81	0.44–1.49	(…)	–	0.81	0.44–1.49
Physically inactive	(…)	–	0.37 ***	0.22–0.61	(…)	–	0.37 ***	0.22–0.63
Maternal education	(…)	–	0.66	0.42–1.02	(…)	–	0.66	0.42–1.02
Paternal education	(…)	–	0.91	0.55–1.47	(…)	–	0.91	0.56–1.48
Fatherless family	(…)	–	0.77	0.51–1.20	(…)	–	0.77	0.50–1.19
No added Fe	(…)	–	0.89	0.57–1.37	(…)	–	0.89	0.58–1.38

OR: Odds ratio. aOR: adjusted OR. (…) Non-observed variables. Overweight: BMI-z from >1 SD to <2 SD. Obesity: BMI-z $\geq$ 2 SD. Physically inactive: $\leq$90 min/week of scheduled exercise. Maternal and paternal education: incomplete high school. * $p < 0.05$; ** $p < 0.01$; *** $p < 0.001$.

Similarly, among students who completed HS, the odds of taking the college entrance exam were significantly lower for those having unhealthy in-home snacks compared to those having healthy in-home snacks (Table 3). After controlling other influences, students who reported consumption of unhealthy in-home snacks were 47% less likely (aOR: 0.53; 95% CI: 0.31–0.88) to take the college entrance exam, compared to students eating healthy snack items. In addition, students eating in-home snacks of unhealthy-to-fair nutritional quality had lower odds of taking the college entrance exam, compared to those with healthier habits, though the association was non-significant. When school snacking was the exposure, the odds of taking the examination for college were also lower in students eating unhealthy snacks (aOR: 0.57; 95% CI: 0.35–0.90) compared to those eating healthy at-school snacks. In all these models, the odds of taking the college entrance exam were significantly associated with sex, maternal education and family structure.

The nutritional quality of snacking was also significantly related with students' final GPA as shown in Figure 3. After accounting for the effect of sex, weight status, physical activity, parental education, family structure and iron supplementation in infancy (Table 4), the group snacking on unhealthy foods at home had a final GPA of 490.0 points, on average, whereas participants having healthy snacks at home had a final GPA of 530.1 points (GPA mean difference = −40.1 points; 95% CI: −59.2; −16.9, $d = 0.43$). When comparing those having unhealthy-to-fair snacks vs. those having healthy snacks at home the GPA mean difference was −27.9 points (95% CI: −43.5; −8.2, $d = 0.30$). It is worth noting that Cohen's d coefficients around 0.20 are considered of interest in educational research when they are based on measures of academic achievement [33]. Lastly, the same pattern was observed when the main exposure was the nutritional quality of at-school snacking.

Table 3. Estimated cross-sectional association between taking the exams for higher education (outcome) and nutritional quality of in-home and at-school snacking (exposure) in students from Santiago, Chile, after adjusting other influences ($n = 571$).

	In-Home Snacking				At-School Snacking			
	OR	95% CI	aOR	95% CI	OR	95% CI	aOR	95% CI
Unhealthy	0.46 **	0.29–0.71	0.53 *	0.31–0.88	0.49 ***	0.32–0.74	0.57 *	0.35–0.90
Unhealthy-to-fair	0.68 *	0.47–0.98	0.75	0.48–1.15	0.71	0.49–1.04	0.81	0.51–1.27
Male	(…)	-	0.66 *	0.45–0.96	(…)	-	0.66 *	0.45–0.97
Overweight	(…)	-	0.99	0.64–1.52	(…)	-	0.99	0.65–1.55
Obesity	(…)	-	0.97	0.56–1.66	(…)	-	0.97	0.57–1.67
Physically inactive	(…)	-	0.85	0.57–1.25	(…)	-	0.84	0.57–1.24
Maternal education	(…)	-	0.63 *	0.42–0.92	(…)	-	0.63 *	0.42–0.92
Paternal education	(…)	-	0.75	0.49–1.13	(…)	-	0.76	0.50–1.15
Fatherless family	(…)	-	0.68 *	0.48–0.99	(…)	-	0.68 *	0.47–0.98
No added Fe	(…)	-	0.84	0.59–1.21	(…)	-	0.84	0.58–1.21

OR: Odds ratio. aOR: adjusted OR. (…) Non-observed variables. Overweight: BMI-z from >1 SD to <2 SD. Obesity: BMI-z $\geq$ 2 SD. Physically inactive: $\leq$90 min/week of scheduled exercise. Maternal and paternal education: incomplete high school. * $p < 0.05$; ** $p < 0.01$; *** $p < 0.001$.

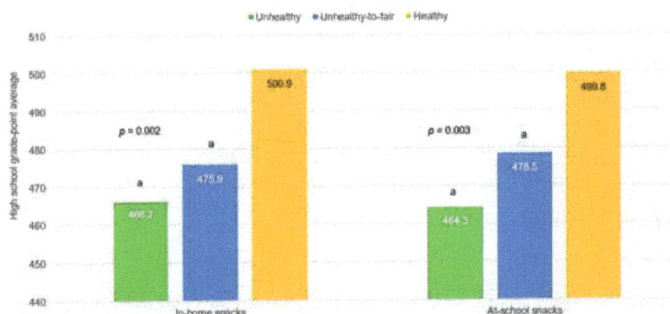

Figure 3. Mean high school grade point average (GPA) by nutritional quality of in-home and at-school snacking ($n = 571$). GPA expressed as standardized score, according to the Chilean Ministry of Education. a, significantly different from the group having healthy snacks at home or at school. p value estimated with Analysis of Variance (ANOVA) with Bonferroni adjustment.

Table 4. Cross-sectional association between academic attainment in high school (outcome) and nutritional quality of in-home snacking and at-school (exposure) in students from Santiago, Chile, after adjusting other influences (n = 571).

	In-Home Snacking			At-School Snacking		
Mean GPA	Mean	Mean		Mean	SD	
Unhealthy (1)	490.0	473.2		473.2	90.2	
Unhealthy-to-fair (2)	502.2	486.8		486.8	89.3	
Healthy (3)	530.1	512.4		512.4	93.6	
Comparison of mean GPA §	Mean diff.	95% CI	d[†]	Mean diff.	95% CI	d[†]
(1) vs. (2)	−12.2	−32.7; 4.6	0.09	−13.6	−33.2; 2.4	0.15
(1) vs. (3)	−40.1 ***	−59.2; −16.9	0.41	−39.2 ***	−57.0; −17.1	0.44
(2) vs. (3)	−27.9 ***	−43.5; −8.2	0.30	−25.6 *	−40.6; −4.9	0.31

GPA: Grade point average (expressed in score according to the Ministry of Education). § ANCOVA: * p < 0.05; *** p < 0.001. Models were adjusted for sex, weight status, familial background and iron supplementation in infancy. [†] Cohen's d coefficients account for the effect of different sample sizes. ESs around 0.20 are of policy interest when they are based on measures of academic achievement [33]. ANCOVA: analysis of covariance.

4. Discussion

4.1. Main Findings

This study explored whether the nutritional quality of in-home and at-school snacking among high school students in Santiago, Chile, was cross-sectionally associated with secondary school academic achievement and the intention to enroll in higher education. Although numerous studies have approached the effects of short-term exposure to a WD on academic outcomes [19], very few have focused on foods consumed during snack times. We found that unhealthy snacking was correlated with lower high school GPA and rate of graduation, as well as a reduced likelihood of taking college admission exams. When controls for sex and other potentially confounding variables (e.g., weight status, physical activity, familial background, etc.) were entered into the models, unhealthy snacking continued to be associated with worse academic results.

Our findings are consistent with previous research that found evidence of a relationship between a healthy diet and academic achievement. The results of a population-based study of 4th and 8th grade Chilean school children—students from subsidized, partially subsidized, and private schools—showed a positive cross-sectional association between performance in language and mathematics as measured by Chile's standardized System for the Assessment of Educational Quality test and the nutritional quality of school snacking, regardless of sex, SES, and other educational influences [17]. Similarly, in a subset (n = 395) of the current sample, Correa et al. [18] observed that, among students taking college entrance exams, unhealthy dietary habits of 16-year-old were associated with lower performance on college examination tests when compared to the performance of students with healthy dietary habits.

Cross-sectional studies conducted in adolescents from other countries also found that participants having healthy dietary habits performed better at school compared to those having unhealthy dietary habits. For instance, the native and foreign language attainment among 14- and 15-year-old Icelandic students, as well as their mathematics achievement, were negatively influenced by poor dietary habits [13,15]. Norwegian 9th and 10th graders with a high intake of sugar-sweetened soft drinks, candies, chocolate, chips, pizza, hot dogs, and hamburgers were up to 6 times more likely to manifest learning difficulties in mathematics. Conversely, a diet of fresh fruits at least once daily reduced the chances of difficulties in these areas [14]. Also in 15- to 17-year-old Norwegian adolescents, high academic achievement was associated with a high intake of fruits and berries, and a low intake of sugar-sweetened beverages [34]. Unfavorable academic performance, as measured by a standardized test, was positively associated with unhealthy dietary patterns in 6- to 13-year-old Taiwanese students. The likelihood of underperforming on the test was 1.63 times higher for students with greater consumption of low-quality foods (e.g., sweets and fried foods) than it was for students with low intake of such items. Fu et al. also showed that students with poor academic performance were less likely to regularly eat foods that are rich in protein, vitamins and minerals [35].

Diet is also an important influence on other determinants of academic success. Among adolescent students from Iceland, having an optimal diet was cross-sectionally associated with decreased odds of behavioral problems in the classroom [36]. Likewise, in 15- and 16-year-old male students from Oslo (Norway), intake of >4 glasses/day of sugar-sweetened soft drinks more than doubled the probability of having behavioral problems at school, compared to students drinking <1 glass of sugary drinks per day [37]. Among female students in Oslo with excessive intake of sugar-sweetened soft drinks, the chances of conduct problems at school were 4.1 times higher compared to the reference group. In males, soft drink consumption was also related to hyperactivity and higher levels of mental distress, both of which are associated with academic difficulties [38].

It is likely that the effect on academic results of excessive consumption of foods high in saturated fats and simple sugars is mediated by the effect of these macronutrients on brain health and cognitive function. In developmental stages such as adolescence, the brain is particularly vulnerable to the effects of excessive intake of saturated fats and simple carbohydrates [5,6]. Diet-induced impairment in learning and hippocampus-dependent memory processes have been widely documented [7,8,39,40]. In addition to reducing production of neurotrophins such as BDNF, other WD-induced effects have been reported on this brain structure, including overexpression of proinflammatory cytokines, mitochondrial damage due to oxidative stress, and altered blood–brain barrier permeability [7,8,10,39]. Also, insulin resistance and hyperleptinemia have been linked to impaired hippocampal synaptic plasticity and poor cognitive functioning [41–43]. Furthermore, evidence suggests that juvenile exposure to a WD may be more harmful than such exposure in adulthood. A 3-week juvenile WD regimen induced similar weight gain and metabolic alterations as did a 12-week adult WD regimen. Juvenile exposure, however, also affected memory consolidation and flexible memory expression while promoting exaggerated pro-inflammatory cytokine expression in the hippocampus after an immune challenge, and it diminished hippocampal neurogenesis [8,39].

While the cross-sectional design of our study prevents definitive conclusions about causality and the direction of the associations depicted here, it is worth noting that research conducted in both animals and humans described short-term effects of Western-type dietary habits on hippocampal-dependent learning and memory. In animals, it is well established that a WD causes rapid impairments of hippocampal-based tasks, with diet-related cognitive effects observed after only 72 h [44,45]. Studies in humans are limited but they confirm that a WD impacts hippocampal memory tasks following a relatively short exposure. Healthy 20-year-old college students from Australia consuming a HFS breakfast (30% saturated fats plus 18% refined sugars), over four consecutive days, showed significantly poorer memory recall compared to control students consuming a healthier breakfast of similar palatability and food types, but significantly lower in saturated fats and refined sugars (5% saturated fats plus 10% sugars). Since these changes in memory performance were linked to shifts in blood glucose across breakfast, authors suggest that this could be one potential mechanism by which a WD affects hippocampal function [46]. In a similar manner, in sedentary men aged 25–45 years, Edwards et al. found decreased power of attention and increased simple reaction time after seven days of consuming a diet comprising 74% kcal. from fat [47]. It is less clear for how long the cognitive effects of a WD will remain and, thus, further investigations should address that question. Although experimental studies in humans show that improvements in memory can occur following reductions in energy intake and fat [48], or shift to a diet low in saturated fats and refined sugars [49], observational longitudinal studies conducted in Anglo-Saxon countries suggest that unhealthy dietary practices in developmental periods have a lasting association with cognitive and educational outcomes that seem to persist over time, regardless of later changes in diet [16,50–52].

Our results also showed that a significant share (73%) of participants in the sample ate snacks of intermediate or poor nutritional value. This is consistent with population surveys conducted nationally and internationally. In Chile, adolescents (aged 14 years to 18 years) ranked first in the consumption of refined sugar (121 g/day) and second in the consumption of saturated fats (12.7 mL-g/day) compared to other age groups. In this age group, the consumption of sugar-sweetened soft drinks was 254 mL/day, according to the latest National Food Consumption Survey [53]. This survey also reported that 97% of children and adolescents aged 6 years to 18 years need to improve the quality of their diets. The World Health Organization's Health Behaviour in School-aged Children (HBSC) survey found that in Scotland, 35% of adolescents eat sweets or chocolate every day, and 18% eat chips every day. In addition, 20% of Scottish female adolescents and 27% of their male counterparts consume sugary soft drinks daily [54]. Among US high schoolers, 22% of males and 17% of females report consumption of sugar-sweetened soft drinks ≥ 2 times per day [55].

4.2. Implications for Practice

Our results are of interest for a number of reasons. Translating research knowledge to practice and policy is much needed in the field of health promotion [56,57]. The idea of testing the connection between diet and cognition using functional cognitive measures such as GPA, graduation rates, and rates of taking college entrance exams was aimed at bridging the gap between research and policymaking. Although evidence on the consequences of unhealthy diets on learning and cognition is growing, the failure to implement effective interventions persists. A more informed approach to this connection can influence healthcare practitioners, educators and parents.

In addition, lower academic results have been associated with several health-risk behaviors in youths. In US adolescent populations, over the past three decades, cross-sectional and longitudinal studies demonstrate links connecting poor academic performance with sedentary lifestyle, alcohol/tobacco abuse, sexually risky behaviors, and violence [58]. All of these risk behaviors have been regarded as important contributors to poor health status in adulthood and multiple social problems. Since the influence of academic performance on future health is known [59], the relationship of diet and academic results may be an important public health tool. It is also important to identify the nutrients and dietary patterns that most influence cognitive health and academic performance.

The fact that adolescents struggle to make healthy dietary choices is not new information. Youthful anomalous health decision-making has been attributed to an aversion to forced choices; the inclination to rely on taste, brands, and convenience as primary drivers of food decisions; and the tendency to discount the value of delayed rewards or penalties [60]. Also, sufficient nutrition knowledge does not necessarily correspond to responsible dietary behavior [61]. Thus, associating healthy dietary choices with school performance can perhaps enhance the value of healthy eating and boost motivation. After all, academic achievement, academic behavior, and academic performance are closely linked to expectations of better postsecondary opportunities and subsequent job status [62,63].

Our results that show an association between a healthy diet and improved cognitive and educational outcomes should be a matter of interest to support nutrition interventions designed for adolescents. To date, the majority of interventions that emphasize the relationship between diet type and cognition and academics have been designed for infants and young children [6,19,52], who are less independent in their food choices. For health promotion purposes, unhealthy dietary habits during adolescence are usually said to be related to early onset of cardiometabolic disorders, including high blood pressure, type-2 diabetes and coronary heart disease, while arguments based on the potential cognitive impact of diet are still lacking. We have seen that adolescents are also exposed to the detrimental cognitive effects of a diet high in saturated fats and refined sugars. Moreover, adolescence is a transitional period with subcortical regions associated with reward-seeking and emotion developing earlier than prefrontal control regions [64]. Greater emotional reactivity and sensitivity may in part explain unhealthy dietary habits among teenagers. Sociocultural changes, the need to fit in, food availability and the quest for independent decision-making also contribute to unhealthy food choices that are common during adolescence [65], making this period one of tremendous importance in terms of cognitive development.

A further implication of these findings is that they can potentially play a major role in health promotion by educational agencies and schools. Dietary habits that comport with food guidelines might help pave the way for students on the path to higher education. Chilean high school students perform far below the Organization for Economic Co-operation and Development (OECD) average in mathematics, reading and science, with less than 2% of 15-year-old scoring in the group of top performers [63]. Evidence shows that students who fail to reach baseline levels of performance in these areas have difficulties with academic readiness, persistence and higher education completion [66]. Nonetheless, 80% of Chilean parents expect their children to obtain a college degree [63].

4.3. Limitations and Strengths

This research provides results that support a connection between nutritious dietary intake and higher academic achievement. Given that most studies have been conducted in the developed world, one strength of this study is that it provides evidence that may be useful for countries undergoing nutritional and epidemiological transitions. Second, the use of a translational research approach to explore the diet–learning–cognition connection and provide applicable results is a positive contribution. Further, to our best knowledge, this is the first study to investigate the association of nutrition and academic achievement on HS students' postsecondary education intentions.

Despite these strengths, several limitations persist that should be considered when interpreting these results. Our sample is not representative of the Chilean adolescent population, as it consisted of adolescents from low and middle SES families. However, data from these socioeconomic groups may be especially important: population-based surveys conducted in Chile show that the prevalence of unhealthy dietary habits, physical inactivity, and excess weight is higher in adolescents from low and middle SES families compared to adolescents from high SES families [53,67]. This means that students from low and middle SES families are more exposed to risk factors for difficulties related to progressing from high school to higher education. Encouraging healthy dietary habits and, in particular, intake of healthy snacks, might smooth the pathway to college. Second, although we accounted for the effect of important confounders (including parental education and family structure), we were not able to consider other key influences, such as family support-related variables, general motivational factors (e.g., achievement motivation), and students' interests in specific subject areas, which may also impact their academic functioning. A third limitation is the cross-sectional nature of the study. Since data on snack quality for each participant was recorded only once, it would be difficult to infer the temporal association between this exposure and the academic outcomes. Thus, only association, and not causation, can be inferred from our study. While our results may be useful to inform new hypotheses, a more complex investigation, such as a longitudinal study or crossover intervention trial, should be conducted to test the temporality of these associations, i.e., that the exposure to Western-type food items precede academic difficulties. Finally, future studies should replicate and extend this analysis in other young populations.

5. Conclusions

Poor nutritional quality snacking at school and at home was associated with poor secondary school academic achievement and lower intention to enroll in higher education. Both types of snacking showed similar associations with these educational outcomes. These results may have important implications for the promotion of healthy lifestyles by educational agencies and schools. Also, associating healthy snacking with educational outcomes can perhaps enhance the value of having responsible health behaviors and boost motivation for a healthy way of life.

Acknowledgments: The authors wish to acknowledge the ongoing commitment of participants and their families. We also thank all the people who contributed to the development of this project, especially, Professors Betsy Lozoff and Marcela Castillo. This study was funded by the National Heart, Blood, and Lung Institute, National Institutes of Health (USA) under grant R01HL088530-2980925, and the National Council for Scientific Research and Technology (CONICYT) (Chile) under grants PAI 79140003 and FONDECYT 1160240. They had no role in the design of the study; in the collection, analyses, or interpretation of data; in the writing of the manuscript, and in the decision to publish the results.

Nutrients **2017**, *9*, 433

Author Contributions: P.C.-B., R.B. and S.G. conceived and designed the study. R.B., P.C.-B. and Y.R. performed the field study. P.C.-B. and R.B. analyzed the data and wrote the paper. Y.R., E.B. and S.G. performed critical analysis of manuscript draft. E.B. and S.G. edited language. All authors read and approved the final manuscript.

Conflicts of Interest: The authors declare no conflict of interest.

References

1. Fraser, B. Latin American countries crack down on junk food. *Lancet* **2013**, *382*, 385–386. [CrossRef]
2. Braithwaite, I.; Stewart, A.; Hancox, R.; Beasley, R.; Murphy, R.; Mitchell, E.A. Fast-food consumption and body mass index in children and adolescents: An international cross-sectional study. *BMJ Open* **2014**, *4*, e005813. [CrossRef] [PubMed]
3. Ministerio de Salud. Global School-Based Health Survey (Chile). Available online: http://www.who.int/chp/gshs/2013_Chile_GSHS_fact_sheet.pdf (accessed on 10 October 2016).
4. Currie, C.; Zanotti, C.; Morgan, A.; Barnekow, V. Social Determinants of Health and Well-Being among Young People. Health Behaviour in School-Aged Children (HBSC) Study: International Report from the 2009/2010 Survey. WHO Regional Office for Europe: Copenhagen. Available online: http://www.euro.who.int/__data/assets/pdf_file/0003/163857/Social-determinants-of-health-and-well-being-among-young-people.pdf (accessed on 2 November 2016).
5. Benton, D. The influence of children's diet on their cognition and behavior. *Eur. J. Nutr.* **2008**, *47*, 25–37. [CrossRef] [PubMed]
6. Nyaradi, A.; Li, J.; Hickling, S.; Foster, J.; Oddy, W. The role of nutrition in children's neurocognitive development, from pregnancy through infancy. *Front. Hum. Neurosci.* **2013**, *7*, 97. [CrossRef] [PubMed]
7. Boitard, C.; Cavaroc, A.; Sauvant, J.; Aubert, A.; Castanon, N.; Layé, S.; Ferreira, G. Impairment of hippocampal-dependent memory induced by juvenile high-fat diet intake is associated with enhanced hippocampal inflammation in rats. *Brain Behav. Immun.* **2014**, *40*, 9–17. [CrossRef] [PubMed]
8. Valladolid-Acebes, I.; Fole, A.; Martín, M.; Morales, L.; Cano, M.; Ruiz-Gayo, M.; Del Olmo, N. Spatial memory impairment and changes in hippocampal morphology are triggered by high-fat diets in adolescent mice. Is there a role of leptin? *Neurobiol. Learn. Mem.* **2013**, *106*, 18–25. [CrossRef] [PubMed]
9. Lynch, M. Long-term potentiation and memory. *Physiol. Rev.* **2004**, *84*, 87–136. [CrossRef] [PubMed]
10. Kanoski, S.; Davidson, T. Western diet consumption and cognitive impairment: Links to hippocampal dysfunction and obesity. *Physiol. Behav.* **2011**, *103*, 59–68. [CrossRef] [PubMed]
11. Beilharz, J.; Maniam, J.; Morris, M. Diet-induced cognitive deficits: The role of fat and sugar, potential mechanisms and nutritional interventions. *Nutrients* **2015**, *7*, 6719–6738. [CrossRef] [PubMed]
12. Blankenship, T.; O'Neill, M.; Ross, A.; Bell, M. Working memory and recollection contribute to academic achievement. *Learn. Individ. Differ.* **2015**, *43*, 164–169. [CrossRef] [PubMed]
13. Sigfúsdóttir, I.; Krisjánsson, A.; Allegrante, J. Health behaviours and academic achievement in Icelandic school children. *Health Educ. Res.* **2007**, *22*, 70–80. [CrossRef] [PubMed]
14. Kristjánsson, A.; Sigfúsdóttir, I.; Allegrante, J. Health behavior and academic achievement among adolescents: The relative contribution of dietary habits, physical activity, body mass index, and self-esteem. *Health Educ. Behav.* **2010**, *37*, 51–64. [CrossRef] [PubMed]
15. Øverby, N.; Lüdemann, E.; Høigaard, R. Self-reported learning difficulties and dietary intake in Norwegian adolescents. *Scand. J. Public Health* **2013**, *41*, 754–760. [CrossRef] [PubMed]
16. Feinstein, L.; Sabates, R.; Sorhaindo, A.; Emmett, P. Dietary patterns related to attainment in school: The importance of early eating patterns. *J. Epidemiol. Commun. Health* **2008**, *62*, 734–739. [CrossRef] [PubMed]
17. Correa-Burrows, P.; Burrows, R.; Orellana, Y.; Ivanovic, D. The relationship between unhealthy snacking at school and academic outcomes: A population study in Chilean schoolchildren. *Public Health Nutr.* **2015**, *18*, 2022–2030. [CrossRef] [PubMed]
18. Correa-Burrows, P.; Burrows, R.; Blanco, E.; Reyes, M.; Gahagan, S. Nutritional quality of diet and academic performance in Chilean students. *Bull. World Health Org.* **2016**, *94*, 185–192. [CrossRef] [PubMed]
19. Burrows, T.; Goldman, S.; Pursey, K.; Lim, R. Is there an association between dietary intake and academic achievement? A systematic review. *J. Hum. Nutr. Diet.* **2016**, *30*, 117–140. [CrossRef] [PubMed]

20. Lozoff, B.; Castillo, M.; Clark, K.; Smith, J.; Sturza, J. Iron supplementation in infancy contributes to more adaptive behavior at 10 years of age. *J. Nutr.* **2014**, *144*, 838–845. [CrossRef] [PubMed]

21. Burrows, R.; Díaz, E.; Schiaraffia, V.; Gattas, V.; Montoya, A.; Lera, L. Dietary intake and physical activity in school age children. *Rev. Med. Chile* **2008**, *136*, 53–63.

22. Gattas, V.; Burrows, R.; Burgueño, M. Validity Assessment of A Food Frequency Questionnaire in Chilean School-Age Children. In Proceedings of the XVI Congress of the Latin-American Society of Pediatric Research and the XXII Pan-American Meeting of Pediatrics, Santiago, Chile, 25–30 April 2007.

23. Ministerio de Salud. *Tablas Chilenas de Composición Química de los Alimentos*; Ministerio de Salud: Santiago, Chile, 2010.

24. Departamento de Evaluación, Medición y Registro Educacional (DEMRE). Prueba de Selección Universitaria. Informe Técnico. Volumen IV. Proceso de Admisión 2016. Unidad de Desarrollo y Análisis. Universidad de Chile. Available online: http://psu.demre.cl/estadisticas/documentos/informes/2016-vol-4-informe-tecnico-admision-2016.pdf (accessed on 19 September 2016).

25. De Onis, M.; Onyango, A.; Borghi, E.; Siyam, A.; Nishida, C.; Siekmann, J. Development of a WHO growth reference for school-aged children and adolescents. *Bull. World Health Org.* **2007**, *85*, 660–667. [CrossRef] [PubMed]

26. Correa-Burrows, P.; Burrows, R.; Orellana, Y.; Ivanovic, D. Achievement in mathematics and language is linked to regular physical activity: A population study in Chilean youth. *J. Sports Sci.* **2014**, *32*, 1631–1638. [CrossRef] [PubMed]

27. Burrows, R.; Correa-Burrows, P.; Orellana, Y.; Almagiá, A.; Lizana, P.; Ivanovic, D. Scheduled physical activity is associated with better academic performance in Chilean school-age children. *J. Phys. Act. Health* **2014**, *11*, 1600–1606. [CrossRef] [PubMed]

28. Godard, C.; Rodríguez, M.; Díaz, N.; Lera, L.; Salazar, G.; Burrows, R. Value of a clinical test for assessing physical activity in children. *Rev. Med. Chile* **2008**, *136*, 1155–1162.

29. Dobow, E.; Boxer, P.; Huesmann, L. Long-term effects of parents' education on children's educational and occupational success: Mediation by family interactions, child aggression, and teenage aspirations. *Merrill Palmer Q.* **2009**, *55*, 224–249. [CrossRef] [PubMed]

30. United Nations Educational, Scientific and Cultural Organization (UNESCO). International Standard Classification of Education. ISCED 2011. Available online: http://www.uis.unesco.org/Education/Documents/isced-2011-en.pdf (accessed on 19 September 2016).

31. Braveman, P.; Cubbin, C.; Egerter, S.; Chideya, S.; Marchi, K.S.; Metzler, M.; Posner, S. Socioeconomic status in health research: One size does not fit all. *JAMA* **2005**, *294*, 2879–2888. [CrossRef] [PubMed]

32. Ginther, D.; Pollak, R. Family structure and children's educational outcomes: Blended families, stylized facts, and descriptive regressions. *Demography* **2004**, *41*, 671–696. [CrossRef] [PubMed]

33. Hedges, L.; Hedberg, E. Intraclass correlation values for planning group-randomized trials in education. *Educ. Eval. Policy Anal.* **2007**, *29*, 60–87. [CrossRef]

34. Stea, T.; Tortsveit, M. Association of lifestyle habits and academic achievement in Norwegian adolescents: A cross-sectional study. *BMC Public Health* **2014**, *14*, 829. [CrossRef] [PubMed]

35. Fu, M.; Cheng, L.; Tu, S.; Pan, W. Association between unhealthful eating patterns and unfavorable overall school performance in children. *J. Am. Diet Assoc.* **2007**, *107*, 1935–1943. [CrossRef] [PubMed]

36. Øverby, N.; Høigaard, R. Diet and behavioral problems at school in Norwegian adolescents. *Food Nutr. Res.* **2012**, *56*. [CrossRef] [PubMed]

37. Lien, L.; Lien, N.; Heyerdahl, S.; Thoresen, M.; Bjertness, E. Consumption of soft drinks and hyperactivity, mental distress, and conduct problems among adolescents in Oslo, Norway. *Am. J. Public Health* **2006**, *96*, 1815–1820. [CrossRef] [PubMed]

38. Polderman, T.; Boomsma, D.; Bartels, M.; Verhulst, F.; Huizink, A. A systematic review of prospective studies on attention problems and academic achievement. *Acta Psychiatr. Scand.* **2010**, *122*, 271–284. [CrossRef] [PubMed]

39. Boitard, C.; Etchamendy, N.; Sauvant, J.; Ferreira, G. Juvenile but not adult exposure to high fat diet impairs relational memory and hippocampal neurogenesis in mice. *Hippocampus* **2012**, *22*, 2095–2100. [CrossRef] [PubMed]

40. Mellendijk, L.; Wiesmann, M.; Kiliaan, A. Impact of nutrition on cerebral circulation and cognition in the metabolic syndrome. *Nutrients* **2015**, *7*, 9416–9439. [CrossRef] [PubMed]

41. Stranahan, A.; Norman, E.; Lee, K.; Mattson, M. Diet-induced insulin resistance impairs hippocampal synaptic plasticity and cognition in middle-aged rats. *Hippocampus* **2008**, *18*, 1085–1088. [CrossRef] [PubMed]
42. Irving, A.; Harvey, J. Leptin regulation of hippocampal synaptic function in health and disease. *Philos. Trans. R. Soc. B Biol. Sci.* **2013**, *369*. [CrossRef] [PubMed]
43. Lee, S.; Zabolotny, J.; Huang, H.; Lee, H.; Kim, Y. Insulin in the nervous system and the mind: Functions in metabolism, memory, and mood. *Mol. Metab.* **2016**, *5*, 589–601. [CrossRef] [PubMed]
44. Murray, A.; Knight, N.; Cochlin, L.; McAleese, S.; Deacon, R.; Rawlins, J.; Clarke, K. Deterioration of physical performance and cognitive function in rats with short-term high-fat feeding. *FASEB J.* **2009**, *23*, 4353–4360. [CrossRef] [PubMed]
45. Beilharz, J.E.; Maniam, J.; Morris, M.J. Short exposure to a diet rich in both fat and sugar or sugar alone impairs place, but not object recognition memory in rats. *Brain Behav. Immun.* **2014**, *37*, 134–141. [CrossRef] [PubMed]
46. Edwards, L.; Murray, A.; Holloway, C.; Clarke, K. Short-term consumption of a high-fat diet impairs whole-body efficiency and cognitive function in sedentary men. *FASEB J.* **2011**, *25*, 1088–1096. [CrossRef] [PubMed]
47. Attuquayefio, T.; Stevenson, R.; Oaten, M.; Francis, H. A four-day Western-style dietary intervention causes reductions in hippocampal-dependent learning and memory and interoceptive sensitivity. *PLoS ONE* **2017**, *12*, e0172645. [CrossRef] [PubMed]
48. Attuquayefio, T.; Stevenson, R. A systematic review of longer-term dietary interventions on human cognitive function: Emerging patterns and future directions. *Appetite* **2015**, *95*, 554–570. [CrossRef] [PubMed]
49. Nilsson, A.; Tovar, J.; Johansson, M.; Radeborg, K.; Björck, I. A diet based on multiple functional concepts improves cognitive performance in healthy subjects. *Nutr. Metab.* **2013**, *10*, 49. [CrossRef] [PubMed]
50. Smithers, L.; Golley, R.; Mittinty, M.; Lynch, J. Do dietary trajectories between infancy and toddlerhood influence IQ in childhood and adolescence? Results from a prospective birth cohort study. *PLoS ONE* **2013**, *8*, e58904. [CrossRef] [PubMed]
51. Theodore, R.; Thompson, J.; Waldie, K.; Mitchell, E. Dietary patterns and intelligence in early and middle childhood. *Intelligence* **2009**, *37*, 506–513. [CrossRef]
52. Nyaradi, A.; Li, J.; Hickling, S.; Whitehouse, A.; Foster, J.; Oddy, W. Diet in the early years of life influences cognitive outcomes at 10 years: A prospective cohort study. *Acta Paediatr.* **2013**, *102*, 1165–1173. [CrossRef] [PubMed]
53. Ministerio de Salud. Encuesta Nacional de Consumo Alimentario. Informe Final de Resultados. Subsecretaría de Salud Pública; Ministerio de Salud: Santiago de Chile. Available online: web.minsal.cl/sites/default/files/ENCA-INFORME_FINAL.pdf (accessed on 27 January 2017).
54. Currie, C.; Van der Sluijs, W.; Whitehead, R.; Currie, D.; Rhodes, G.; Neville, F.; Inchley, J. HBSC 2014 Survey in Scotland National Report. Child and Adolescent Health Research Unit (CAHRU). University of St Andrews: Fife. Available online: www.hbsc.org/news/index.aspx?ni=3272 (accessed on 27 January 2017).
55. Kann, L.; Kinchen, S.; Shankil, S.; Zaza, S. Youth risk behavior surveillance. United Sates 2013. *MMWR CDC Surveill. Summ.* **2014**, *63*, 29–35.
56. Spoth, R.; Rohrbach, L.; Greenberg, M.; Hawkins, J. Addressing core challenges for the next generation of type 2 translation research and systems: The translation science to population impact (TSci impact) framework. *Prev. Sci.* **2013**, *14*, 319–351. [CrossRef] [PubMed]
57. Biglan, A. The ultimate goal of prevention and the larger context for translation. *Prev. Sci.* **2016**. [CrossRef] [PubMed]
58. Bradley, B.; Greene, A. Do health and education agencies in the United States share responsibility for academic achievement and health? A review of 25 years of evidence about the relationship of adolescents' academic achievement and health behaviors. *J. Adolesc. Health* **2013**, *52*, 523–532. [PubMed]
59. Baker, D.; Leon, J.; Smith-Greenaway, E.; Collins, J.; Movit, M. The education effect on population health: A reassessment. *Popul. Dev. Rev.* **2011**, *37*, 307–332. [CrossRef] [PubMed]
60. Just, D.; Mancino, L.; Wansink, B. *Could Behavioral Economics Help Improve Diet Quality for Nutrition Assistance Program Participants?* US Department of Agriculture: Washington, DC, USA.
61. Kersting, M.; Sichert-Hellert, W.; Vereecken, C.; Sette, S. Food and nutrient intake, nutritional knowledge and diet-related attitudes in European adolescents. *Int. J. Obes.* **2008**, *32*, 35–41. [CrossRef] [PubMed]

62. Centers for Disease Control and Prevention, National Center for Chronic Disease Prevention and Health Promotion. Health and Academic Achievement. Available online: http://www.cdc.gov/healthyschools/health_and_academics/pdf/health-academic-achievement.pdf (accessed on 2 November 2016).
63. Organization for Economic Cooperation and Development, Program for International Students Assessment. Programme for International Students Assessment 2012 Results in Focus. What 15-Year-Old Know and What They Can Do with What They Know. Available online: http://www.oecd.org/pisa/keyfindings/pisa-2012-results.htm (accessed on 7 December 2016).
64. Casey, B.; Jones, R.; Hare, T. The adolescent brain. *Ann. N. Y. Acad. Sci.* **2008**, *1124*, 111–126. [CrossRef] [PubMed]
65. Pedersen, S.; Grønhøj, A.; Thøgersen, J. Following family or friends. Social norms in adolescent healthy eating. *Appetite* **2015**, *86*, 54–60. [CrossRef] [PubMed]
66. Hakkarainen, A.; Holopainen, L.; Savolainen, H. Mathematical and reading difficulties as predictors of school achievement and transition to secondary education. *Scand. J. Educ. Res.* **2013**, *57*, 488–506. [CrossRef]
67. Ministerio de Educación. Informe de resultados Estudio Nacional Educación Física 2013. Agencia de Calidad de la Educación. Available online: http://archivos.agenciaeducacion.cl/biblioteca_digital_historica/resultados/2013/result8b_edfisica_2013.pdf (accessed on 2 November 2016).

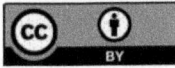

nutrients

MDPI

Article

Dietary Patterns among Vietnamese and Hispanic Immigrant Elementary School Children Participating in an After School Program

Megan A. McCrory [1,*], Charles L. Jaret [2], Jung Ha Kim [2] and Donald C. Reitzes [2]

[1]   Department of Health Sciences, Programs in Nutrition, Sargent College of Health
      and Rehabilitation Sciences, Boston University, Boston, MA 02215, USA
[2]   Department of Sociology, College of Arts and Sciences, Georgia State University, Atlanta, GA 30302, USA;
      cjaret@gsu.edu (C.L.J.); jhkim@gsu.edu (J.H.K.); dreitzes@gsu.edu (D.C.R.)
*   Correspondence: mamccr@bu.edu; Tel.: +1-617-353-2739

Received: 25 February 2017; Accepted: 1 May 2017; Published: 5 May 2017

Abstract: Immigrants in the U.S. may encounter challenges of acculturation, including dietary habits, as they adapt to new surroundings. We examined Vietnamese and Hispanic immigrant children's American food consumption patterns in a convenience sample of 63 Vietnamese and Hispanic children in grades four to six who were attending an after school program. Children indicated the number of times they consumed each of 54 different American foods in the past week using a food frequency questionnaire. We ranked each food according to frequency of consumption, compared the intake of foods to the USDA Healthy Eating Pattern, and performed dietary pattern analysis. Since the data were not normally distributed we used two nonparametric tests to evaluate statistical significance: the Kruskal–Wallis tested for significant gender and ethnicity differences and the Wilcoxon signed-rank test evaluated the food consumption of children compared with the USDA recommended amounts. We found that among USDA categories, discretionary food was most commonly consumed, followed by fruit. The sample as a whole ate significantly less than the recommended amount of grains, protein foods, and dairy, but met the recommended amount of fruit. Boys ate significantly more grains, proteins, and fruits than did girls. Dietary pattern analysis showed a very high sweet snack consumption among all children, while boys ate more fast food and fruit than girls. Foods most commonly consumed were cereal, apples, oranges, and yogurt. Ethnicity differences in food selection were not significant. The high intake of discretionary/snack foods and fruit, with low intake of grains, vegetables, protein, and dairy in our sample suggests Vietnamese and Hispanic immigrant children may benefit from programs to improve diet quality.

Keywords: food preferences; food habits; diet/standards; gender factors; acculturation

1. Introduction

Immigrants in the U.S. may encounter challenges of acculturation, including dietary habits, as they adapt to new surroundings in the host country [1]. Studies show a health paradox in that early in their arrival, immigrants may be healthier than their U.S. counterparts, but later go on to develop health risks as they adapt to a more Western lifestyle [2]. In general, a higher level of acculturation is associated with greater risk for chronic diseases [3,4]. The impact of acculturation may in part be responsible for the large disparities in rates of obesity and chronic disease among U.S. minority immigrants [5]. In the U.S., African Americans and Hispanics are at higher risk for obesity, diabetes [6], and heart disease [7] than Caucasians. Few studies have been conducted among Asian Americans. A recent U.S. national survey showed that although non-Hispanic Asians generally are not as unhealthy as other U.S. adults, there was great diversity in the health of different Asian American groups [8].

In particular, 16.8% of Vietnamese adults were considered to be in fair or poor health, compared to 8.1–12.2% for other Asian American groups and 12.4% for all U.S. adults [8].

Dietary choices during childhood are important for health during childhood and later life [9,10]. Therefore, the dietary intake of immigrant children is important for their health as adults. Relatively few studies have been conducted on the dietary intake of immigrant children. As reviewed recently [11], Asian American youth as a whole have high intakes of fruits, vegetables, and white rice, as well as high fat and high sugar foods, and as a result of acculturation their diets consist of both traditional Asian foods and American foods. "Asian Americans" include many different Asian cultures, each having different diets, but relatively few studies have been done on specific Asian subgroups so it is difficult to make firm conclusions about each. In one study of Vietnamese, Hispanic, African American and Caucasian adolescents residing in Worcester, Massachusetts, Vietnamese youth had higher fruit and vegetable intake and lower dairy intake compared to Caucasians, while Hispanic youth had a lower intake of fruits and vegetables, but dairy did not differ from that of Caucasians [12]. In another study of California youth, Mexican and other Hispanic children did not differ substantially in dietary practices, whereas among seven Asian American subgroups, Filipino, Korean, Vietnamese, and Japanese children were more likely to consume fast food than Chinese children [13]. Yet, Vietnamese, Koreans, and Filipinos were also likely to consume more vegetables than the Chinese. In the same study, there was no significant gender difference in consumption among Hispanic youth, but among Asian Americans, girls had significantly lower vegetable intake, and non-significantly lower fruits, fruit juice, and fast food intake. In a study of Korean Americans, there was a shift away from Korean foods to more American foods, but the quality of diet did not vary by acculturation status [14]. However, a study of South Asian immigrants in Canada showed a mix of positive and negative outcomes: the more acculturated ate more fruits and vegetables and less deep fried food, but also more convenience food, red meat, and high-sugar foods [15].

The purposes of this study were to examine the quality of food selection in a convenience sample of school-aged immigrant Vietnamese and Hispanic girls and boys based on their answers on a simple food intake questionnaire, and to test for differences by gender and ethnicity. We defined the quality of food selection in two ways: (1) consistency with the USDA Healthy Eating Pattern [16]; and (2) dietary pattern analysis to determine which foods listed on the questionnaire were eaten in similar patterns (e.g., if children who ate a lot of chocolate candy also frequently ate cookies and cake; or if those who rarely ate apples also did not eat other fruits).

2. Materials and Methods

2.1. Study Design

The data used in this study were from a survey, "My Food Choices," conducted by the Asian American Community Research Institute of the Center for Pan Asian Community Services, Inc. (CPACS) in Atlanta, GA, USA. We obtained the data with permission from CPACS. CPACS is the oldest and largest grassroots community organization in the Southeast serving Asian immigrant and refugee families and their descendants [17]. A considerable number of Hispanic children also participate in its after-school programs. As of December 2015, over 40 percent of all children and youth programs participants at CPACS were Hispanic [18,19].

2.2. Participants and Recruitment

The survey was conducted at three of CPACS's after-school program sites in January and February of 2012. CPACS's purpose in conducting the survey was to determine the types of foods and beverages readily available and consumed by the children attending its after-school programs. The children participating in these programs were either Vietnamese or Hispanics living in a low-income immigrant community. All children who participated in the survey were fourth, fifth, and sixth graders, eligible for free lunch at school and had at least one immigrant or refugee parent/guardian.

Because the survey targeted young children, CPACS sent a bi-lingual letter to each child's parents to obtain informed consent for their child's participation in the survey. Data were collected from only the children with parental approval to participate in the survey. A total of 63 children (approximately 90% of those who were eligible) completed the survey. On-site teachers or tutors recorded site information and assigned a unique identification number to all collected surveys. The present research team obtained the questionnaires in Fall 2015. Because the questionnaires were de-identified, the Institutional Review Board at Georgia State University determined the project was not human subjects research as per U.S. Dept. of Health and Human Services.

2.3. Instruments

The "My Food Choices" questionnaire was designed by CPACS staff. The questionnaire consisted of 54 questions, each asking about the frequency of consumption of a type or class of food, e.g., "carrots," "fried chicken or nuggets," or "yogurt." The foods and beverages included on the questionnaire were typical American foods that may be consumed by children at home, school, or restaurants, and represented examples from all food groups (fruits, vegetables, dairy, meat and beans, cereals, sweets). Many of the foods on the questionnaire were often served to the children at CPACS, or in their school cafeteria. A sample question is shown in Appendix A (Figure A1). Next to the name of each food type was a small photo of a serving of the food or a package containing it. For each food type the questionnaire asked: "In the last week, how many times did you eat/drink?". The possible responses were: zero, one, two, three, four, five, six, and seven or more times. The children read and completed the questionnaire without assistance from CPACS staff or parents. Children took approximately 15–20 min to complete the questionnaire.

2.4. Data Analysis

The data were analyzed using SPSS, version 20 (IBM, Armonk, NY, USA). Prior to analysis, a number of steps were taken. First, missing data were filled in when possible using multiple regression analysis and discriminant analysis as described below. Variables were also examined for normality. None of the variables were normally distributed (based on the Shapiro-Wilk statistic and on skewness and kurtosis), therefore the data are described by reporting the median and interquartile range (Q1, Q3), and further analyses were carried out using nonparametric procedures. In addition, while the original 54-item questionnaire had water as one of the food items, this item was excluded from analysis (except to describe consumption frequency) because water, although a required nutrient, does not fit into one of the U.S. Department of Agriculture's (USDA) food groups [16].

We used the nonparametric Wilcoxon signed-rank test to determine whether there was a statistically significant difference between their actual food consumption and the USDA recommended amounts. Although we were interested in testing for differences by gender within each ethnicity, the small number of Vietnamese (n = 15) compared to Hispanic (n = 48) children in our sample made it statistically impractical to examine a gender by ethnicity interaction effect. Therefore, our main focus was to test for gender and ethnicity differences. The nonparametric Kruskal–Wallis test was performed to test for differences in food intake between boys and girls. In supplemental analyses, we tested the independent associations of gender and ethnicity with food intake by using ANOVA with gender as a fixed factor and ethnicity as a covariate, modeling only the main effects and not the interaction effects. The results of these analyses were not qualitatively different from those generated by the nonparametric tests. For all analyses, statistical significance was set at α = 0.05.

2.4.1. Response Rate and Procedures for Filling in Missing Data

Overall, children's response rate on questionnaire was very good, with only 50 of the 3402 potential responses (1.5%) to the food items left unanswered. Where possible, we obtained an estimated value to replace a missing value by utilizing a multiple regression equation to predict how frequently a child ate that food item. A multiple regression model for a food item on which there was missing data was created by using other food items to predict the frequency of consumption of the food item in question. If the best multiple regression model could predict actual consumption of that food item with a high degree of accuracy (i.e., R^2 of 0.60 or higher and low standard error), then it was used to predict the child's food consumption for that item. If the multiple regression equation was of lessor quality or if the child had more than five missing values on food consumption items, then no estimate was made and a "missing value" code in the data analysis of that food item was retained.

In three cases, data on the child's gender was missing and in one case the child's ethnicity was missing. In these cases, discriminant analysis proved highly accurate in distinguishing boys from girls and Vietnamese from Hispanics. Specifically, by identifying a small subset of food items on which consumption levels of boys (or Hispanics) were very different than girls (or Vietnamese), discriminant analysis was able to correctly classify 86.2% of known boys (25 out of 29) boys and 89.7% of known girls (26 out of 29). This discriminant analysis classified two children with missing data on gender as female, while the third case retained a missing value code because it had too much missing data on food consumption items used in the discriminant analysis. Discriminant analysis also correctly classified 83.3% of known Vietnamese children (10 out of 12) and 87.2% of known Hispanic (41 out of 47), and that analysis led to a classification of "Hispanic" for the one case with missing data on ethnicity. Thus, the demographic composition of this sample was: 26 Hispanic boys, 22 Hispanic girls, 5 Vietnamese boys, and 9 Vietnamese girls (one Vietnamese child had missing data for his/her gender).

2.4.2. Determination of Adherence to the USDA Dietary Guidelines for Americans

We categorized each of the food items according to USDA food groups (Table 1). Note that the categorization was not mutually exclusive, i.e., a food could appear in one or more of the groups (e.g., macaroni and cheese was assigned to both the grains and the dairy categories). This is because many foods contain components that belong to different food groups, as described by the USDA [20]. We then compared the actual number of servings per week of vegetables, fruits, grains, dairy, and proteins food groups, as well as oils and discretionary foods consumed by the children with the USDA recommended number of servings for 10-year-old children (which we estimated to be the average age of the children in our sample) based on the USDA Healthy Eating Pattern [16]. To perform this analysis, we assumed that the portion of each food consumed was equivalent to one serving. We calculated the recommended number of servings per week in each food group by multiplying the daily number of recommended servings by seven days per week.

Table 1. Classification of food frequency questionnaire items into USDA food groups.

Food Group	Food Items
Fruits	fruit juice, bananas, apples, grapes, pears, oranges, raisins, mixed fruit, peaches
Vegetables	green beans, other beans, carrots, greens, broccoli, sweet potatoes, French fries or tater tots, other potatoes, corn, tossed salad, yellow squash, tomatoes, vegetable soup
Grains	cereal, honey buns, pretzels, spaghetti, macaroni and cheese, fried rice, other rice, rice and gravy, hamburger, pizza, cookies, snack cake, cake
Protein Foods	peanut butter, hot chicken wings, chicken not fried, fried chicken or chicken nuggets, fish sticks, hamburger, cheese-burger, pizza
Dairy	low fat milk, whole milk, yogurt, cheese, macaroni and cheese, cheeseburger, pizza, ice cream
Oils	chips, hot chicken wings, fried chicken or chicken nuggets, fish sticks, fried rice, French fries or tater tots, salad, mayonnaise
Discretionary	fruit-flavored drinks, soda, cereal, honey buns, chips, yogurt, rice and gravy, mayonnaise, ice cream, cookies, snack cake, chocolate candy, cake, jam, jelly or syrup

2.4.3. Factor Analysis to Determine Dietary Patterns

We performed factor analysis on the 53 food items (excluding water) with quartimax rotation. We used quartimax rather than varimax rotation because we were more interested in learning which foods load most strongly on a factor (quartimax rotation) than minimizing the number of foods associated with each factor (varimax rotation). Thirteen factors with eigenvalues over 1.00 were produced (accounting for 80.1% of the variance), but the most substantively interesting were the first five factors (which account for 58.1% of total variance). These five factors are shown in Table 2. Factor loadings for food items used to compute each factor score are shown in bold.

Table 2. Dietary patterns based on factor analysis of Vietnamese and Latino children's food selections ($n = 63$).

	Veggies Plus	Sweet Snacks	Fruit	Fast Food	Other Veggies
fish sticks	**0.797**	0.162	0.050	0.094	−0.072
broccoli	**0.784**	0.112	0.124	0.062	0.228
carrots	**0.770**	0.081	0.309	0.138	−0.002
other beans	**0.747**	0.044	0.145	0.077	−0.027
green beans	**0.709**	0.136	−0.069	0.046	0.158
sweet potatoes	**0.681**	0.212	−0.091	0.181	0.321
rice & gravy	**0.657**	0.249	−0.143	0.198	−0.039
pretzels	**0.653**	0.087	0.437	0.135	0.107
spaghetti	**0.599**	0.335	0.147	0.171	0.117
snack cakes	0.169	**0.824**	0.102	0.199	−0.032
cookies	0.292	**0.789**	0.220	0.087	−0.113
mayonnaise	0.163	**0.781**	0.034	0.056	0.067
chocolate candy	0.102	**0.768**	0.117	0.280	0.003
ice cream	0.184	**0.734**	0.120	0.373	−0.145
cake	0.178	**0.653**	0.139	0.091	0.364
jam, jelly, syrup	−0.022	**0.647**	0.141	−0.108	0.325
chips	−0.050	**0.625**	0.270	0.199	0.034
popcorn	0.210	**0.584**	0.115	0.169	0.060
fruit-flavored drink	−0.103	**0.570**	0.034	0.231	−0.129
oranges	0.016	0.221	**0.816**	0.107	0.030
apples	0.156	0.363	**0.728**	0.075	0.001
bananas	0.217	0.419	**0.726**	0.070	0.063
fruit juice	0.236	0.004	**0.622**	−0.133	−0.202
grapes	0.360	0.340	**0.589**	−0.054	−0.052
peaches	0.522	−0.062	**0.575**	0.283	−0.055
hamburgers	0.216	0.303	0.142	**0.816**	0.064
pizza	0.253	0.371	0.049	**0.782**	−0.013
hot wings	0.284	0.296	−0.005	**0.701**	−0.112
french fries/tater tots	0.216	0.165	−0.013	**0.680**	−0.036
fried chicken/nuggets	0.196	0.355	0.125	**0.641**	0.114
yellow squash	0.374	0.226	0.036	0.002	**0.761**
tomatoes	0.341	0.020	−0.003	0.008	**0.711**
tossed salad	0.208	−0.010	−0.104	−0.004	**0.618**
greens	0.502	−0.081	−0.001	−0.081	**0.350**
Eigenvalue	15.86	5.60	3.82	3.09	2.40
%Variance	29.93	10.57	7.21	5.83	4.53

The factor loadings used to compute each factor score are shown in boldface type.

3. Results

On the first factor ("Veggies Plus"), foods with the highest factor loadings were mainly vegetables (beans, carrots, broccoli, sweet potatoes) plus rice with gravy and three unexpected foods: fish sticks, spaghetti, and pretzels. Children who ranked high on the Veggies Plus factor ate a relatively healthy diet, with low consumption of soda, fruit-flavored drinks, and chips. Factor 2 ("Sweet Snacks") reflected the least healthy foods, with items like snack cakes, cookies, chips, and ice cream loading strongly on this factor. Children with high scores on the Sweet Snacks factor ate very little greens, peaches, salad, and pears. Factor 3 ("Fruit") represented fruit consumption, with items like oranges, bananas, apples, and fruit juice having the highest factor scores. Those with high scores on the Fruits factor ate little vegetable soup, salad, or hot wings, and do not drink soda. The foods loading strongest on factor 4 ("Fast Food") were hamburgers, pizza, hot wings, French fries or tater tots, and fried chicken/nuggets. Those who were high on the Fast Food factor also often ate cheeseburgers and ice cream and infrequently ate fruit, cereal, and vegetables other than corn. The less often eaten vegetables (yellow squash, vegetable soup, tossed salad, and greens) comprised factor 5 ("Other Veggies"), and it partially reflected a healthy diet, since children scoring high on this factor ate little ice cream or cookies, but they also ate little chicken, fruit, and cereal. To produce an index for each of these factors, we summed children's scores on the food items specified in boldface type in Table 2. The reliability of these indexes is quite good, as Cronbach's alphas are: factor 1 (vegetables plus) = 0.91; factor 2 (sweets) = 0.91; factor 3 (fruits) = 0.87; factor 4 (fast food) = 0.89; and factor 5 (less popular veggies) = 0.79.

In general, this sample of immigrant children's food consumption responses clustered at the low end of the range (Table 3). For 17 of the 54 foods listed, 16 had a median of 0 and one had a median of 1, while 20 other items (including carrots, hamburgers, fried chicken or nuggets, and other beans) were eaten only once per week. Cereal was the most often eaten food (its median was four times per week, as was milk for low-fat and whole milk combined). Certain fruits (e.g., apples, oranges, grapes, bananas) were eaten fairly often, but other fruits (pears, peaches, and raisins) were infrequently eaten by most immigrant children. Most protein sources like hamburgers, fried chicken, peanut butter, and chicken were each consumed one or fewer times per week. Concerning beverages, water was most often consumed, followed by fruit-flavored drinks, fruit juice, low fat milk and whole milk, and sodas were consumed the least often. Snack foods like chips, cookies, and ice cream were among the most commonly consumed items at twice per week each, while others of these types of snack foods including snack cakes, cake, pretzels, and honey buns were consumed fairly infrequently.

Table 3. Food consumption frequency (per week) for a sample of Vietnamese and Hispanic immigrant children (*n* = 63).

Food	Median (Times/Week)	Interquartile Range	Type of Food	Median (Times/Week)	Interquartile Range
water	>6	4–7	popcorn	1.0	0–3
cereal	4.0	2–7	fried chicken or nuggets	1.0	0–3
apples	3.0	2–7	hot chicken wings	1.0	0–3
oranges	3.0	2–5	peanut butter	1.0	0–3
yogurt	3.0	0–5	macaroni & cheese	1.0	0–3
grapes	2.0	1–6	other beans	1.0	0–3
bananas	2.0	1–5	fried rice	1.0	0–3
chips	2.0	1–5	other rice	1.0	0–3
fruit-flavored drinks	2.0	1–5	cheese	1.0	0–2
pizza	2.0	1–4	other potatoes	1.0	0–2
cookies	2.0	0–5	mayonnaise	0.5	0–3
fruit juice	2.0	0–4	peaches	0.0	0–4
ice cream	2.0	0–5	greens	0.0	0–2
low fat milk	2.0	0–4	cheeseburger	0.0	0–2
mixed fruit	2.0	0–5	green beans	0.0	0–3
broccoli	2.0	0–4	pretzels	0.0	0–2
whole milk	2.0	0–4	jam, jelly, or syrup	0.0	0–2
chocolate candy	1.0	0–5	chicken not fried	0.0	0–2
French fries or tater tots	1.0	0–4	honey buns	0.0	0–2
carrots	1.0	0–4	tomatoes	0.0	0–2
hamburgers	1.0	0–3	tossed salad	0.0	0–2
snack cakes	1.0	0–4	raisins	0.0	0–1
spaghetti	1.0	0–4	sweet potatoes	0.0	0–1
soda	1.0	0–3	vegetable soup	0.0	0–2
pears	1.0	0–3	fish sticks	0.0	0–1
corn	1.0	0–3	yellow squash	0.0	0–1
cake	1.0	0–3	rice with gravy	0.0	0–1

3.1. Consumed vs. Recommended Number of Servings in USDA Food Groups

Figure 1 shows the median and interquartile range for consumption per week of foods grouped into USDA categories compared with the recommended number of servings per week, arranged in descending order of the recommendation for all children, boys, girls, Vietnamese, and Hispanic children. The sample as a whole ate significantly less than the recommended amount of grains, protein foods, and dairy, but met the recommended amount of fruit. Examining USDA food group consumption by gender, while the median consumption was higher in boys than in girls for all food groups, the differences were significant for grains, protein foods, and fruits (all $p < 0.05$), and marginally nonsignificant for dairy, oils, and discretionary foods (p-values ranged from 0.056 to 0.09). Results were similar when analyzed by ANOVA, controlling for ethnicity (Table S1). In addition, compared with the recommended number of servings, boys' median consumption was significantly lower for grains and protein foods, and significantly higher for fruits, while girls' median consumption was significantly lower for grains, protein foods, and dairy, and significantly higher for fruits. For both boys and girls, the highest number of servings came from discretionary foods, followed by grains and fruits. Of the food groups, fruit consumption was relatively high, with 67% of the sample reaching the recommended value (75% of boys and 58% of girls). A relatively high number of boys also reached the recommended number of servings for dairy (58%) and vegetables (50%), while only 31% and 20% of boys reached the recommended number of servings for grains and protein foods, respectively. Only 35% of girls reached the recommended number of servings for vegetables, and 23, 10, and 6% of girls consumed the recommended number of dairy, grain, and protein servings, respectively.

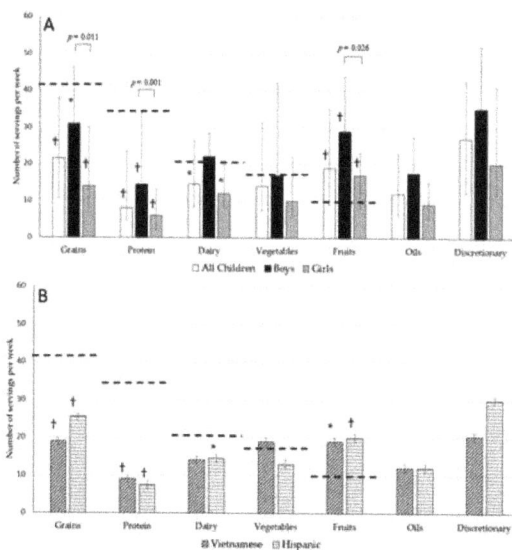

Figure 1. Reported median number of servings per week consumed in USDA food groups versus recommended values in a sample of fourth, fifth, and sixth grade Vietnamese and Hispanic immigrant children (n = 63) for (**A**) all children, boys, and girls; and (**B**) Vietnamese and Hispanic children. Error bars show interquartile range (25th and 75th percentiles). Dotted horizontal lines represent USDA recommended number of servings per week for 10-year-old boys and girls [16]. Symbol next to vertical bar indicates significant difference between number of servings consumed compared with the USDA recommendation (* for $p < 0.05$; † for $p < 0.01$). p-values are shown for Kruskal–Wallis test for significant differences between boys and girls; p-values for gender differences in consumption of other food groups were 0.058 for dairy, 0.117 for vegetables, 0.056 for oils, and 0.09 for discretionary. Differences by ethnicity were not significant (p-values ranged from 0.398 to 0.993).

In contrast, the figure also shows that there were no significant differences in food group intake by ethnicity. Results were similar when analyzed by ANOVA, controlling for gender (Table S1). While a majority of Vietnamese and Hispanic children met or exceeded the recommended number of servings of fruits ($p < 0.05$ and $p < 0.01$, respectively), they consumed a significantly lower number of servings of grains and protein foods ($p < 0.01$). In fact, only 8% and 14% of Vietnamese children met or exceeded the recommended amount of grains and proteins, respectively; while only 23% and 13% of Hispanic children ate the recommended amount of grains and protein foods. Most Vietnamese and Hispanic children also consumed a lower number of dairy servings compared with the recommendation, but this difference was significant only for Hispanic children ($p < 0.05$). The recommended number of vegetable servings was met by 62% of Vietnamese but only 38% of Hispanic children.

3.2. Dietary Patterns Discerned by Factor Analysis

Dietary patterns from factor analysis for all of the children in our sample, as well as by ethnicity and gender, are shown in Table 4. For all children, foods in the Sweet Snacks and Fruits factors were most frequently consumed, followed by foods in the Veggies Plus factor, then the Fast Food and Other Veggies Factors. Dietary patterns did not differ significantly by ethnicity, although Hispanic children consumed foods in Sweet Snacks much more frequently and Other Veggies much less frequently than did Vietnamese children. When examined by gender, however, frequency of consumption in each factor was higher for boys than for girls. This gender difference reached statistical significance for Fruits and Fast Food factors, and was marginally nonsignificant for the Veggies Plus factor.

Table 4. Median (Q1, Q3) consumption frequency per week of factor analysis-derived dietary patterns for a sample of Vietnamese and Hispanic immigrant children ($n = 63$).

	All Children	Ethnicity Analysis			Gender Analysis		
		Vietnamese ($n = 15$)	Hispanic ($n = 48$)	Kruskal–Wallis *p*-Value [1]	Boys ($n = 31$)	Girls ($n = 31$)	Kruskal–Wallis *p*-Value [1]
Sweet Snacks	19.0 (7, 34)	12.5 (7, 20)	22.0 (7, 39)	0.160	23.0 (8, 39)	13.0 (7, 26)	0.157
Fruits	15.0 (8, 26)	13.0 (7, 22)	15.5 (8, 29)	0.262	21.0 (9, 33)	13.0 (7, 22)	0.043
Veggies Plus	7.0 (4, 20)	7.0 (4, 13)	7.5 (4, 21)	0.951	11.0 (5, 37)	6.0 (3, 15)	0.069
Fast Food	6.0 (3, 16)	8.0 (3, 15)	6.0 (2, 21)	0.853	9.5 (4, 23)	4.0 (2, 14)	0.029
Other Veggies	2.0 (0, 8)	7.5 (1, 10)	2.0 (0, 7)	0.185	2.0 (0, 14)	2.0 (0, 8)	0.648

[1] Probabilities are statistical significance of Kruskal–Wallis test for differences in consumption of foods in each factor by ethnicity and gender. One Vietnamese child whose gender was unknown was not included in the gender analysis.

4. Discussion

We examined dietary patterns based on USDA food groups and dietary pattern analysis (factor analysis) in a convenience sample of Vietnamese and Hispanic school-aged immigrant children attending after-school programs. Several findings are especially interesting. On the positive side, most children in this sample ate the recommended number of servings per week of fruit, and approximately half of the boys ate the recommended number of servings of vegetables and dairy foods. Also, given the concern that many children drink too much soda, another positive finding was that the frequency of soda consumption was low (median was only once per week and interquartile range was 0 to 3). On the negative side, many of the children in our sample reported that for several food groups, their diets were below the recommended number of servings. Indeed, 87% of the sample was below the weekly amount in protein foods, 80% below in grains, 60% below in dairy, and 57% below the recommended weekly servings of vegetables. In addition, we found high levels of consumption of sweet snacks and fast food. Differences between the two ethnicities were not significant, but boys consumed significantly more servings per week of grains, protein, and fruits than girls. These findings suggest a generally unhealthy diet in these immigrant children, and that they may benefit from programs and interventions to improve diet quality.

Our finding of relatively high fruit consumption and low consumption of vegetables and diary is consistent with previous studies that find immigrants' adoption of American diets and eating patterns is typically not a wholly healthy change [21–23] and it may put them at risk of unhealthy outcomes [24–26]. In particular, our results in Vietnamese children which showed high consumption frequencies of fruit and vegetables and a low consumption frequency of dairy are in general agreement with previous studies [12,13,27], but there is some disagreement on consumption of meat (which falls into the protein foods group) between our study and another [27]. In addition, the findings of previous studies in Hispanic children with regard to these food groups are mixed [12,13], making comparisons with our results difficult and also mixed. Both ethnicities in our study had a relatively high intake of discretionary foods, which was not high in Vietnamese children in previous research [12] but was high in another study in Hispanic children [13]. Comparison of our data with previous studies must be done with caution due to methodological variations across the studies including differences in sample size, age groups, family income, acculturation status, and secular trends in U.S. food supply since the data across studies were collected from 1986 to 2013. Potentially, the generally unhealthy diet of children in our sample might be attributable to low family incomes (given that all the children qualified for free school lunches) and/or that traditional Vietnamese and Hispanic diets may be lower in protein and dairy foods than Western diets. We note that this survey was not a full inventory of all American foods eaten (nor did it cover traditional Vietnamese or Latin American foods), so it did not include some potential sources of protein (e.g., eggs, pork, or fish other than fish sticks). Therefore, it is possible that the low intake of protein foods is not as severe as these data imply. Nonetheless, the apparent low consumption of protein and other healthy foods found here merits further research. Taken together, our findings highlight the need for extensive investigation of the dietary practices of immigrant groups in general and children in particular. We need to discover whether continued eating of traditional foods by immigrants or their children can alleviate deficits in consumption of healthy food categories, or if they can shift to healthier choices of American foods. Also, we need to investigate how low income, the spatial location of good grocery stores, and the cultural meanings of traditional and American foods affect immigrants' food choices.

Further, we found interesting differences in food consumption by gender. For most food groups, especially proteins, grains, and fruits, boys reported more servings than girls. Several factors may account for this gender difference in food consumption. First, although within this age group, the recommedations for energy intake and the recommended number of servings in each food group do not differ between boys and girls [16], in US national survey data, boys report a higher energy intake than girls [28]. Therefore, it may be expected that the boys in our sample would report consuming more servings of any or all of the food groups than girls. In addition, there may be some behavioral and cultural factors that potentially contributed to the gender differences in intake observed in our study. Specifically, here may be traditional cultural gender norms that favor boys and place higher value on the good health of boys and men over girls and women [29]. In addition, studies show that immigrant parents allow sons more freedom to explore and adopt American cultural behaviors but often discourage or prohibit it for daughters, preferring that they maintain traditional customs [30,31]. This could help explain the more frequent consumption of American food by boys in our sample. It is also possible that gender norms encourage boys to be more assertive in interpersonal interactions [32] and therefore encourage boys to ask for and expect more servings of food than girls. Similarly, greater food consumption may be perceived as more masculine and as a means of confirming a male masculine identity, as well as a sense of personal empowerment [33]. In stark contrast, traditional gender norms may highlight petite body images for girls and associate positive self-meanings to girls who eat less and are slim in appearance [34,35]. The gender difference in our study may suggest the need for more in-depth study of the relationship between gender norms and the gender-related meanings assigned to food, both within Western culture and the traditional cultures of immigrant groups.

There are several limitations to this study. Beginning with the sample, the respondents were not randomly selected. However, we took advantage of the data which had been collected by CPACS as an opportunity to quantify the diet quality of immigrant children, a population whose diet and health have been understudied. A larger number of Vietnamese respondents would have enabled us to more directly investigate ethnic and cultural differences in food selection. In addition, about 10% of the children who were eligible to complete the survey did not participate, and there could have been differences between children who participated and those who did not, including age, grade level, and family income differences. Concerning the latter, however, any income differences were small, and unlikely to have created bias in the sample since all children were from families whose income was below the U.S. poverty line. Similarly, a question on the survey asking the respondent's age would have allowed us to control for age differences in our analysis of gender and independently investigate possible age effects. Another limitation is that while we have data on the number of times a child ate each pictured food, we do not know the actual amount of food consumed per serving. Further, the food items pictured in the questionnaire were all typically American and did not include traditional ethnic foods. The 54 foods included on the questionnaire were a subset of all of the actual (or potential) foods that the children in this sample may eat. Although many of the foods listed on the questionnaire were served to the children in their after school programs at CPACS and thus were believed to have been appropriately included, it is possible that a questionnaire containing a longer or different list of foods could have produced results that differed from our findings. In addition, the food consumption data were self-reported (rather than a precise measurement of the volume of food eaten) and therefore are subject to social desirability bias. The study was conducted in January and February, and did not take into account potential effects of seasonality on the results. The study is also limited by its lack of data on children's families and other demographic information. While all the children in this study were eligible for free lunch at school and had at least one parent/guardian who is an immigrant or refugee, a more complete analysis would have included variables such as total family income, English-speaking ability, parents' and children's immigration status, and their length of time in the United States. These limitations mean that we must be cautious in drawing conclusions from our findings. Nevertheless, this research may be a useful initial step in learning about the nutritional status of these two important groups of immigrant children, and can inform future, more in-depth studies on this topic.

5. Conclusions

While our sample size was relatively small and non-random, the results of the present study suggest that further study of the diets and food consumption of immigrant and refugee children is an important direction for continued research. First and foremost, the link between food consumption and health outcomes needs to be directly investigated with more comprehensive measures of the children's diets, health status, and health risks. Further studies should also compare children from different racial and ethnic groups, as well as the possible independent effects of immigration status and social background factors on food selection and health outcomes. The results also may have implications for helping Hispanic, Vietnamese, and other immigrant children. Educational and outreach programs in partnership with community organizations and religious institutions should focus on encouraging families to serve healthful traditional foods, especially those that increase portions of grains and proteins. In this regard, the food consumption of boys and girls may need to be recognized as different with special efforts to offer girls more servings of nutritious foods, and for boys to moderate their consumption of discretionary food such as candy and other high calorie snacks.

Supplementary Materials: The following are available online at www.mdpi.com/2072-6643/9/5/460/s1, Table S1: Independent associations of gender and ethnicity with USDA food groups and dietary patterns from factor analysis in a sample of Vietnamese and Hispanic children (*n* = 63).

Acknowledgments: The study was not funded by outside sources. We thank CPACS for the use of the survey data, and Zoe Elizabeth Fawcett for technical assistance.

Author Contributions: J.H.K. conceived and designed the study; J.H.K. administered the questionnaire; C.L.J. analyzed the data; M.A.M., C.L.J. and D.C.R. wrote and edited the paper; J.H.K. edited the paper. All authors interpreted the results, provided substantive comments, and read and approved the final manuscript.

Conflicts of Interest: M.A.M., C.L.J. and D.C.R. declare no conflicts of interest. J.H.K. was employed by CPACS at the time of data collection, but was no longer employed by CPACS when the data were analyzed and the manuscript was written. CPACS had no role in the analyses or interpretation of data, in the writing of the manuscript, and in the decision to publish the results.

Appendix A

In the last week, how many times did you eat oranges?

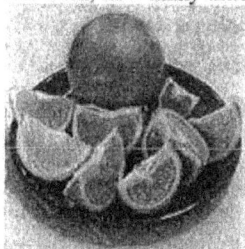

a. 0 times last week

b. 1 time last week

c. 2 times last week

d. 3 times last week

e. 4 times last week

f. 5 times last week

g. 6 times last week

h. 7 or more times last week

Figure A1. Sample question from 54 item food frequency questionnaire. The full questionnaire is available from the authors upon request.

References

1. Wang, Y.; Min, J.; Harris, K.; Khuri, J.; Anderson, L.M. A systematic examination of food intake and adaptation to the food environment by refugees settled in the United States. *Adv. Nutr.* **2016**, *7*, 1066–1079. [CrossRef] [PubMed]

2. Rosas, L.G.; Guendelman, S.; Harley, K.; Fernald, L.C.; Neufeld, L.; Mejia, F.; Eskenazi, B. Factors associated with overweight and obesity among children of Mexican descent: Results of a binational study. *J. Immigr. Minor. Health* **2011**, *13*, 169–180. [CrossRef] [PubMed]

3. Kobel, S.; Lammle, C.; Wartha, O.; Kesztyus, D.; Wirt, T.; Steinacker, J.M. Effects of a randomised controlled school-based health promotion intervention on obesity related behavioural outcomes of children with migration background. *J. Immigr. Minor. Health* **2017**, *19*, 254–262. [CrossRef] [PubMed]

4. Wang, S.; Quan, J.; Kanaya, A.M.; Fernandez, A. Asian Americans and obesity in California: A protective effect of biculturalism. *J. Immigr. Minor. Health* **2011**, *13*, 276–283. [CrossRef] [PubMed]

5. Wang, M.C. Obesity and Asian Americans: Prevalence, risk factors, and future research directions. In *Handbook of Asian American Health*; Yoo, G.J., Le, M.-N., Oda, A.Y., Eds.; Springer: New York, NY, USA, 2013.

6. Goran, M.I.; Ball, G.D.; Cruz, M.L. Obesity and risk of type 2 diabetes and cardiovascular disease in children and adolescents. *J. Clin. Endocrinol. Metab.* **2003**, *88*, 1417–1427. [CrossRef] [PubMed]

7. Chen, J.L.; Weiss, S.; Heyman, M.B.; Lustig, R. Risk factors for obesity and high blood pressure in Chinese American children: Maternal acculturation and children's food choices. *J. Immigr. Minor. Health* **2011**, *13*, 268–275. [CrossRef] [PubMed]

8. Bloom, B.; Black, L.I. Health of non-Hispanic Asian adults: United States, 2010–2014. *NCHS Data Brief* **2016**, *247*, 1–8.

9. Kelder, S.H.; Perry, C.L.; Klepp, K.I.; Lytle, L.L. Longitudinal tracking of adolescent smoking, physical activity, and food choice behaviors. *Am. J. Public Health* **1994**, *84*, 1121–1126. [CrossRef] [PubMed]

10. Qi, Y.; Niu, J. Does childhood nutrition predict health outcomes during adulthood? Evidence from a population-based study in China. *J. Biosoc. Sci.* **2015**, *47*, 650–666. [CrossRef] [PubMed]

11. Diep, C.S.; Foster, M.J.; McKyer, E.L.; Goodson, P.; Guidry, J.J.; Liew, J. What are Asian-American youth consuming? A systematic literature review. *J. Immigr. Minor. Health* **2015**, *17*, 591–604. [CrossRef] [PubMed]

12. Wiecha, J.M.; Fink, A.K.; Wiecha, J.; Hebert, J. Differences in dietary patterns of Vietnamese, White, African-American, and Hispanic adolescents in Worcester, Mass. *J. Am. Diet. Assoc.* **2001**, *101*, 248–251. [CrossRef]

13. Guerrero, A.D.; Ponce, N.A.; Chung, P.J. Obesogenic dietary practices of Latino and Asian subgroups of children in California: An analysis of the California Health Interview Survey, 2007–2012. *Am. J. Public Health* **2015**, *105*, e105–e112. [CrossRef] [PubMed]

14. Lee, S.K.; Sobal, J.; Frongillo, E.A., Jr. Acculturation and dietary practices among Korean Americans. *J. Am. Diet. Assoc.* **1999**, *99*, 1084–1089. [CrossRef]

15. Lesser, I.A.; Gasevic, D.; Lear, S.A. The association between acculturation and dietary patterns of South Asian immigrants. *PLoS ONE* **2014**, *9*, e88495. [CrossRef] [PubMed]

16. U.S. Department of Health and Human Services; U.S. Department of Agriculture. *2015–2020 Dietary Guidelines for Americans*, 8th ed.; USDA: Washington, DC, USA, 2015.

17. Center for Pan Asian Community Services. Available online: http://www.cpacs.org (accessed on 29 December 2016).

18. Center for Pan Asian Community Services. *2013–2014 Annual Report*; CPACS: Atlanta, GA, USA, 2014.

19. Center for Pan Asian Community Services. *2014–2015 Annual Report*; CPACS: Atlanta, GA, USA, 2015.

20. Bowman, S.A.; Clemens, J.C.; Friday, J.E.; Theorig, R.C.; Mosfegh, A.J. *Food Patterns Equivalents Database 2011–12: Methodology and User Guide*; U.S. Department of Agriculture, Agricultural Research Service, Beltsville Human Nutrition Research Center, Food Surveys Research Group: Beltsville, MD, USA, 2014.

21. Creighton, M.J.; Goldman, N.; Pebley, A.R.; Chung, C.Y. Durational and generational differences in Mexican immigrant obesity: Is acculturation the explanation? *Soc. Sci. Med.* **2012**, *75*, 300–310. [CrossRef] [PubMed]

22. Lara, M.; Gamboa, C.; Kahramanian, M.I.; Morales, L.S.; Bautista, D.E. Acculturation and Latino health in the United States: A review of the literature and its sociopolitical context. *Annu. Rev. Public Health* **2005**, *26*, 367–397. [CrossRef] [PubMed]

23. Park, S.Y.; Murphy, S.P.; Sharma, S.; Kolonel, L.N. Dietary intakes and health-related behaviours of Korean American women born in the USA and Korea: The Multiethnic Cohort Study. *Public Health Nutr.* **2005**, *8*, 904–911. [CrossRef] [PubMed]

24. Cho, Y.; Frisbie, W.P.; Hummer, R.A.; Rogers, R.G. Nativity, duration of residence, and health of Hispanic adults in the United States. *Int. J. Migr. Rev.* **2004**, *38*, 184–211. [CrossRef]

25. Jasti, S.; Lee, C.H.; Doak, C. Gender, acculturation, food patterns, and overweight in Korean immigrants. *Am. J. Health Behav.* **2011**, *35*, 734–745. [CrossRef] [PubMed]

26. Yang, E.J.; Chung, H.K.; Kim, W.Y.; Bianchi, L.; Song, W.O. Chronic diseases and dietary changes in relation to Korean Americans' length of residence in the United States. *J. Am. Diet. Assoc.* **2007**, *107*, 942–950. [CrossRef] [PubMed]

27. Betts, N.M.; Weidenbenner, A. Dietary intakes, iron status, and growth status of Southeast Asian refugee children. *Nutr. Res.* **1986**, *6*, 509–515. [CrossRef]

28. U.S. Department of Agriculture, Agricultural Research Service. *What We Eat in America, NHANES 2013–2014, Individuals 2 Years and over (Excluding Breastfed Children), Day 1*; USDA: Washington, DC, USA, 2016.

29. Vlassoff, C. Gender differences in determinants and consequences of health and illness. *J. Health Popul. Nutr.* **2007**, *25*, 47–61. [PubMed]

30. Espiritu, Y.L. *We Don't Sleep around Like White Girls Do: Family, Culture, and Gender in Filipina American Lives*; University of California Press: Berkeley, CA, USA, 2003.

31. Zhou, M.; Bankston, C.L. *Growing Up American: How Vietnamese Children Adapt to Life in the United States*; Russel Sage: New York, NY, USA, 1998.

32. Costa, P.T., Jr.; Terracciano, A.; McCrae, R.R. Gender differences in personality traits across cultures: Robust and surprising findings. *J. Personal. Soc. Psychol.* **2001**, *81*, 322–331. [CrossRef]

33. Turner, K.; Ferguson, S.; Craig, J.; Jeffries, A.; Beaton, S. Gendered identity negotiations through food consumption. *Young Consum.* **2013**, *14*, 280–288. [CrossRef]
34. Wardle, J.; Robb, K.A.; Johnson, F.; Griffith, J.; Brunner, E.; Power, C.; Tovee, M. Socioeconomic variation in attitudes to eating and weight in female adolescents. *Health Psychol.* **2004**, *23*, 275–282. [CrossRef] [PubMed]
35. McGinnis, J.M.; Gootman, J.A.; Kraak, V.I. *Food Marketing to Children and Youth: Threat or Opportunity*; National Academies Press: Washington, DC, USA, 2006; pp. 91–132.

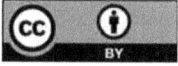

nutrients

MDPI

Article

Association between Picky Eating Behaviors and Nutritional Status in Early Childhood: Performance of a Picky Eating Behavior Questionnaire

Kyung Min Kwon [1], Jae Eun Shim [2,3,*], Minji Kang [4] and Hee-Young Paik [1,4]

[1] Department of Food and Nutrition, College of Human Ecology, Seoul National University, 1 Gwanak-ro, Gwanak-gu, Seoul 08826, Korea; ckyme@snu.ac.kr (K.M.K.); hypaik@snu.ac.kr (H.-Y.P.)

[2] Department of Food and Nutrition, Daejeon University, 62 Daehak-ro, Dong-gu, Daejeon 34520, Korea

[3] Daejeon Dong-gu Center for Children's Food Service Management, Daejeon University, 62 Daehak-ro, Dong-gu, Daejeon 34520, Korea

[4] Research Institute of Human Ecology, College of Human Ecology, Seoul National University, 1 Gwanak-ro, Gwanak-gu, Seoul 08826, Korea; mjkang@snu.ac.kr

* Correspondence: jshim@dju.kr; Tel.: +82-42-280-2469

Received: 4 April 2017; Accepted: 2 May 2017; Published: 6 May 2017

Abstract: Picky eating behaviors are frequently observed in childhood, leading to concern that an unbalanced and inadequate diet will result in unfavorable growth outcomes. However, the association between picky eating behaviors and nutritional status has not been investigated in detail. This study was conducted to assess eating behaviors and growth of children aged 1–5 years from the Seoul Metropolitan area. Primary caregivers completed self-administered questionnaires and 3-day diet records. Differences in the nutrient intake and growth indices between picky and non-picky eaters were tested by analysis of covariance. Children "eating small amounts" consumed less energy and micronutrients (with the exception of calcium intake), but picky behaviors related to a "limited variety" resulted in a significant difference regarding nutrient density for some micronutrients. Children with the behavior of "eating small amounts" had a lower weight-for-age than that of non-picky eaters; especially, the older children with the behaviors of "eating small amounts" or "refusal of specific food groups" had lower height-for-age compared with non-picky eaters. These results suggest that specific picky eating behaviors are related to different nutrient intake and unfavorable growth patterns in early childhood. Thus, exploration of potential interventions according to specific aspects of picky eating and their efficacy is required.

Keywords: picky eating; early childhood; diet; growth

---

1. Introduction

Picky eating is a frequent eating problem in childhood that concerns many parents [1–4]. In young children, picky eating can contribute to a poor dietary intake and growth status [2,4–6] and may have long-term effects [7–10]. A recent review presented conflicting reports on dietary intake patterns in picky eating children: some studies reported an increased intake of energy or energy-dense foods including snacks and sweets, while most studies reported a limited variety of food intake with reduced energy consumption [11]. Both patterns could cause inappropriate changes in the nutrient composition of the diet and are related to unfavorable growth (i.e., poor growth and overweight) and subsequent health problems [11–14].

However, previous approaches to evaluating picky eaters are insufficient to explain the conflicting reports on dietary intake patterns, and investigate the association with growth outcomes. In previous studies, caregivers of picky-eating children reported various problems with feeding them: eating insufficient amounts, avoiding new foods, preferring foods prepared in specific ways, or having a strong preference for particular foods [2,4,6,8,15–18]. Picky eating is a complex concept composed of several types of eating behaviors [19]; nevertheless, picky eating has generally been measured by a single simple question based on parents' perceptions of feeding difficulty or pickiness [2,18], or by a list of questions about eating behaviors and feeding practices [4,7,16,20,21]. The differences in measurements regarding picky eating focusing on one aspect or approaches using measurement tools consisting of mixed concepts leads to confusion and problems in interpretation [22].

Two recent studies have tried to present a clear definition of picky eating, and have characterized children's picky eating behaviors with two attributes based on previously-reported aspects of picky eating behaviors: eating small amounts of food, and eating a limited variety of foods [19,23]. In the studies, "limited variety" consisted of three sub-constructs of "unwillingness to try new food", "rejection of specific food groups" (i.e., fruits, vegetables, meats, and fish), and "preference for specific food preparation methods". To find critical behaviors in child growth, the association of the four aspects of picky behaviors and growth in young children was examined at a medical clinic for picky eaters [23]. The medical clinic study measured the level of the four aspects of picky eating behaviors using similar questions to the present study (i.e., the same questions for the measurement of "eating small amounts" and "neophobic behavior", 9 vs. 12 food groups for "refusal of specific food groups", and 7 vs. 9 food groups for preference for specific food preparation method). In the study, negative association between "eating small amounts" and height-for-age was observed. Difference in nutrient intake and the relations with growth outcomes in a community setting have not yet been examined.

Thus, the present study investigated the picky eating behaviors of the four constructs in children aged 1 to 5 years at the community level. Further, the performance using the four-construct scale was evaluated qualitatively by examining how the four different aspects of picky eating were associated with dietary intake and growth. It is hypothesized that each aspect would have a specific pattern in dietary intake and growth.

2. Materials and Methods

2.1. Study Participants

This study is a cross-sectional survey targeting children aged 1 to 5 years from the Seoul Metropolitan Area of Korea. Participants were recruited between September 2014 and July 2015. Convenience sampling was employed to recruit volunteers by using flyers, public announcements, and online announcements at Community Health centers, a pharmacy, and an online caregiver's community. Voluntarily participating primary caregivers of the children were asked to complete the survey questionnaire. Participants were enrolled after the caregivers were given a full explanation of the purpose and protocols of the research in person. The Seoul National University Institutional Review Board approved the study protocol (IRB No. 1407/001-034), and all primary caregivers provided written informed consent.

2.2. Measurements

2.2.1. Picky Eating Behaviors

Picky eating behaviors were assessed using survey questions from previous studies [19,23]. Caregivers were asked to respond to the frequency of each question using a five-point response scale of 1 (almost never) to 5 (almost always). The higher scores demonstrated greater picky eating behavior, so the reverse-described questions were transposed. Self-administered surveys were reviewed by a trained dietitian and confirmed by interview. The four specific picky eating behaviors and the related questions were:

- Eating small amounts, with the question of "How often do you attempt to persuade your child to eat a food?", and two reversed-described questions: "In general, at the end of a meal how often has your child eaten the amount you think he/she should eat?" and "Does your child have a good appetite?"

- Neophobic behavior, with two reverse-described questions: "How often does your child try new and unfamiliar foods at home?", and "How willing is your child to enjoy new and unfamiliar food when offered?"
- Refusal to eat specific food groups, using the question on 12 food groups: "How often does your child refuse the following foods: beans, vegetables, mushrooms, seaweeds, meat, fish, shrimp, shellfish, eggs, fruits, milk, and yogurt?"
- Preference for a specific food preparation method, with the question on nine food groups: "Does your child eat any of the following foods only if prepared in a specific way: beans, vegetables, mushrooms, seaweeds, meat, fish, shrimp, shellfish, and eggs?"

It was assumed that the children have potential picky eating characters if the response score to each question was higher than neutral. "Eating small amounts" and "neophobic behavior" were summated rating scales. Therefore, the children whose mean score of responses was >3 were classified as "picky eaters" for "eating small amounts" and "neophobic behavior". The internal consistency of items on these constructs was measured using the Cronbach's coefficient α ($\alpha = 0.80$ for "eating small amounts" and $\alpha = 0.73$ for "neophobic behavior"). Whether children refused a food group or whether children had preference for a specific preparation method to a food group was also determined by a response score > 3. However, "refusal to eat specific food groups" and "preference for a specific food preparation method" were not summated rating scales. The constructs consisted of multiple questions about behaviors to different food groups. Therefore, "refusal to eat specific food groups" and "preference for a specific food preparation method" were evaluated based on the number of foods refused and number of foods with specific preparation method preferred, respectively. The cut-off number was set based on the mean numbers of food groups with responses more than neutral (1.8 for refused food groups and 1.2 for preference for a specific food preparation method). Therefore, children who refused more than two food groups were classified as picky eaters of "refusal to eat specific food groups" and children with a preference for a specific food preparation method in any food group were categorized as picky eaters of "preference for a specific food preparation method". If certain food groups had never been tried, the food groups were not counted when "refusal to eat specific food groups" or "preference for a specific food preparation method" was evaluated. Children who had any one of the sub-constructs, "neophobic behavior", "refusal to eat specific food groups", and "preference for a specific food preparation method" were defined as children with 'limited variety'. Children who had any one of the picky eating main constructs, "eating small amounts" and "limited variety", were classified as picky eaters.

2.2.2. Dietary Intakes

Non-consecutive 3-day diet records were used to collect the dietary intake data of each subject. To minimize errors in portion size, the caregivers were asked to record the intake amount by using two-dimensional measurement tools. The protocol for coding diet records was prepared by a research dietitian supervisor. Based on the protocol, trained dietitian interviewers reviewed the data by telephone interview. For children who were still being breastfed, the intake of breastmilk was assessed according to the reported feeding time; the amount being fed was considered to be 1 fl. oz. (29.6 mL) for every 5 min [24]. All dietary data were converted to nutrient intake values using the DES-KOREA (Diet Evaluation System, 2011, Human Nutrition Lab at Seoul National University, Republic of Korea), which is a web-based dietary assessment program [25,26]. The DES incorporates a recipe and nutrient database. The recipe database contains 3916 recipes for common Korean dishes, and the nutrient database contains 4222 food items [27,28]. The mean daily intake, the energy distribution for macronutrients, the nutrient density (intake/1000 kcal of energy) for micronutrients, and the total dietary fiber were evaluated.

2.2.3. Growth Indices

Primary caregivers were asked to measure the weight and height of their children at the local hospital or community health center and report the values to the research dietitian by mail. Confirmation was made through telephone interviews. The height data for children aged ≤24 months were converted into lengths by adding 0.7 cm, following the WHO (World Health Organization) child growth standards [29]. The height/length and weight values were converted into z-scores for weight-for-age, height-for-age (length-for-age), and BMI (body mass index)-for-age, compared with the WHO child growth standards for 0–60 months [29] and the WHO growth reference data for 61–228 months [30].

2.2.4. Covariates

A questionnaire investigating the children's eating behaviors, feeding practices, and care environment was administered, and data were obtained by self-reporting via the caregivers of the participating children. The sociodemographic characteristics included information pertaining to the caregivers, such as age, education level of both parents (≤high school, college graduate, graduate school), and monthly household income (≤$2800, $2800 to $3900, and ≥$3900), and information pertaining to the children, such as age and sex. In addition, Nutrition Plus participation (a nutrition supplemental program for women, infants and children in Korea) and infant feeding practices were investigated. Infant feeding practice was evaluated according to the duration of breastfeeding, the introduction of formula or milk, and the introduction of supplementary foods. This information was transformed into binary variables, including breastfeeding initiation, exclusive breastfeeding during the first 3 months and 6 months of life, and early introduction of supplementary foods before 6 months of age [31].

2.3. Statistical Analysis

The data of sociodemographic characteristics and the prevalence of picky eating habits were presented as numbers and proportions for categorical variables or as means and standard deviations for numeric variables. The differences in nutrient intake and z-scores of growth indices between picky eaters and non-picky eaters in each construct were tested by analysis of covariance to adjust for the child's age and sex and the education level of both parents, after examination of covariates as potential confounders [32]. All the statistical analyses were performed using SAS (version 9.3, 2011, SAS Institute Inc., Cary, NC, USA), and the statistical significance was determined at 0.05.

3. Results

3.1. Sociodemographic Characteristics of Study Participants

Among the 221 children of the caregivers who initially volunteered and were eligible for the study, 14 with missing data from their diet records and 1 who had consecutive food records were excluded. An additional 22 participants were excluded because of food restrictions due to food allergies, a vegetarian diet, or religious beliefs, leaving 184 children with complete data.

As shown in Table 1, participants generally lived in well-educated middle-class families. Approximately 39% of children participated in Nutrition Plus. The growth indices of all participants were within the normal ranges.

Table 1. Selected characteristics of children aged 1 to 5 years and their caregivers (*n* = 184).

Variables	
Characteristics of children	
Age (year), mean ± SD	2.8 ± 1.4
Sex, % boy	48.9
	n (%)
Infant feeding practice	
Breastfeeding initiation	177 (96.2)
Exclusive breastfeeding under 3 months of life	166 (90.2)
Exclusive breastfeeding under 6 months of life	93 (50.5)
Introduction of complementary foods [a] before 6 months of age	55 (29.9)
Nutrition Plus [b] participation	
Yes	72 (39.1)
No	112 (60.9)
Picky eating behavior [c]	129 (70.1)
Eating small amount	55 (29.9)
Limited variety [d]	123 (66.9)
Neophobic behavior	60 (32.6)
Refusal of specific food groups	81 (44.0)
Preference for a specific food preparation method	91 (49.5)
	mean ± SD
Growth status (*z*-score)	
Weight for age	0.1 ± 0.8
Height for age	−0.3 ± 1.1
BMI for age	0.3 ± 1.0
Characteristics of caregivers and the household	
Age (year), mean ± SD	34.9 ± 3.8
	n (%)
Education level of father	
≤High school	18 (9.8)
University	137 (74.5)
Graduate school	29 (15.8)
Education level of mother	
≤High school	29 (15.8)
University	135 (73.4)
Graduate school	20 (10.9)
Household income	
≤$2800	76 (41.3)
$2800 to $3900	58 (31.5)
≥$3900	50 (27.2)

[a] All foods except breast milk and formula; [b] A Nutrition supplemental program for women, infant, and children in Korea; [c] Children who had any one of the picky eating constructs: 'eating small amounts' and 'limited variety'; [d] Children who had any one of the sub- constructs of limited variety: 'neophobic behavior', 'refusal to eat specific food groups', and 'preference for a specific food preparation method'.

3.2. Proportion of Picky Eaters

The proportion of participants with the behavior of "eating small amounts" was 29.9% and with the "limited variety" was 66.9%; with the "preference for a specific food-preparation method" was 49.5%, with the "refusal to eat specific food groups" was 44.0%, with the "neophobic behavior" was 32.6% (Table 1). In addition, compared with the younger children, the older children aged 4 to 5 years showed higher rates of eating behaviors related to a variety of foods, especially "neophobic behavior" (47.5% vs. 25.6%, *p* = 0.0032). Most children showed more than one kind of picky behavior: of the children with the behavior of "eating small amounts", 67.3% also displayed a "refusal to eat specific food groups" and 43.6% "neophobic behavior"; of the children with "neophobic behavior", 40.0% exhibited "eating small amounts" and 75.0% a "refusal to eat specific food groups"; of the children with a "refusal to eat specific food groups", 45.7% exhibited "eating small amounts" and 55.6% "neophobic behavior"; of the children with "preference for a specific food-preparation method", 63.7% exhibited a "refusal to eat specific food groups"; 9.8% of the children exhibited all of these picky eating behaviors, while 29.9% had none of the picky eating behaviors (data not shown).

The proportions of children who refused each food groups and who preferred specific preparation for each food groups are shown in Figures 1 and 2. The three most frequently refused food groups were shellfish, beans, and vegetables, and the three least refused food groups were fish, fruits, and eggs. Children required foods to be prepared in a certain way—mainly for shellfish and beans. Only 3% of children required eggs to be prepared in a certain way. Fish was not likely to be refused; however, it was required to be prepared in a certain way.

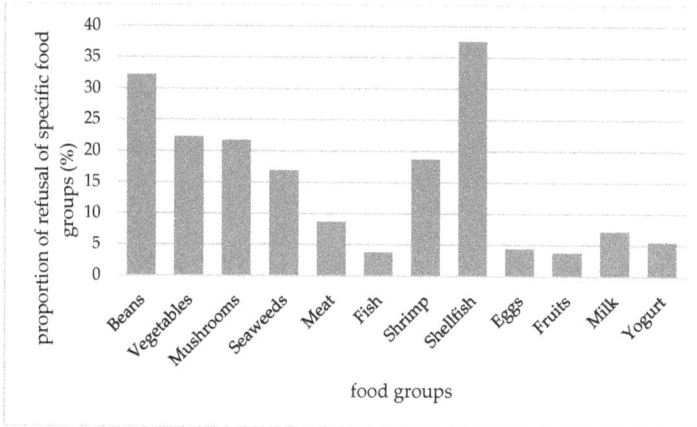

Figure 1. The proportion of children who usually refused a specific food group. The descriptive statistics for the distribution of number of food groups refused as follows: mean $\pm$ SD = 1.8 $\pm$ 1.9, Q_1 = 0, median = 1, and Q_3 = 3.

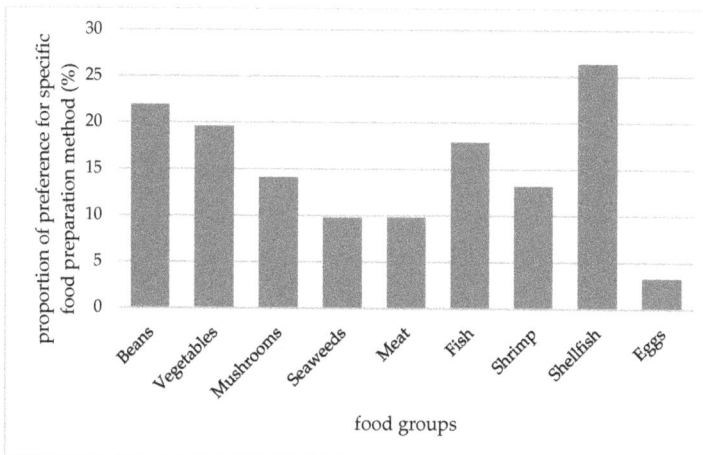

Figure 2. The proportion of children who usually requested food preparation in a certain way for each food group. The descriptive statistics for the distribution of number of food groups with specific preparation as follows: mean $\pm$ SD = 1.2 $\pm$ 1.8, Q_1 = 0, median = 0, and Q_3 = 1.

3.3. Comparison of the Dietary Intake and Growth Indices between Picky Eaters and Non-Picky Eaters

3.3.1. Dietary Intake

The characteristics of the dietary intake of picky eaters—as compared to non-picky eaters—varied with each eating behavior (Table 2). Children considered to be "eating small amounts" had a significantly lower intake of energy and all micronutrients, with the exception of calcium intake. With respect to the picky eating behavior of a limited variety, there was no significant difference in energy intake between picky and non-picky eaters. The children with "neophobic behavior" consumed less dietary fiber per 1000 kcal of energy intake than did their counterparts. Picky eaters with a "refusal of specific food groups" consumed less micronutrients, with the exception of calcium and niacin intake. There was also a significant difference in nutrient density with some micronutrients. The "preference for a specific food preparation method" was related to lower intakes of iron and vitamin A.

3.3.2. Growth Indices

The comparison of growth indices between picky eaters and non-picky eaters are presented in Table 3. Picky eaters "eating small amounts" had lower z-scores for weight-for-age ($p = 0.0010$) and BMI-for-age ($p = 0.0278$) but lower scores for height-for-age, with marginal significance ($p = 0.054$). Picky eaters "eating small amounts" aged 4 to 5 years had significantly lower z-scores for all three growth indices. Picky eaters with "refusal of specific food groups" were related with lower height-for-age in this age group.

Table 2. Comparison of nutrient intakes between picky eaters and non-picky eaters according to specific picky eating behaviors (n = 184).

	Eating Small Amounts			Neophobic Behavior			Refusal of Specific Food Groups			Preference for Specific Food Preparation Method		
	Yes (n = 55)	No (n = 129)	p [a]	Yes (n = 60)	No (n = 124)	p [a]	≥2 (n = 81)	0–1 (n = 103)	p [a]	≥1 (n = 91)	0 (n = 93)	p [a]
						mean ± standard deviation						
Mean daily dietary intake												
Energy (kcal)	1155 ± 340	1340 ± 348	0.0005	1299 ± 393	1278 ± 336	0.6959	1261 ± 364	1304 ± 348	0.2210	1265 ± 361	1304 ± 350	0.1273
Protein (% Energy)	16 ± 3	16 ± 2	0.8880	16 ± 2	16 ± 2	0.0745	16 ± 2	16 ± 2	0.8004	16 ± 2	16 ± 2	0.4553
Lipid (% Energy)	24 ± 5	24 ± 5	0.4794	24 ± 6	24 ± 5	0.4390	24 ± 5	24 ± 5	0.6578	23 ± 5	24 ± 5	0.8095
Carbohydrate (% Energy)	60 ± 6	61 ± 6	0.5902	60 ± 6	61 ± 6	0.1876	60 ± 6	61 ± 6	0.7830	61 ± 6	60 ± 5	0.9370
Calcium (mg)	416 ± 146	449 ± 217	0.2252	440 ± 209	438 ± 194	0.3546	404 ± 157	466 ± 223	0.0919	411 ± 162	466 ± 227	0.0705
Iron (mg)	8 ± 3	10 ± 4	0.0073	9 ± 3	10 ± 4	0.0938	9 ± 3	10 ± 5	0.0198	9 ± 3	10 ± 5	0.0146
Vit. A (µg RE)	393 ± 205	460 ± 239	0.0370	382 ± 187	468 ± 245	0.0859	386 ± 187	483 ± 252	0.0064	404 ± 199	475 ± 254	0.0231
Thiamin (mg)	0.66 ± 0.24	0.78 ± 0.26	0.0116	0.78 ± 0.29	0.72 ± 0.25	0.5680	0.71 ± 0.27	0.76 ± 0.25	0.0367	0.74 ± 0.26	0.75 ± 0.26	0.1562
Riboflavin (mg)	0.9 ± 0.3	1.0 ± 0.3	0.0072	1.0 ± 0.3	1.0 ± 0.3	0.6564	0.9 ± 0.3	1.0 ± 0.3	0.0444	0.9 ± 0.3	1.0 ± 0.3	0.1868
Niacin (mg)	8 ± 3	9 ± 3	0.0018	9 ± 4	9 ± 3	0.2177	9 ± 3	9 ± 3	0.1640	9 ± 3	9 ± 3	0.1754
Vit. C (mg)	77 ± 55	94 ± 61	0.0380	83 ± 64	92 ± 57	0.1119	82 ± 57	95 ± 61	0.0274	89 ± 67	90 ± 52	0.4510
Total Dietary Fiber (g)	11 ± 4	13 ± 5	0.0122	12 ± 5	12 ± 4	0.1032	12 ± 5	13 ± 5	0.0110	12 ± 5	13 ± 5	0.0980
Nutrient density (intake/1000 kcal)												
Calcium (mg)	371 ± 113	332 ± 111	0.2044	336 ± 102	347 ± 117	0.2556	327 ± 103	357 ± 118	0.3166	328 ± 93	359 ± 127	0.1935
Iron (mg)	7 ± 2	7 ± 3	0.2711	7 ± 1	7 ± 3	0.1159	7 ± 1	8 ± 3	0.0524	7 ± 2	8 ± 3	0.0696
Vit. A (µg RE)	349 ± 172	348 ± 172	0.4670	301 ± 151	371 ± 177	0.1554	315 ± 154	375 ± 181	0.0514	325 ± 146	371 ± 192	0.1247
Thiamin (mg)	0.56 ± 0.12	0.58 ± 0.12	0.3715	0.60 ± 0.13	0.56 ± 0.11	0.1805	0.56 ± 0.13	0.58 ± 0.11	0.0335	0.58 ± 0.11	0.57 ± 0.12	0.6568
Riboflavin (mg)	0.8 ± 0.2	0.8 ± 0.2	0.6383	0.8 ± 0.1	0.8 ± 0.2	0.2690	0.7 ± 0.1	0.8 ± 0.2	0.1702	0.7 ± 0.1	0.8 ± 0.2	0.6353
Niacin (mg)	7 ± 1	7 ± 2	0.0758	7 ± 1	7 ± 1	0.0683	7 ± 1	7 ± 1	0.3064	7 ± 1	7 ± 2	0.7212
Vit. C (mg)	68 ± 35	71 ± 42	0.2579	64 ± 42	72 ± 39	0.1617	65 ± 38	73 ± 42	0.0769	69 ± 42	70 ± 38	0.6559
Total Dietary Fiber (g)	9 ± 3	10 ± 2	0.4781	9 ± 2	10 ± 3	0.0167	9 ± 2	10 ± 3	0.0074	10 ± 2	10 ± 3	0.3655

[a] P-value adjusted for age, sex, and education level of both parents. RE: retinol equivalent.

Table 3. Comparison of growth indices between picky eaters and non-picky eaters according to specific picky eating behaviors (n = 184).

	Eating Small Amounts			Neophobic Behavior			Refusal of Specific Food Groups			Preference for Specific Food Preparation Method		
Total subjects (n = 184)	Yes (n = 55)	No (n = 129)	p [a]	Yes (n = 60)	No (n = 124)	p [a]	≥2 (n = 81)	0–1 (n = 103)	p [a]	≥1 (n = 91)	0 (n = 93)	p [a]
Growth status (z-score)												
Weight-for-age	−0.2 ± 0.9	0.2 ± 0.8	0.0010	0.1 ± 0.9	0.1 ± 0.8	0.9797	0.0 ± 0.9	0.1 ± 0.7	0.4137	0.1 ± 0.8	0.0 ± 0.8	0.2268
Height-for-age	−0.5 ± 1.1	−0.2 ± 1.1	0.0545	−0.5 ± 1.3	−0.2 ± 1.0	0.1057	−0.3 ± 1.1	−0.2 ± 1.1	0.8774	−0.1 ± 1.1	−0.4 ± 1.1	0.0275
BMI-for-age	0.0 ± 1.3	0.4 ± 0.9	0.0278	0.5 ± 1.1	0.2 ± 1.0	0.1329	0.2 ± 0.9	0.3 ± 1.1	0.4653	0.2 ± 0.9	0.3 ± 1.2	0.4831
Children aged 1 to 3 years (n = 125)	Yes (n = 42)	No (n = 83)	p [a]	Yes (n = 32)	No (n = 93)	p [a]	≥2 (n = 52)	0–1 (n = 73)	p [a]	≥1 (n = 61)	0 (n = 64)	p [a]
Growth status (z-score)												
Weight-for-age	−0.1 ± 0.9	0.2 ± 0.8	0.0911	0.0 ± 1.0	0.1 ± 0.8	0.8962	0.1 ± 1.0	0.1 ± 0.7	0.6288	0.1 ± 0.9	0.0 ± 0.8	0.5295
Height-for-age	−0.4 ± 1.2	−0.2 ± 1.2	0.3665	−0.7 ± 1.5	−0.1 ± 1.0	0.0657	−0.2 ± 1.2	−0.3 ± 1.2	0.3806	−0.1 ± 1.2	−0.4 ± 1.2	0.1739
BMI-for-age	0.1 ± 1.3	0.3 ± 0.9	0.2833	0.6 ± 1.2	0.1 ± 1.0	0.0575	0.2 ± 0.8	0.2 ± 1.2	0.8383	0.2 ± 0.9	0.3 ± 1.3	0.6564
Children aged 4 to 5 years (n = 59)	Yes (n = 13)	No (n = 46)	p [a]	Yes (n = 28)	No (n = 31)	p [a]	≥2 (n = 29)	0–1 (n = 30)	p [a]	≥1 (n = 30)	0 (n = 29)	p [a]
Growth status (z-score)												
Weight-for-age	−0.6 ± 0.7	0.2 ± 0.7	0.0007	0.1 ± 0.8	0.0 ± 0.8	0.9373	−0.2 ± 0.8	0.2 ± 0.8	0.0750	0.1 ± 0.8	0.0 ± 0.8	0.3427
Height-for-age	−0.8 ± 0.7	−0.1 ± 0.8	0.0049	−0.2 ± 0.9	−0.3 ± 0.7	0.8754	−0.5 ± 0.9	−0.1 ± 0.7	0.0450	−0.1 ± 0.8	−0.4 ± 0.8	0.1434
BMI-for-age	−0.2 ± 0.9	0.4 ± 0.9	0.0194	0.3 ± 0.9	0.3 ± 0.9	0.9966	0.2 ± 0.9	0.4 ± 0.9	0.8184	0.2 ± 1.0	0.4 ± 0.9	0.7406

[a] P-value adjusted for age, sex, and education level of both parents. BMI: body mass index.

4. Discussion

Research on picky eating faces difficulties due to a lack of widely-accepted definitions and appropriate measurement tools. Different definitions used by different researchers may indicate that picky eating behavior is not simple, but rather has complex characteristics that cannot be defined by one single aspect. Thus, in the present study, different aspects of picky eating were clarified and then measured and evaluated separately for their associations with nutritional status. The results suggested that picky eating behavior consists of different constructs showing specific nutrient intake and growth patterns, and the measurement tool could be used to investigate picky eating behaviors and the associated outcomes.

The present study adopted the previous approach to measure the two main constructs of "eating small amounts" and "limited variety" in picky eating behaviors, and the three sub-constructs of "neophobic behavior", "refusal of specific food groups", and "preference for a specific preparation method" in "limited variety" [19,23]. "Eating small amounts" refers to consuming insufficient food, and "limited variety" includes "neophobic behavior", which refers to avoiding new foods and a "refusal of specific food groups" as well as a "preference for a specific preparation method", which refers to children's likes and dislikes of specific foods and certain recipes for each food [19,23]. While children show more than one construct behavior simultaneously and the classification of children overlapped, this approach could find a specific association between children's eating behaviors and diet and growth.

Children "eating small amounts" consumed less energy and nutrients and had lower scores for growth indices compared with non-picky eaters in the present study. The frequently reported behaviors of picky eating children were spitting food out, eating avoidance, or throwing food, which may lead to "eating small amounts" [33]. Additionally, caregivers who experienced feeding difficulties reported that their children had a low appetite [34]. These fussy behaviors—which lead to consuming less food—were related to dietary problems in the present study. In previous studies, children classified as picky eaters had lower intakes of energy and nutrients, such as vitamin E, folate, and dietary fiber [2,4,5,17], and the children had slower growth rates and gained less weight [2,6,12]. However, the previous studies did not try to identify which specific picky eating behaviors were associated with the nutrient intakes and the growth outcomes.

A longitudinal study reported that children who are picky eaters are more likely to have a low BMI-for-age [12]. The risk was likely to increase when the picky eating problem continued as the children became older [30]. In the present study, it was observed that association between growth indices and picky eating behaviors was more prominent in the older children than in the younger children. Moreover, in the present study, the children with picky eating habits in the older age group had shorter heights and lower BMIs than those in the younger age group, indicating the need for further examination whether unfavorable long-term growth outcomes would be induced by picky eating behaviors.

In other studies, food neophobia and food rejection were related with limited preference for all food groups—especially vegetables and fruits [35,36]. In the present study, picky eaters with behaviors related to choosing a limited variety of foods had a lower quality of diet for some micronutrients, but not energy. However, the "refusal of some food groups" was related to lower height-for-age among children aged 4 to 5 years in this study. This suggests the necessity for further investigation on long-term problems induced by food avoidance, in terms of the negative influence of micronutrient deficiency on linear growth. Younger picky eaters with "neophobic behavior" were likely to have a lower z-score for height-for-age ($p = 0.0657$) and a higher z-score for BMI-for-age ($p = 0.0575$). If food neophobia is not appropriately countered at the period of introduction of complementary food, some food groups may remain refused throughout the life. Thus, in younger children, food neophobia and the long-term impact on growth may be concerns, even though energy consumption is not compromised.

It has been reported that the main reason for rejecting foods is distaste and dislike of color [37,38]. Cooking changes the color, taste, and texture of foods. Many of the children with "preference for a specific food preparation" had the picky eating behavior of "refusal of some food groups", while their dietary intake and growth indices were not compromised. The most dramatic change of children's food choice was fish. It indicated that if children could find an appropriate preparation for disliked foods then they might choose to eat the foods with the preparation. These findings imply that an appropriate food preparation method that positively influences food intake would be helpful for the prevention of poor growth. The impact of "preference for a specific food preparation method" needs to be assessed in further studies.

However, there are some limitations to this study. It was conducted as a cross-sectional study of a well-educated, small-scale sample living in a metropolitan area. Thus, this study was not free from counter causality (i.e., smaller children with less appetite behaving in a way to be classified as picky eaters), and generalizability of the results is limited. Potential confounders were not fully evaluated and controlled for; a few socio-demographic characteristics were controlled for, but other potential covariates such as the child's characteristics and child feeding practices were not. The study variables were measured by the caregiver's report, which represented personal values and expectations. Additionally, separate evaluation of "refusal to eat specific food groups" and "preference for a specific food preparation method" was a novel approach in this area. Therefore, evidence for relevant question forms and response cut-off criteria was scarce. Mean numbers of food groups were adopted as cut-off values, but might seem to be arbitrary. Currently, the two sub-constructs were not absolutely diagnosed, but relatively; nevertheless, association with growth status was observed. Especially strength of the association was dependent on the duration of picky eating behaviors. Further examinations in various populations and exploration of the association with growth outcome through a relevant study design (i.e., a cohort study) could accumulate evidence for more relevant criteria. In addition, the dietary intake of the children was estimated by parents, and the influence of childcare was not considered. Finally, analysis of the association between picky eating behaviors and the adequacy of nutrient intake and growth was stratified by age group; however, the significance of the association was marginal due to the small sample size.

Despite these limitations, the findings from this study should enhance understanding of the association between eating and growth patterns in children. A child's picky eating behavior has several aspects, although they tend to overlap somewhat. Moreover, different aspects of the behaviors seemed to have a different meaning in terms of a child's nutritional status. Further study is required to confirm the causality of the observed associations. Investigations of the development of specific picky eating behaviors and long-term outcomes induced by the specific picky eating behaviors are also required. In addition, various attempts to improve the accuracy of classification of the picky eating behaviors are also required.

5. Conclusions

This study established concepts for—and measurement of—picky eating behaviors, and assessed the association of picky eating with diet and growth in early childhood. The specific measurement—which consisted of the categories "eating small amounts", "neophobic behavior", "refusal of specific food groups", and "preference for a specific food preparation method"—properly explained the characteristics of various picky eating problems in early childhood. The results of this study suggest that picky eating behaviors—especially eating small amounts of food—are related to insufficient nutrient intake, creating an unfavorable growth pattern. However, the long-term impacts of a diet with limited variety need to be identified.

Acknowledgments: This research was supported by Basic Science Research Program through the National Research Foundation of Korea (NRF) funded by the Ministry of Science, ICT & Future Planning (NRF-2013R1A1A2057600 and NRF-2016R1D1A1B03931820).

Author Contributions: J.S. conceived and designed the research; K.K. and M.K. performed the research; K.K., N.K., H.P. and J.S. analyzed the data; H.P. contributed reagents/materials/analysis tools; K.M.K. and J.S. wrote the paper.

Conflicts of Interest: The authors declare no conflict of interest.

Appendix A. Children's Picky Eating Behavior Questionnaire

Eating Small Amounts

1. In general, at the end of a meal how often has your child eaten the amount you think he/she should eat?

Almost Never				Almost Always
1	2	3	4	5

2. How often do you attempt to persuade your child to eat a food?

Almost Never				Almost Always
1	2	3	4	5

3. Does your child have a good appetite?

Very Bad				Very Good
1	2	3	4	5

Limited Variety

Neophobic Behavior

4. How often does your child try new and unfamiliar foods at home?

Almost Never				Almost Always
1	2	3	4	5

5. How willing is your child to enjoy new and unfamiliar food when offered?

Very Unwilling				Very Willing
1	2	3	4	5

Refusal of Specific Food Groups

6. How often does your child refuse the following foods: beans, vegetables, mushrooms, seaweeds, meat, fish, shrimp, shellfish, eggs, fruits, milk, and yogurt?

Food	Almost Never 1	2	3	4	Almost Always 5	Not Applicable
Beans	☐	☐	☐	☐	☐	☐
Vegetables	☐	☐	☐	☐	☐	☐
Mushrooms	☐	☐	☐	☐	☐	☐
Seaweeds	☐	☐	☐	☐	☐	☐
Meat	☐	☐	☐	☐	☐	☐
Fish	☐	☐	☐	☐	☐	☐
Shrimp	☐	☐	☐	☐	☐	☐
Shellfish	☐	☐	☐	☐	☐	☐
Eggs	☐	☐	☐	☐	☐	☐
Fruits	☐	☐	☐	☐	☐	☐
Milk	☐	☐	☐	☐	☐	☐
Yogurt	☐	☐	☐	☐	☐	☐

Preference for a Specific Food Preparation Method

7. Does your child eat any of the following foods only if prepared in a specific way: beans, vegetables, mushrooms, seaweeds, meat, fish, shrimp, shellfish, and eggs?

Food	Almost Never 1	2	3	4	Almost Always 5	Not Applicable
Beans	☐	☐	☐	☐	☐	☐
Vegetables	☐	☐	☐	☐	☐	☐
Mushrooms	☐	☐	☐	☐	☐	☐
Seaweeds	☐	☐	☐	☐	☐	☐
Meat	☐	☐	☐	☐	☐	☐
Fish	☐	☐	☐	☐	☐	☐
Shrimp	☐	☐	☐	☐	☐	☐
Shellfish	☐	☐	☐	☐	☐	☐
Eggs	☐	☐	☐	☐	☐	☐

References

1. Jacobi, C.; Schmitz, G.; Agras, W.S. Is picky eating an eating disorder? *Int. J. Eat. Disord.* **2008**, *41*, 626–634. [CrossRef] [PubMed]
2. Carruth, B.R.; Ziegler, P.J.; Gordon, A.; Barr, S.I. Prevalence of picky eaters among infants and toddlers and their caregivers' decisions about offering a new food. *J. Am. Diet. Assoc.* **2004**, *104*, S57–S64. [CrossRef] [PubMed]
3. Li, Y.; Shi, A.P.; Wan, Y.; Hotta, M.; Ushijima, H. Child behavior problems: Prevalence and correlates in rural minority areas of China. *Pediatr. Int.* **2001**, *43*, 651–661. [CrossRef] [PubMed]
4. Galloway, A.T.; Fiorito, L.; Lee, Y.; Birch, L.L. Parental pressure, dietary patterns, and weight status among girls who are "picky eaters". *J. Am. Diet. Assoc.* **2005**, *105*, 541–548. [CrossRef] [PubMed]
5. Dubois, L.; Farmer, A.P.; Girard, M.; Peterson, K. Preschool children's eating behaviours are related to dietary adequacy and body weight. *Eur. J. Clin. Nutr.* **2007**, *61*, 846–855. [CrossRef] [PubMed]
6. Wright, C.M.; Parkinson, K.N.; Shipton, D.; Drewett, R.F. How do toddler eating problems relate to their eating behavior, food preferences, and growth? *Pediatrics* **2007**, *120*, e1069–e1075. [CrossRef] [PubMed]
7. Ashcroft, J.; Semmler, C.; Carnell, S.; van Jaarsveld, C.H.M.; Wardle, J. Continuity and stability of eating behaviour traits in children. *Eur. J. Clin. Nutr.* **2008**, *62*, 985–990. [CrossRef] [PubMed]
8. Mascola, A.J.; Bryson, S.W.; Agras, W.S. Picky eating during childhood: a longitudinal study to age 11 years. *Eat. Behav.* **2010**, *11*, 253–257. [CrossRef] [PubMed]
9. Kotler, L.A.; Cohen, P.; Davies, M.; Pine, D.S.; Walsh, B.T. Longitudinal relationships between childhood, adolescent, and adult eating disorders. *J. Am. Acad. Child. Adolesc. Psychiatry* **2001**, *40*, 1434–1440. [CrossRef] [PubMed]
10. Taylor, C.M.; Northstone, K.; Wernimont, S.M.; Emmett, P.M. Macro-and micronutrient intakes in picky eaters: A cause for concern? *Am. J. Clin. Nutr.* **2016**, *104*, 1647–1656. [CrossRef] [PubMed]
11. Taylor, C.M.; Wernimont, S.M.; Northstone, K.; Emmett, P.M. Picky/fussy eating in children: Review of definitions, assessment, prevalence and dietary intakes. *Appetite* **2015**, *95*, 349–359. [CrossRef] [PubMed]
12. Dubois, L.; Farmer, A.; Girard, M.; Peterson, K.; Tatone-Tokuda, F. Problem eating behaviors related to social factors and body weight in preschool children: A longitudinal study. *Int. J. Behav. Nutr. Phys. Act.* **2007**, *4*, 9. [CrossRef] [PubMed]
13. Rivera, J.A.; Hotz, C.; Gonzalez-Cossio, T.; Neufeld, L.; Garcia-Guerra, A. The effect of micronutrient deficiencies on child growth: A review of results from community-based supplementation trials. *J. Nutr.* **2003**, *133*, 4010S–4020S. [PubMed]
14. Nicklas, T.A.; Baranowski, T.; Cullen, K.W.; Berenson, G. Eating Patterns, Dietary Quality and Obesity. *J. Am. Coll. Nutr.* **2001**, *20*, 599–608. [CrossRef] [PubMed]
15. Wardle, J.; Guthrie, C.A.; Sanderson, S.; Rapoport, L. Development of the Children's Eating Behaviour Questionnaire. *J. Child Psychol. Psychiatry* **2001**, *42*, 963–970. [CrossRef] [PubMed]

16. Davies, W.H.; Ackerman, L.K.; Davies, C.M.; Vannatta, K.; Noll, R.B. About Your Child's Eating: Factor structure and psychometric properties of a feeding relationship measure. *Eat. Behav.* **2007**, *8*, 457–463. [CrossRef] [PubMed]

17. Carruth, B.R.; Skinner, J.; Houck, K.; Moran, J.; Coletta, F.; Ott, D. The Phenomenon of "Picky Eater": A Behavioral Marker in Eating Patterns of Toddlers. *J. Am. Coll. Nutr.* **1998**, *17*, 180–186. [CrossRef] [PubMed]

18. Jacobi, C.; Agras, W.S.; Bryson, S.; Hammer, L.D. Behavioral validation, precursors, and concomitants of picky eating in childhood. *J. Am. Acad. Child. Adolesc. Psychiatry* **2003**, *42*, 76–84. [CrossRef] [PubMed]

19. Shim, J.E.; Kim, J.; Mathai, R.A.; Team, S.K.R. Associations of infant feeding practices and picky eating behaviors of preschool children. *J. Am. Diet. Assoc.* **2011**, *111*, 1363–1368. [CrossRef] [PubMed]

20. Galloway, A.T.; Lee, Y.; Birch, L.L. Predictors and consequences of food neophobia and pickiness in young girls. *J. Am. Diet. Assoc.* **2003**, *103*, 692–698. [CrossRef] [PubMed]

21. Van der Horst, K. Overcoming picky eating. Eating enjoyment as a central aspect of children's eating behaviors. *Appetite* **2012**, *58*, 567–574. [CrossRef] [PubMed]

22. Dovey, T.M.; Staples, P.A.; Gibson, E.L.; Halford, J.C. Food neophobia and "picky/fussy" eating in children: A review. *Appetite* **2008**, *50*, 181–193. [CrossRef] [PubMed]

23. Shim, J.E.; Yoon, J.H.; Kim, K.; Paik, H.Y. Association between picky eating behaviors and growth in preschool children. *J. Nutr. Health* **2013**, *46*, 418. [CrossRef]

24. Fisher, J.O.; Butte, N.F.; Mendoza, P.M.; Wilson, T.A.; Hodges, E.A.; Reidy, K.C.; Deming, D. Overestimation of infant and toddler energy intake by 24-h recall compared with weighed food records. *Am. J. Clin. Nutr.* **2008**, *88*, 407–415. [PubMed]

25. Jung, H.J.; Han, S.N.; Song, S.; Paik, H.Y.; Baik, H.W.; Joung, H. Association between adherence to the Korean Food Guidance System and the risk of metabolic abnormalities in Koreans. *Nutr. Res. Pract.* **2011**, *5*, 560–568. [CrossRef] [PubMed]

26. Jung, H.J.; Lee, S.N.; Kim, D.; Noh, H.; Song, S.; Kang, M.; Song, Y.J.; Paik, H.Y. Improvement in the technological feasibility of a web-based dietary survey system in local settings. *Asia Pac. J. Clin. Nutr.* **2015**, *24*, 308–315. [PubMed]

27. Rural Development Administration. *Studies on Developing the Software Program for Dietary Evaluation in Rural Area*; Rural Development Administration: Suwon, Korea, 2000; pp. 383–454. (In Korean)

28. Korea Centers for Disease Control and Prevention. *Development of Open-Ended Dietary Assessment System for Korean Genetic Epidemiological Cohorts*; Korea Centers for Disease Control and Prevention: Suwon, Korea, 2008. (In Korean)

29. Group WHOMGRS. WHO Child Growth Standards based on length/height, weight and age. *Acta Paediatr.* **2006**, *95*, 76–85.

30. De Onis, M.; Onyango, A.W.; Borghi, E.; Siyam, A.; Nishida, C.; Siekmann, J. Development of a WHO growth reference for school-aged children and adolescents. *Bull. World Health Org.* **2007**, *85*, 660–667. [CrossRef] [PubMed]

31. Gartner, L.M.; Morton, J.; Lawrence, R.A; Naylor, A.J.; O'Hare, D.; Schanler, R.J.; Eidelman, A.I. American Academy of Pediatrics Section on Breastfeeding. Breastfeeding and the use of human milk. *Pediatrics* **2005**, *115*, 496–506. [PubMed]

32. Margetts, B.M.; Nelson, M. Overview of the principles of nutritional epidemiology. In *Design Concepts in Nutritional Epidemiology*; Margetts, B.M., Nelson, M., Eds.; Oxford University Press: New York, NY, USA, 1997; pp. 3–38.

33. Lewinsohn, P.M.; Holm-Denoma, J.M.; Gau, J.M.; Joiner, T.E.; Striegel-Moore, R.; Bear, P.; Lamoureux, B. Problematic eating and feeding behaviors of 36-month-old children. *Int. J. Eat. Disord.* **2005**, *38*, 208–219. [CrossRef] [PubMed]

34. Wright, C.M.; Parkinson, K.N.; Drewett, R.F. How does maternal and child feeding behavior relate to weight gain and failure to thrive? Data from a prospective birth cohort. *Pediatrics* **2006**, *117*, 1262–1269. [CrossRef] [PubMed]

35. Russell, C.G.; Worsley, A. A population-based study of preschoolers' food neophobia and its associations with food preferences. *J. Nutr. Educ. Behav.* **2008**, *40*, 11–19. [CrossRef] [PubMed]

36. Cooke, L.; Wardle, J.; Gibson, E.L. Relationship between parental report of food neophobia and everyday food consumption in 2–6-year-old children. *Appetite* **2003**, *41*, 205–206. [CrossRef]

37. Addessi, E.; Galloway, A.T.; Visalberghi, E.; Birch, L.L. Specific social influences on the acceptance of novel foods in 2–5-year-old children. *Appetite* **2005**, *45*, 264–271. [CrossRef] [PubMed]
38. Koivisto, U.K.; Sjoden, P.G. Reasons for rejection of food items in Swedish families with children aged 2–17. *Appetite* **1996**, *26*, 89–103. [CrossRef] [PubMed]

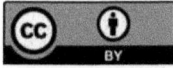

nutrients

MDPI

Article

The Association between Parent Diet Quality and Child Dietary Patterns in Nine- to Eleven-Year-Old Children from Dunedin, New Zealand

Brittany Davison [1], Pouya Saeedi [1], Katherine Black [1], Harriet Harrex [1], Jillian Haszard [1], Kim Meredith-Jones [2], Robin Quigg [3], Sheila Skeaff [1], Lee Stoner [4], Jyh Eiin Wong [5] and Paula Skidmore [1,*]

[1] Department of Human Nutrition, University of Otago, Dunedin 9054, New Zealand; brittany_davison@hotmail.com (B.D.); pouya.saeedi@otago.ac.nz (P.S.); katherine.black@otago.ac.nz (K.B.);harriet.harrex@otago.ac.nz (H.H.); jillian.haszard@otago.ac.nz (J.H.); sheila.skeaff@otago.ac.nz (S.S.)
[2] Department of Medicine, University of Otago, Dunedin 9054, New Zealand; kim.meredith-jones@otago.ac.nz
[3] Cancer Society Social and Behavioural Research Unit, Department of Preventive and Social Medicine, Dunedin School of Medicine, University of Otago, Dunedin 9054, New Zealand; robin.quigg@otago.ac.nz
[4] Department of Exercise and Sports Science, University of North Carolina, Chapel Hill, NC 27519, USA; stonerl@email.unc.edu
[5] School of Healthcare Sciences, Faculty of Health Sciences, Universiti Kebangsaan Malaysia, Kuala Lumpur 50300, Malaysia; wjeiin@ukm.edu.my
* Correspondence: paula.skidmore@otago.ac.nz; Tel.: +64-(03)-479-8374; Fax: +64-(03)-479-7958

Received: 14 March 2017; Accepted: 4 May 2017; Published: 11 May 2017

Abstract: Previous research investigating the relationship between parents' and children's diets has focused on single foods or nutrients, and not on global diet, which may be more important for good health. The aim of the study was to investigate the relationship between parental diet quality and child dietary patterns. A cross-sectional survey was conducted in 17 primary schools in Dunedin, New Zealand. Information on food consumption and related factors in children and their primary caregiver/parent were collected. Principal component analysis (PCA) was used to investigate dietary patterns in children and diet quality index (DQI) scores were calculated in parents. Relationships between parental DQI and child dietary patterns were examined in 401 child-parent pairs using mixed regression models. PCA generated two patterns; 'Fruit and Vegetables' and 'Snacks'. A one unit higher parental DQI score was associated with a 0.03SD (CI: 0.02, 0.04) lower child 'Snacks' score. There was no significant relationship between 'Fruit and Vegetables' score and parental diet quality. Higher parental diet quality was associated with a lower dietary pattern score in children that was characterised by a lower consumption frequency of confectionery, chocolate, cakes, biscuits and savoury snacks. These results highlight the importance of parental modelling, in terms of their dietary choices, on the diet of children.

Keywords: children; parents; diet quality; dietary patterns

1. Introduction

Good dietary habits need to be developed during childhood, not only to improve short-term health and but also to avoid carrying unhealthy habits into adulthood, which is also associated with negative health outcomes in long term, such as increased risk of cardiovascular disease [1,2]. One key area associated with children's dietary intake is the influence of parental diet [3–5]. Previous research in this area initially focused heavily on the relationships between parental and child consumption of fruit and vegetables [6]. More recent studies have looked at different food groups and/or nutrients, including a review that showed associations between child and parent intake of energy and total fat [7–9]. However, it is unrealistic to assume that foods are eaten in isolation. Instead, it is important to recognise that people consume meals and that there are synergistic relationships between food and nutrients [10]. To consider the diet as a whole, dietary patterns can be used. These take into account the combinations of foods consumed and have been increasingly used alongside individual dietary intake data. Dietary patterns can be derived theoretically or empirically [11].

Theoretical dietary patterns are used to determine how closely people adhere to a diet. For example, the Healthy Eating Index (HEI) is used to measure how well an individual's diet conforms to the US Healthy Food Pyramid [12]. Empirically derived dietary patterns use statistical techniques, such as principal component analysis (PCA), to derive data driven patterns specific to the population of interest [11]. There is little research investigating the relationship between parent and child dietary patterns, particularly with regards to empirically derived dietary patterns. Only three studies have investigated the association between parent and child diet quality, all of which used theoretical methods to determine dietary patterns [7,13,14]. All found positive relationships between parent and child diet quality.

The limited current literature provides an indication that dietary quality is associated between parents and children, although theoretically derived patterns based on the national nutrition guidelines differ between countries. Consequently, any significant relationships found using a particular country specific index may not be applicable to other populations. Secondly, there is a lack of research investigating the relationship between parent and child diets using empirically derived dietary patterns. The objective of the current study was to determine whether a higher parent DQI score based on the New Zealand Food and Nutrition Guidelines is associated with more healthful dietary patterns in New Zealand children aged 9–11.

2. Materials and Methods

2.1. Study Design and Participants

The present study analysed data collected as part of the Physical activity, Exercise, Diet And Lifestyle Study (PEDALS), which was a cross-sectional survey conducted in Dunedin, New Zealand between April and December 2015. Thirty out of 55 primary schools in the greater Dunedin area were invited to participate. The remaining schools were not invited as they had less than 15 Year 5 and 6 pupils on the school roll. In New Zealand, Year 5 and 6 students are typically between 9–11 years old. School principals were sent study invitation packs and if they agreed to participate, the research team visited the school to present at a Year 5 and 6 assembly. Eligible students were given packs to take home, containing letters of information and consent forms for themselves and their parents. Written parental consent and written child assent were both required in order for both the child and parent to participate. The study was conducted in accordance with the Declaration of Helsinki, and all procedures involving human subjects were approved by the University of Otago Human Ethics Committee

2.2. Data Collection

Participating children completed two questionnaires during class time, with assistance for reading questions given from the research team when necessary. The first questionnaire contained questions about the child (date of birth, age, sex, and year at school), their food and drink consumption, and known correlates of these. The second questionnaire focused on physical activity and its correlates. Trained research assistants also measured children's height, weight, waist circumference, handgrip strength, body composition, blood pressure and arterial stiffness. Cardiovascular fitness was assessed using the 20 metre shuttle run test. Child participants also received accelerometers to wear for seven days. The children were given two further questionnaires and an accelerometer to take home to their primary caregiver/parent/guardian. The parent questionnaire covered similar topics to the children's questionnaires. Questions on ethnicity, socio-economic status (SES), height, weight, education and health behaviours were also included. SES was assessed using the New Zealand Deprivation Index Score (NZDep13), which combines nine variables from the 2013 census, reflecting eight dimensions of deprivation, including owning a house and access to a car [15]. The deprivation index is an ordinal scale ranging from one (least deprived) to ten (most deprived). School decile is determined by the deprivation level, as measured by NZDep13, of students attending the school, with the lowest decile rating reflecting the 10% of schools nationwide with students mostly from high deprivation areas. School decile was divided into 'Low' (Deciles 1 to 4) 'Middle' (Deciles 5 to 8) and 'High' (Deciles 9 and 10).

The PEDALS Food Frequency Questionnaire (FFQ) was used to assess the children's usual dietary intake. This was a 28-item non-quantitative FFQ, which incorporates questions from the Health Behaviour in School-Age Children Questionnaire [16]. The PEDALS FFQ has been shown to have acceptable relative validity and reproducibility in this age group [16]. The food items included were fruits, vegetables, milk (standard (full fat), light/semi-skimmed (contains around 1.5 g fat per 100 mL) and trim/skimmed (contains around 0.1 g fat per 100 mL), cheese, yoghurt, ice cream, processed meats, other meats, fish, fruit juice, fizzy drinks (diet and standard), breakfast cereals, bread (white and brown/wholemeal), rice, pasta, potato, potato chips, hot chips, biscuits, bakery food, snack bars, lollies/sweets, chocolate, tomato sauce/ketchup and sandwich spreads. Participants reported their usual intake from seven categories ranging from 'Never' to 'Every day, more than once.'

Included in the second parent questionnaire was a dietary habits questionnaire (DHQ), which was used to assess parental dietary intake and eating habits, and was used in the 2008–2009 Adult Nutrition Survey in New Zealand [17]. This DHQ focused on food choices made over the previous four weeks. Nineteen questions were included, beginning with ten questions assessing intake of red and processed meat, chicken, fish and shellfish, hot chips, soft drinks and energy drinks, fruit juice and confectionery. Participants reported consumption from one of six categories: never; less than once a week; one to two times per week; three to four times a week; five to six times a week; seven or more times per week. There were five questions on dietary practices, such as removing fat from meat and chicken, adding salt to food, and choosing low fat and salt varieties over standard varieties. Lastly, there were four questions on type of milk, butter or margarine, bread and cooking fat used most often. Information was also collected on the highest level of education obtained by the parent participant and answers were collapsed into three groups—Secondary education until around minimum school leaving age (15 to 16 years) or equivalent, further secondary school completion (usually around 18 years), and post-secondary education.

Missing data were imputed for certain questions from the questionnaires. For responses to be imputed, at least 75% of each set of questions, where a question had at least four sub-questions, needed to have been completed and 'worst-case scenario' responses were entered. For these analyses, the only data that were imputed were for the FFQ and the DHQ. The FFQ was considered a question, and each item within it a sub-question. Thirty-five data points (0.25% of the total) were imputed for the entire FFQ dataset. The DHQ was also considered a question, and each item within it a sub-question. Seventy-two data points (0.85% of the total) were imputed for the entire DHQ dataset.

2.3. Statistical Analysis

Participants (child and parent pair) were excluded if they did not have complete information on all variables of interest for this analysis. For descriptive analyses, ethnicity was categorised into three groups, as in previous New Zealand surveys [17]: 'Māori'; 'Pacific People'; and 'New Zealand European and Other' (NZEO) were prioritised in that order. NZEO includes those who identify as New Zealand European, as well as other groups that were too small for individual analysis, such as Indian and Korean. Due to the small number of Māori and Pacific Island participants in the sample, ethnicity was further condensed to two groups: 'Māori and Pacific People' and 'NZEO' when included in multivariate analysis. Child body mass index (BMI) was calculated using measured height and weight, z-scores calculated using World Health Organisation (WHO) growth charts and categorised using the WHO categorization [18]. Self-reported height and weight were used to calculate parent BMI. A BMI < 25 was categorized as healthy, 25–29.9 was overweight, and ≥ 30 was obese. Twenty-eight food items from the PEDALS FFQ were aggregated into 21 groups based on similarity in nutritional profile. Children's dietary pattern scores were derived using PCA with varimax orthogonal rotation. Determining the number of components (patterns) was based on eigenvalues >1 and identification of the elbow in the scree plot [19]. Once the patterns had been identified, food groups within these patterns with factor loadings ≥0.2 were considered significant when naming the patterns. Skew was removed from the distribution of the scores and then scores were standardized. A dietary quality index (DQI) for parents was calculated from the DHQ data. This was slightly modified from that developed by Wong et al. for New Zealand adolescents aged 16–18 years [20]. The only modifications made to the adult index, compared to the published adolescent index, were the exclusion of the items assessing frequency of consumption of confectionery, fruit juice, processed meat, and type of cooking fat (which loaded very lowly on the index), and the inclusion of two items assessing frequency of adding salt and consumption of reduced-salt foods. This adult DQI showed good validity in the 3993 adult participants from the 2008–2009 New Zealand Adult Nutrition Survey (unpublished data). A 5-point scoring system was used, with scores ranging from 0 to 4. A response that matched a more positive dietary habit was assigned a higher score. The total diet quality score was a summation of scores from 15 items and ranged from 0 to 60.

Mixed regression models were used to investigate associations, with school as a random effect. These were used to determine the difference between boys' and girls' dietary pattern scores and male and female parent DQI scores. Both unadjusted and adjusted models were run for the association between parent DQI score and child dietary patterns. Adjustment was made for parent age, sex and BMI; child age, sex, ethnicity and BMI z-score; and level of deprivation (NZDep13). We also ran an additional model that included parental education, but as the addition of this variable made no difference to any results this is not shown.

Interaction terms between the DQI score and (a) who completed the DQI (mother or father) and (b) sex of the child were included to determine whether associations between dietary patterns and DQI were moderated by the sex of the parent or the child. If an interaction term was significant, then stratified results were also determined. If not significant, then the interaction term was removed from the model. Regression coefficients (95% CI) and *P* values are presented. Two-sided *p* values of < 0.05 were considered statistically significant. All statistical analysis used Stata 14.1 (StataCorp, College Station, TX, USA).

3. Results

Overall, complete demographic, questionnaire and anthropometric data was obtained from 401 child–parent pairs. Figure 1 provides an overview of school, student and parent recruitment. Seventeen of 30 invited schools took part, with 470 students available on data collection days. Of these, 468 students took part in PEDALS. The majority of students (57%) attended high decile schools (8–10) (Table 1). The mean age of the child participants was 10.2 years. The majority of child participants were of NZEO ethnicity, with 9% identifying as Māori and 3% as Pacific People. Based on the WHO BMI categories, 16% of child participants were overweight and 11% were obese. Parent participants were on average 41.6 years old and the majority of those completing the parental questionnaires were female (83.5%). Overall, 50% of parents were overweight or obese (70% of fathers and 46% of mothers). Forty-seven percent of fathers and 44% of mothers were in the lowest NZDep13 categories (1–3).

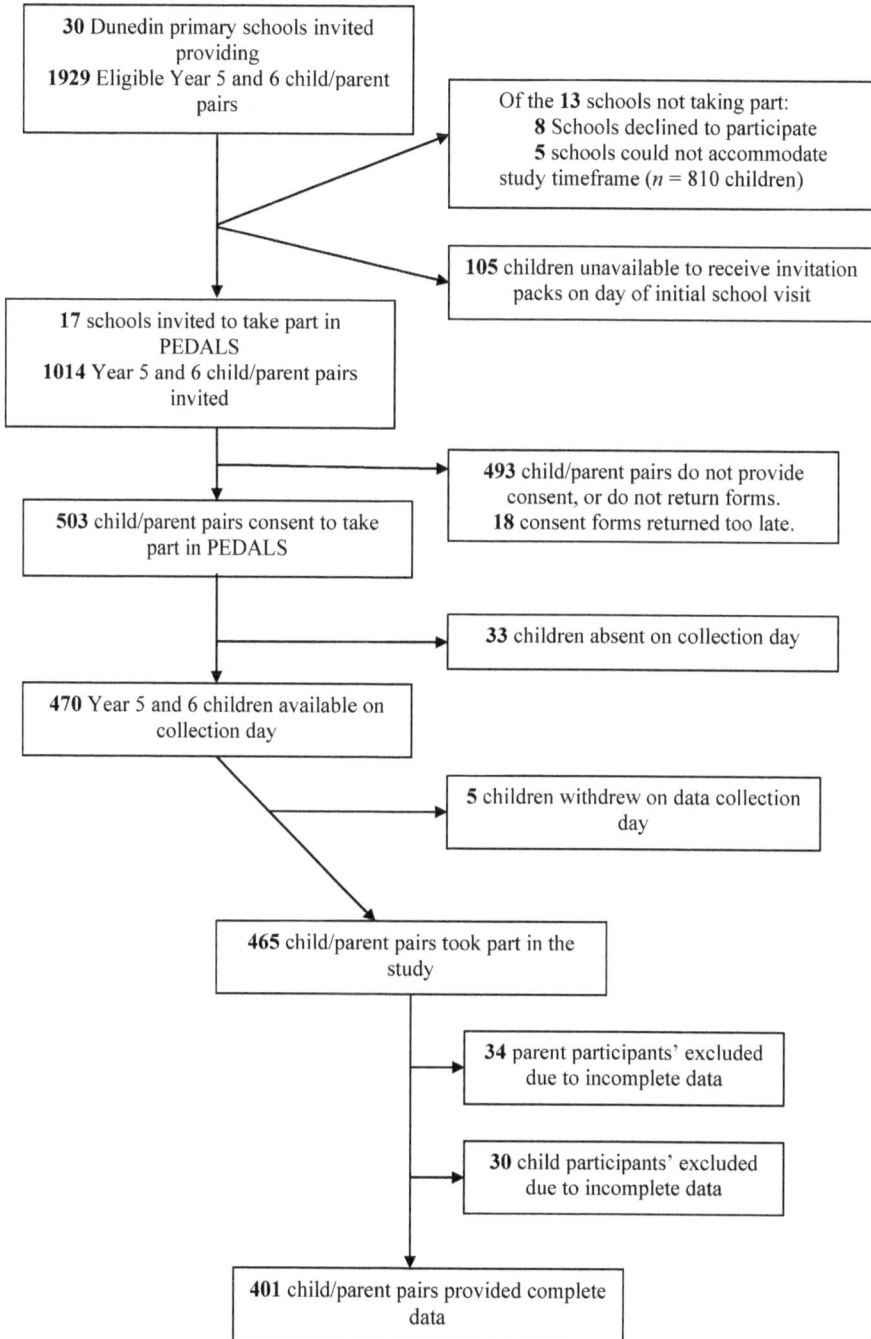

Figure 1. Recruitment flowchart for PEDALS.

Table 1. Characteristics of child and parent PEDALS participants.

Characteristic	Total Children (n = 401)		Boys (n = 198)		Girls (n = 203)		Total Parents (n = 401)		Fathers (n = 66)		Mothers (n = 335)	
	n	(%)	n	(%)	n	(%)	n	(%)	n	(%)	n	(%)
Age (years) *	10.2	0.6	10.3	0.6	10.2	0.6	41.6	5.5	43.5	6.3	41.3	5.3
Ethnicity												
Māori	36	9	23	12	13	6	21	5	2	3	19	6
Pacific	11	3	4	2	7	4	4	1	0	0	4	1
NZEO	354	88	171	86	183	90	376	94	64	97	312	93
BMI †												
Underweight/normal	292	73	144	73	148	73	201	50	20	30	181	54
Overweight	66	16	27	13	39	19	133	33	33	50	100	30
Obese	43	11	27	14	16	8	67	17	13	20	54	16
School Year												
Year 5	227	57	104	53	123	61			37	56	190	57
Year 6	174	43	94	47	80	39			29	44	145	43
School decile												
Low (1–3)	26	6	13	7	13	6			6	9	20	6
Medium (4–7)	147	37	67	34	80	39			28	42	119	36
High (8–10)	228	57	118	59	110	55			32	49	196	58
NZDep13 §												
Low (1–3)	180	45	99	50	81	40			31	47	149	44
Medium (4–6)	151	38	66	33	85	42			18	27	133	40
High (7–10)	70	17	33	17	37	18			17	26	53	16
DQI score ‖ (range from 0–60)							43	7	40	6	44	7

* Presented as mean and standard deviation; † World Health Organisation (WHO) criteria used to derive and allocate BMI categories; ‡ Ratings given to schools in New Zealand to determine government funding; deciles range from 1 (low) to 10 (high). The lower the decile, the more funding received; § The New Zealand Deprivation Index 2013; ‖ Diet Quality Index.

Fruits and vegetables were consumed at least once every day by 66% and 56% of children, respectively. Four percent of children consumed fizzy drinks, 4% consumed diet fizzy drinks, 5% consumed lollies/sweets and 5% consumed chocolate every day. Three percent of parents consumed fizzy drink and 5% consumed confectionery every day. Only 1% or less consumed red meat, hot chips or processed meat every day. Standard milk was the most commonly consumed milk by parents (42%) and light grain bread was the most commonly consumed bread (48%).

PCA produced two dietary patterns that explained 37% of the total variance. The patterns were a 'Snacks' pattern and a 'Fruit and Vegetables' pattern (Table 2). The 'Snacks' pattern loaded positively for ice cream, non-dairy drinks, white bread, pasta and noodles, salty snacks, sweet baked items, lollies/sweets, sweet snacks and sandwich spreads. The 'Fruit and Vegetables' pattern loaded positively for fruits, vegetables, trim milk, standard milk, cheese, yoghurt, processed meats, other meats, breakfast cereals and brown/wholemeal bread.

Boys had a significantly higher 'Snacks' pattern score compared to girls 0.13 (SD = 1.0) compared to −0.12 (SD = 1.0), $p = 0.005$. There was no significant difference between boys and girls for 'Fruit and Vegetables' pattern scores ($p = 0.384$). The mean parent DQI score was 43 (SD = 7), with a possible highest score of 60. The mean score for mothers was 44 (SD = 7), four points higher than the mean father score of 40 (SD = 6) ($p < 0.001$). After adjustment for confounders there was a significant inverse relationship between the 'Snacks' pattern score and parent DQI scores, with a one unit increase in parental diet quality score associated with a 0.03SD (CI: 0.02, 0.04) decrease in the child 'Snacks' pattern score (Table 3). There was no significant relationship between the 'Fruit and Vegetables' pattern and DQI score. None of the included interaction terms included in the models were significant (data not shown).

Table 2. Factor loadings (orthogonal varimix rotation) of food items/groups in two identified dietary patterns in 9–11 year-old children in PEDALS.

Food Items/Group	Snacks	Fruit and Vegetables
Fruits	−0.10	0.33
Vegetables (including potato) *	−0.01	0.36
Trim milk (green) [including on cereals, milo, hot chocolate]	−0.03	0.31
Milk (blue) [including on cereals, milo, hot chocolate]	0.02	0.29
Cheese	0.00	0.33
Yoghurt	0.01	0.33
Ice cream	0.28	0.02
Processed meat (such as meat pies, sausage, sausage roll, salami, luncheon, bacon, ham)	0.12	0.25
Other meats (such as mince, beef, chicken)	0.12	0.27
Fish (including canned tuna or salmon, fish cakes, fish fingers, fish pie, battered fish)	0.18	0.14
Non-dairy drinks †	0.31	0.02
Breakfast cereals	0.00	0.25
White bread	0.26	−0.05
Brown /Wholemeal bread	−0.12	0.32
Rice, rice based dishes	0.16	0.10
Pasta (such as spaghetti, macaroni), noodles	0.24	0.12
Salty snacks ‡	0.40	−0.05
Biscuits, cakes, muffins, doughnuts, fruit pies	0.35	−0.04
Lollies/sweets	0.33	−0.09
Sweet snacks §	0.33	0.02
Spreads ‖	0.29	0.02
Eigen value	5.36	2.60
Variance explained	25.5%	12.4%

* Vegetables: "vegetables" + "Potato (such as mashed, boiled)"; † Non-dairy drinks: "Fruit juice (such as Orange juice, Apple juice, Raro, Refresh, Keri, Twist, Ribena"; + "Diet fizzy drinks (such as Diet Coke, Pepsi Max, Sprite Zero and any other "light" or "sugar free" varieties)" + "Fizzy drinks (such as Coke, Pepsi, Sprite, L&P, Fanta, Ginger Beer)"; ‡ Salty snacks: "Potato chips, potato snacks, corn chips" + "Hot chips, wedges, French fries"; § Sweet snacks: "Snack bars (such as muesli bar, fruit bar, rice bubble bar)" + "Chocolate, Chocolate bars"; ‖ Spreads: "Tomato sauce, Ketchup" + "Peanut butter, Nutella" + "Jam, honey".

Table 3. Associations between children dietary patterns and parent Diet Quality Index Scores.

		DQI Score				
		Unadjusted			Adjusted *	
	β	(95% CI)	*p*	β	(95% CI)	*p*
'Snacks'	−0.04	−0.05, −0.02	<0.001	−0.03	−0.04, −0.02	<0.001
'Fruit and Vegetables'	0.01	−0.002, 0.03	0.091	0.01	−0.001, 0.03	0.060

* Adjusted for parent age, sex and BMI, and child age, sex, ethnicity and BMI z-score, and level of deprivation (NZDep13).

4. Discussion

This is the first study globally to investigate the relationship between parental and child dietary patterns using theoretical and empirical methods of derivation, respectively. The results indicate that there is an inverse association between parent diet quality and the child 'Snacks' pattern.

In this study, 66% of children consumed fruit at least once daily, whereas only 4% had fizzy drinks every day, suggesting that this sample of children had relatively healthy diets. However, it cannot be concluded whether or not the children were reaching the recommended three servings of vegetables and two servings of fruit per day as this information cannot be derived from a non-quantitative FFQ. Data from a nationally representative New Zealand study conducted in 2008–2009 shows that only 30% of 5–9 years old and less than 38% of 10–14 years old were achieving both recommendations [21]. As the sample from the current study had relatively low levels of deprivation and the children were mainly from the NZEO group, it is possible that a higher proportion of children were having five servings of fruit and vegetables per day compared to the national average. However, this is purely speculation, given the nature of the FFQ used in this study.

Two dietary patterns were derived from the child FFQ data using PCA: 'Snacks' and 'Fruit and Vegetables'. Though empirically derived dietary patterns are specific to the population of interest, similarities across studies are commonly seen, allowing for comparisons between populations. The 'Snacks' pattern and 'Fruit and Vegetables' patterns derived in this study resemble patterns in other studies with similar aged children across the Western world [22–24]. Whilst the naming of the patterns varies, the foods contributing the most to these patterns are comparable. For example, Oellingrath et al. [23] derived a 'Varied Norwegian' pattern in 924 children aged 9–10 years, which is similar to the 'Fruit and Vegetables' pattern derived in this study. Food groups that loaded positively in both of these patterns included fruit, vegetables, potatoes, cheese, yoghurt and brown bread. The results from this study show that boys have a higher 'Snacks' score compared to the girls. This finding is also similar to the Oellingrath et al. study [23] who found that boys had a higher score for their 'Snacking' pattern. It is not surprising that in both studies, boys had a more frequent consumption of treat and junk type foods that taste good due to their high fat and/or sugar content, as previous research has suggested that taste is a major influence in boys' food preference and food choice [24]. Conversely, girls report to be more influenced by how healthy foods are than how they taste [25,26].

In the current study, parents' diet quality was negatively associated with the children's 'Snacks' pattern. This suggests that if parents have a poorer quality diet, their children's overall diet consists of a more frequent consumption of less healthful foods. Though there are no other studies investigating the relationship between theoretically and empirically derived dietary patterns in parents and children, there is other evidence to suggest that diet quality are closely positively related between parents and children [7,13]. We found that adjustment for parental education had no real effect on any analyses but this is likely to be due to that fact that 71% of participating parents had post-secondary school level education.

Using an a priori dietary score to measure dietary quality in children is controversial, as some investigators believe further validation and longitudinal research is needed before these can be used in epidemiological studies [27]. The rationale behind this is that it is unknown which study designs and settings are most appropriate when utilising a priori scores to determine paediatric disease risk [27]. The use of PCA, and derivation of multiple also allows for investigation of the relationship between parental diet quality and different aspects of the child diet.

It is likely that the overall diets of 9–12 year-old children are associated with their parent's diets due to the lack of autonomy children have at this age in regard to dietary choices. Children in this age range consume at least two-thirds of their meals at home and are provided with nearly all of their food by their parents [13]. The literature convincingly suggests that many individual foods consumed by children are influenced by their parent's intakes [6–9]. At this age, parents are considered to be one of the strongest influences on children's diets [28–30]. It is therefore interesting that in the current study only certain combinations of foods and drinks that loaded strongly in the patterns were significantly associated with parent diet quality ('Snacks' pattern), while others were not ('Fruit and Vegetables' pattern). It may be that associations are attenuated as some parental questionnaires were completed by the child's male caregiver. The non-quantitative nature of the child FFQ may also explain these results. However, it may also be because the snack type foods are the ones that children may have more autonomy over, rather than those provided in main meals.

It is important to remember that the cross-sectional nature of this study means that directions of relationships cannot be measured. However, if we could assume that the parental diet influences the diet of their child, then improving parent diet quality has the potential to positively change children's diets. Data from the 2014–2015 New Zealand Health Survey shows that approximately 64% of adults consume three or more servings of vegetables daily and 57% consume two or more servings of fruit daily [31]. If more New Zealand parents can reach these targets, then the likelihood of their children also doing this may be increased. However, given the fact that significant relationships were only seen for the "Snacks" pattern, a focus on reducing consumption of less healthy foods by parents may be a more effective strategy.

As children grow into adolescents, the association between parents' and children's diets may weaken due to increased autonomy and greater influences outside of the home, such as school, jobs and social activities [32]. Previous research showing that the odds ratio for healthy diet agreement between parents and children falling from 4.05 for 2–10 years old, to 1.55 for children and adolescents older than 10 years [9]. Such findings highlight how the influences of children's diets change during the transition from childhood to adolescence, making this a key time to optimise food intake. Previous research shows that while dietary habits track from childhood into adolescence and adulthood [1], healthy eating habits also decline, particularly during the transition from childhood to adolescence [33]. Therefore, by providing a family environment that optimizes the development of healthy eating before adolescence, the effects of a decline in healthy eating during adolescents may be less marked. More recent research [34] has also shown that parental influence is also associated with healthier diet behaviours in adolescence. However, it may well be that this is due to maintenance or adaptation of already learned behaviours, rather than learning new behaviours.

Some limitations of this study include the use of a FFQ to measure the children's dietary intake, which only measures frequency, not amounts. In addition to this, the FFQ was relatively short with only 28 items, meaning the entire diet may not have been extensively covered. Despite this, the FFQ was found to be a valid tool for ranking participants according to food group intake [15] and was an appropriate method for this study, where multiple questionnaires were being administered. The DHQ was previously validated in almost 4000 adults so was suitable to be used in this study (unpublished data). Furthermore, although the sample of participants in PEDALS is representative of the Dunedin population it is not nationally representative, as there is a lower proportion of Māori and Pacific people in Dunedin, compared to the whole of New Zealand [33]. This is also reflected in the high proportion of those from higher decile schools and areas of low neighbourhood deprivation and the lower levels of overweight and obesity compared to national level data [35]. However, the schools who were not chosen to take part, or who declined participation, were not markedly different in decile from those who participated and the majority of schools not participating were those of higher deciles. Also, the sample is representative of the population of the South Island of New Zealand [35] and as the majority of New Zealanders are of 'New Zealand European or Other' ethnicity, the results of the current study are likely to be applicable to the majority of New Zealand children.

This study has several strengths, in particular the use of dietary patterns, rather than selected food groups. This is advantageous as dietary patterns look at the diet as a whole. All PCA analyses require some potentially subjective decisions to be made, but this was minimised through the use of standardised methods to group foods and naming patterns in a similar way to previous studies. Sufficient children were recruited into the PEDALS Study to meet the requirements for PCA. At least ten participants per food group entered into PCA are required in order to obtain robust results [36] and the study sample more than met this. Lastly, all questionnaires used were previously tested and validated in similar populations to this sample.

5. Conclusions

The current study found an association between parental diet quality and selected children's dietary patterns. Parents with a poor diet quality were more likely to have children that had a frequent consumption of 'Snacks'. This highlights the need for further investigation into the relationship between parent and child dietary patterns, as poor childhood diet quality remains prevalent in large parts of the world.

Acknowledgments: The authors would like to thank all participating schools for providing appropriate space for us to carry out our data collection, access to the students during class time, and assisting with supervision of students during data collection. We also thank all students and parents who participated in the study and all those who were involved in data collection and processing. PEDALS was funded by the National Heart Foundation of New Zealand (Grant number 1618) and The University of Otago (Grant number ORG 0114-1015).

Author Contributions: B.D., P.S., S.S., K.B. and J.H. were responsible for the development of this particular study and performing data analyses. P.S. is the principal investigator for the overall PEDALS project and was responsible for conception and design of the project and oversaw questionnaire design, data collection and data processing. S.P., H.H., K.M.J., R.Q., L.S. and J.E.W. contributed to the design of the project, including questionnaire design, data collection and processing. B.D. wrote the first draft, under the supervision of PMLS. All authors provided critical review and revision of the manuscript and have read and approved the final version of the manuscript.

Conflicts of Interest: The authors declare no conflict of interest. The founding sponsors had no role in the design of the study; in the collection, analyses, or interpretation of data; in the writing of the manuscript, and in the decision to publish the results.

References

1. Craigie, A.M.; Lake, A.A.; Kelly, S.A.; Adamson, A.J.; Mathers, J.C. Tracking of obesity-relatedbehaviours from childhood to adulthood: A systematic review. *Maturitas* **2011**, *70*, 266–284. [CrossRef] [PubMed]

2. Kaikkonen, J.E.; Mikkilä, V.; Raitakari, O.T. Role of childhood food patterns on adult cardiovascular disease risk. *Curr. Atheroscler. Rep.* **2014**, *16*, 1–15. [CrossRef] [PubMed]

3. Patrick, H.; Nicklas, T.A. A review of family and social determinants of children's eating patterns and diet quality. *J. Am. Coll. Nutr.* **2005**, *24*, 83–92. [CrossRef] [PubMed]

4. Crockett, S.J.; Sims, L.S. Environmental influences on children's eating. *J. Nutr. Educ.* **1995**, *27*, 235–249. [CrossRef]

5. Wardle, J.; Cooke, L. Genetic and environmental determinants of children's food preferences. *Br. J. Nutr.* **2008**, *99*, S15–S21. [CrossRef] [PubMed]

6. Pearson, N.; Biddle, S.J.H.; Gorely, T. Family correlates of fruit and vegetable consumption in children and adolescents: A systematic review. *Public Health Nutr.* **2009**, *12*, 267–283. [CrossRef] [PubMed]

7. Robinson, L.N.; Rollo, M.E.; Watson, J.; Burrows, T.L.; Collins, C.E. Relationships between dietary intakes of children and their parents: A cross-sectional, secondary analysis of families participating in the Family Diet Quality Study. *J. Hum. Nutr. Diet.* **2015**, *28*, 443–451. [CrossRef] [PubMed]

8. Wolnicka, K.; Taraszewska, A.M.; Jaczewska-Schuetz, J.; Jarosx, M. Factors within the family environment such as parents' dietary habits and fruit and vegetable availability have the greatest influence on fruit and vegetable consumption by Polish children. *Public Health Nutr.* **2015**, *18*, 2705–2711. [CrossRef] [PubMed]

9. Wang, Y.; Beydoun, M.A.; Li, J.; Liu, Y.; Moreno, L.A. Do children and their parents eat a similar diet? Resemblance in child and parental dietary intake: Systematic review and meta-analysis. *J. Epidemiol. Community Health* **2011**, *65*, 177–189. [CrossRef] [PubMed]

10. Michels, K.B.; Schulze, M.B. Can dietary patterns help us detect diet–disease associations? *Nutr. Res. Rev.* **2005**, *18*, 241–248. [CrossRef] [PubMed]

11. Newby, P.K.; Tucker, K.L. Empirically derived eating patterns using factor or cluster analysis: A review. *Nutr. Rev.* **2004**, *62*, 177–203. [CrossRef] [PubMed]

12. Lazarou, C.; Newby, P.K. Use of dietary indexes among children in developed countries. *Adv. Nutr.* **2011**, *2*, 295–303. [CrossRef] [PubMed]

13. Beydoun, M.; Wang, Y. Parent-child dietary intake resemblance in the United States: Evidence from a large representative survey. *Soc. Sci. Med.* **2009**, *68*, 2137–2144. [CrossRef] [PubMed]

14. Robson, S.M.; Couch, S.C.; Peugh, J.L.; Glanz, K.; Zhou, C.; Sallis, J.F.; Saelens, B.F. Parent diet quality and energy intake are related to child diet quality and energy intake. *J. Acad. Nutr. Diet.* **2016**, *116*, 984–990. [CrossRef] [PubMed]

15. Atkinson, J.; Salmond, C.; Crampton, C. *NZDep2013 Index of Deprivation User's Manual*; University of Otago: Wellington, New Zealand, 2014.

16. Saeedi, P.; Skeaff, S.A.; Eiin Wong, J.; Skidmore, P.M.L. Reproducibility and relative validity of a short food frequency questionnaire in 9–10 year-old children. *Nutrients* **2016**, *8*, 1–13. [CrossRef] [PubMed]

17. A Focus on Nutrition: Key Findings of the 2008/09 New Zealand Adult Nutrition Survey. Available online: https://www.health.govt.nz/system/files/documents/publications/a-focus-on-nutrition-v2.pdf (accessed on 14 March 2017).

18. de Onis, M.; Onyango, A.W.; Borghi, E.; Siyam, A.; Nishida, C.; Siekmann, J. Development of a WHO growth reference for school-aged children and adolescents. *Bull. World Health Organ.* **2007**, *85*, 660–667. [CrossRef] [PubMed]

19. Osborne, J.; Costello, A. Best practices in exploratory factor analysis: Four recommendations for getting the most from your analysis. *Pan-Pacific Manag. Rev.* **2009**, *12*, 131–146.

20. Wong, J.E.; Skidmore, P.M.L.; Williams, S.M.; Parnell, W.R. Healthy dietary habits score as an indicator of diet quality in New Zealand Adolescents. *J. Nutr.* **2014**, *144*, 937–942. [CrossRef] [PubMed]

21. A National Survey of Children and Young People's Physical Activity and Dietary Behaviours in New Zealand: 2008/09. Available online: https://www.health.govt.nz/system/files/documents/publications/cyp-physical-activity-dietary-behaviours-08-09-keyfindgs.pdf (accessed on 14 March 2017).

22. Aranceta, J.; Perez Rodrigo, C.; Ribas, L.; Serra-Majem, L. Sociodemographic and lifestyle determinants of food patterns in Spanish children and adolescents: The enKid study. *Eur. J. Clin. Nutr.* **2003**, *57*, S40–S44. [CrossRef] [PubMed]

23. Oellingrath, I.M.; Svendsen, M.V.; Brantsæter, A.L. Eating patterns and overweight in 9- to 10-year-old children in Telemark County, Norway: A cross-sectional study. *Eur. J. Clin. Nutr.* **2010**, *64*, 1272–1279. [CrossRef] [PubMed]

24. Nu, C.T.; MacLeod, P.; Barthelemy, J. Effects of age and gender on adolescents' food habits and preferences. *Food Qual. Prefer.* **1996**, *7*, 251–262. [CrossRef]

25. Sweeting, H.N. Gendered dimensions of obesity in childhood and adolescence. *Nutr. J.* **2008**, *7*, 1–14. [CrossRef] [PubMed]

26. Weible, D. Gender-driven food choice: Explaining school milk consumption of boys and girls. *J. Consum. Policy* **2013**, *36*, 403–423. [CrossRef]

27. Marshall, S.; Burrows, T.; Collins, C.E. Systematic review of diet quality indices and their associations with health-related outcomes in children and adolescents. *J. Hum. Nutr. Diet.* **2014**, *27*, 577–598. [CrossRef] [PubMed]

28. Brug, J.; Tak, N.; te Velde, S.; Bere, E.; de Bourdeaudhuij, I. Taste preferences, liking and other factors related to fruit and vegetable intakes among schoolchildren: Results from observational studies. *Br. J. Nutr.* **2008**, *99*, S7–S14. [CrossRef] [PubMed]

29. Davison, K.K.; Birch, L.L. Childhood overweight: A contextual model and recommendations for future research. *Obes. Rev.* **2001**, *2*, 159–171. [CrossRef] [PubMed]

30. Koui, E.; Jago, R. Associations between self-reported fruit and vegetable consumption and home availability of fruit and vegetables among Greek primary-school children. *Public Health Nutr.* **2008**, *11*, 1142–1148. [CrossRef] [PubMed]

31. Ministry of Health. *Tier 1 Statistics 2014/15: New Zealand Health Survey*; Ministry of Health: Wellington, New Zealand, 2015.

32. Videon, T.M.; Manning, C.K. Influences on adolescent eating patterns: The importance of family meals. *J. Adolesc. Health* **2003**, *32*, 365–373. [CrossRef]

33. Birch, L.; Savage, J.S.; Ventura, A. Influences on the development of children's eating behaviours: From infancy to adolescence. *Can. J. Diet. Pract. Res* **2007**, *68*, S1–S56.

34. Draper, C.E.; Grobler, L.; Micklesfield, L.K.; Norris, S.A. Impact of social norms and social support on diet, physical activity and sedentary behaviour of adolescents: A scoping review. *Child Care Health Dev.* **2015**, *41*, 654–667. [CrossRef] [PubMed]

35. 2013 Census QuickStats about Culture and Identity. Available online: http://www.stats.govt.nz/Census/2013-census/profile-and-summary-reports/quickstats-culture-identity.aspx (accessed on 14 March 2017).

36. Floyd, F.; Wildaman, K. Factor analysis in the development and refinement of clinical assessment instruments. *Psychol. Assess.* **1995**, *7*, 286–299. [CrossRef]

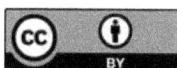

nutrients

MDPI

Article

Food Sources of Energy and Nutrients in Infants, Toddlers, and Young Children from the Mexican National Health and Nutrition Survey 2012

Liya Denney [1,*], Myriam C. Afeiche [1], Alison L. Eldridge [1] and Salvador Villalpando-Carrión [2,3]

[1] Nestlé Research Center, Lausanne 1000, Switzerland; myriam.afeichezehil@rdls.nestle.com (M.C.A.); alison.eldridge@rdls.nestle.com (A.L.E.)

[2] Children's Hospital of Mexico Federico Gómez, National Institute of Health, Mexico City 06720, Mexico; salvador.villalpando@MX.nestle.com

[3] Nestlé Infant Nutrition, Mexico City 11520, Mexico

* Correspondence: liya.denney@rdls.nestle.com; Tel.: +41-21-785-8954

Received: 16 March 2017; Accepted: 8 May 2017; Published: 13 May 2017

Abstract: Food sources of nutrients in Mexican children are not well known. To fill the knowledge gap, dietary intake was assessed in 2057 children using a 24-h dietary recall. All reported foods and beverages were assigned to one of 76 food groups. Percent contribution of each food group to nutrient intake was estimated for four age groups: 0–5.9, 6–11.9, 12–23.9, and 24–47.9 months. Breast milk, infant formula, and cow's milk were the top sources of energy and nutrients, especially in younger groups. Among infants aged 6–11.9 months, the top food sources of energy included soups and stews, cookies, fruit, tortillas, eggs and egg dishes, and traditional beverages. The same foods plus sweetened breads, dried beans, and sandwiches and tortas were consumed as the top sources of energy among toddlers and young children. Milk, soups, and stews were the top contributors for all nutrients and tortillas, eggs, and egg dishes were among the top contributors for iron and zinc. This study showed that low nutrient-dense cookies, sweetened breads, and traditional beverages were among the core foods consumed early in life in Mexico. This compromises the intake of more nutritious foods such as vegetables and fortified cereals and increases the risk of obesity.

Keywords: ENSANUT 2012; infants; toddlers; young children; food sources; energy; nutrients

1. Introduction

Proper nutrition throughout infancy and early childhood is not only vital for optimal growth and development but also helps to lay the foundation for a child's future health [1,2]. The diet in infancy and early childhood is marked by high nutrient needs [3], a transition from an all-milk diet to family foods in the first year of life [4], and the development of food preferences that may affect long-term food choices later in life [5].

The quality of a child's nutrition is shaped by decisions made by parents and caregivers as well as the social and economic environment. At present, Mexico is facing malnutrition characterized by stunting and micronutrient deficiencies in young children from low-income families, iron deficiency anemia in young children, widespread obesity in all age groups, and a high prevalence of non-communicable chronic diseases [6–10]. As for young children, recent studies from the 2012 Mexican National Health and Nutrition Survey (Encuesta Nacional de Salud y Nutrición; ENSANUT 2012) have observed shortcomings in infant and child feeding practices [11]. Examples include a low prevalence of breastfeeding, low consumption of iron-rich foods, and high consumption of sugar-sweetened beverages and sweet foods [12,13]. These shortcomings very likely contribute to the imbalanced nutrient intakes reported in recent dietary surveys, including inadequate intakes of iron, calcium, vitamin D, vitamin E, folate, and fiber and excessive intakes of energy, added sugars, saturated fat, and sodium [14–18].

Quantitative assessment of food sources of energy and nutrients can show what foods are important contributors of nutrients in the population's diet. This knowledge can assist healthcare professionals to form targeted measures to correct shortcomings. Up to now, detailed quantitative analyses on the dietary sources of nutrients in Mexico have been lacking. One recent study conducted in Mexican children under two years of age reported food sources of energy but not nutrients [12]. To fill the knowledge gap, the aim of this study was to describe and identify the principal sources of energy and nutrients in the diets of infants, toddlers, and young children from the ENSANUT 2012.

2. Materials and Methods

2.1. Study Population

ENSANUT is a cross-sectional, population-based survey that characterizes the health and nutritional status of the Mexican population [19]. The survey used a multi-stage, stratified, and clustered sampling system drawn to represent all states, four geographic regions, and socioeconomic strata in Mexico. The data were collected from 50,528 Mexican households, with a response rate of 87% [19]. A total of 2057 children from birth to four years of age were used in the current analysis. The data are presented for four age groups: infants 0–5.9 months (n = 182), infants 6–11.9 months (n = 229), toddlers 12–23.9 months (n = 538), and young children 24–47.9 months (n = 1108). The survey protocol and data collection instruments were approved by the Ethics Committee of the Mexican National Institute of Public Health (Instituto Nacional de Salud Pública). Written informed consent was obtained from each eligible person 18 years and older or from the parent or caregiver of participants under 18 years. The characteristics of the study population have been described previously [13]. Briefly, the majority of children (70%) lived in urban areas. Of the primary caregivers, most often the mother (85%) had an elementary and/or secondary education; 70% were unemployed and 47% were married.

2.2. Dietary Data Collection

One 24-h dietary recall was collected for each child through a face-to-face interview by trained interviewers with the parent or caregiver. The interviewers asked about all foods and beverages and the amount consumed of each item for the previous 24-h period. Custom recipes or standard recipes developed by the National Institute of Public Health were used to estimate the ingredients in mixed food items. The amount of each food item or ingredient consumed was estimated using common household measurement aids (including spoons, cups, slices, handfuls, etc.) and the information was then converted to grams and milliliters depending on the type of food or beverage consumed. To improve dietary recall data, the ENSANUT 2012 implemented an automated five-step multiple-pass method and collected data on both weekdays and weekend days [16].

Quality control of the dietary intake data was conducted in two stages, as reported previously by Lopez-Olmedo and colleagues [16]. Briefly, in the first stage, the foods reported by a participant were reviewed and information including coding, quantity reported, recipe ingredients, and the context in which the meal or feeding episode took place was scrutinized. In the second stage, energy and nutrient intakes were reviewed to identify implausible values. The ratio of daily energy intake to estimated energy requirement was calculated for each person and each day and transformed to a logarithmic scale to remove outliers below -3 SDs and above $+3$ SDs. Excessive micronutrient intakes were defined as those that exceeded 1.5 times of the 99th percentile of the observed intake distribution of the nutrient in the corresponding sex and age group [16].

Breast milk consumption was estimated based on the child's age in months and the total amount of other milk (infant formula and cow's milk) reported over the course of the recall day [20,21]. For exclusively breastfed infants aged birth to 5.9 months, an average intake of 780 mL/day of human milk was assumed; for partially breastfed infants, the amount of human milk was computed as

Nutrients **2017**, *9*, 494

780 mL/day minus the amount of infant formula/other milks consumed. For infants aged six to 11 months fed human milk as the sole milk source, the amount of human milk was assumed to be 600 mL/day. For partially breastfed infants, the amount of human milk was computed as 600 mL/day minus the amount of infant formula/other milks consumed. For breastfed young children aged 12 to 17 months, the amount of human milk was computed as 89 mL per feeding occasion. For breastfed young children aged 18 to 23 months, the amount of human milk was computed as 59 mL per feeding occasion [20,21].

2.3. Analytic Methods

Energy and nutrient intakes were estimated based on the food composition database from the National Institute of Public Health in Mexico (67% foods) [22] and the food composition tables from the United States Department of Agriculture's Nutrient Database for Dietary Studies (33% of foods). [23]. To calculate added sugars, the intake of each food was linked at the ingredient level (single foods, standardized recipes) or dish level (custom recipes) to the U.S. Department of Agriculture's National Nutrient Database for Standard Reference [23] and then further linked to the MyPyramid Equivalents Database [24]. Teaspoon equivalents in the Food Patterns Equivalents Database were converted to grams with the use of the ratio 4.2 g/teaspoon. Vitamin A was estimated in retinol activity equivalents using the following formula [25]: Retinol activity = μg retinol + $\frac{1}{2}$ (μg beta-carotene equivalents/6).

To investigate food sources of energy and nutrients, a list of 76 food groups was formed based on previous dietary intake studies in young children in the USA (Table 1) [26–28]. Two trained Mexican dietary research specialists and a nutrition scientist at Nestlé adjusted food groups to incorporate local food culture and reflect the relative role of specific types of foods and beverages in the diets of infants, toddlers, and young children living in Mexico [13]. Some common food mixtures were estimated "as consumed", such as soups, stews, and mixed dishes, and considered a single food item. All foods, beverages, and nutrient supplements were assigned to one of the 76 food groups (Table 1).

Table 1. Food group classifications *.

Milk and Milk Products	**Vegetables**	Pasta mixed dishes
Breast milk	Baby food (vegetables)	**Sweets**
Infant formula (iron fortified powder or fluid)	Dark green/dark green mixtures	Cookies
Cow's milk (fluid, powdered, flavored, whole or reduced-fat)	White potatoes or starchy/starchy mixtures	Cakes
Cheese	Deep yellow/deep yellow mixtures	Pies & pastries
Yogurt (baby food yogurt or yogurt)	Vegetables (all other/other mixtures)	Sweetened breads (sweet rolls, doughnuts, muffins)
Meat/Poultry/Fish/Meat Alternates	100% vegetable juice	Candy
Baby food (meat)	**Fruit**	Mexican desserts
Meats (chicken, turkey or beef)	Baby food (fruit) (apples and apple mixture, bananas and banana mixtures, pear and pear mixtures, other fruit/fruit mixtures)	Ice cream/frozen yogurt/puddings
Fish/shellfish	Canned fruit	Sugars
Game	Fresh or frozen fruit (bananas, berries, nectarines & peaches, pears, melons, guava, other fruit)	Syrups
Hot dogs/cold cuts/bacon/sausage	100% baby fruit juice	Preserves/jelly
Organ meats	100% fruit juice	Fruit-flavored drinks
Pork/ham	**Mixed Dishes**	Carbonated sodas
Dried beans	Beans & rice, chili, bean mixtures with or without meat	Sweetened tea and coffee
Eggs & egg dishes	Beef or pork with vegetables and /or rice/pasta/potatoes	Artificially sweetened powdered beverages
Peanut/nuts/seeds	Chicken or turkey with vegetables and /or rice/pasta/potatoes	Yakult (skimmed milk fermented with *Lactobacillus casei*)
Vegetarian meat substitutes	Fish or shellfish with vegetables and/or rice/pasta/potatoes	Traditional beverages (*atoles, licuados or aguas frescas*)
Grains and Grain Products	Soups & stews	**Other**
Infant cereal	Meat tacos	Butter
Breakfast cereals (plain cereal, cereal flakes, corn flakes or oatmeal)	Vegetable & cheese tacos	Sour cream (whole or reduced fat)
Bread/rolls/biscuits/bagels	Enchiladas	Salty snacks (grain snacks and those made from starchy vegetables)
Tortillas (plain)	Tortillas with fillings/toppings	Condiments, herbs and seasonings
Bars/cereal/granola	Tamales	Salad dressing
Crackers/pretzels/rice cakes	Sandwiches & tortas	Water
Pancakes/waffles/French toast	Wheat-based pasta mixed dishes	Mineral water
Pasta	Pizza	Salsas, *moles, adobo*
Rice	Rice-based mixed dishes	Supplements (fortified or vitamins)

* The food classification scheme was adapted from the one developed by for the Feeding Infants and Toddlers Study [26] and modified to include commonly consumed foods among Mexican children. All foods and beverages were classified into these 76 mutually exclusive categories.

2.4. Statistical Analysis

Stata (StataCorp. 2015 Stata Statistical Software: Release 14. College Station, TX, USA: StataCorp LP) was used to create data files, assign individual foods and beverages to food groups, and calculate the contribution of each food group to the overall intake of energy and nutrients. The weighted percentage contribution of each food group for all infants, toddlers, and young children was calculated by adding the amount of a given nutrient provided by each food group for all individuals and dividing by the total intake of that nutrient consumed by all individuals from all foods and beverages. All estimates incorporated appropriate sample weights to reflect nationally representative results. Only food groups that contributed over 1% of the nutrient intake are presented in this study. Sources of energy and nutrients were assessed separately and are presented for the four age groups mentioned above.

3. Results

Food sources of energy and 14 nutrients in the diets of infants, toddlers, and young children are presented in Table 2 through 16. In each table, the food groups listed present at least 80% of the total energy or nutrient intake.

3.1. Energy, Macronutrients, and Fiber

Different types of milk were the top sources of energy across all age groups but the relative contribution reduced markedly with age. Breast milk, infant formula, and cow's milk were the first, second, and third sources of energy, collectively contributing 89% of total energy among infants 0–5.9 months (Table 2). These milk sources were still the top three sources of energy among infants 6–11.9 months but the total contribution was lower (53%) as more non-milk foods were consumed. Among toddlers 12–23.9 months, cow's milk was the first source of energy, infant formula was the third, and breast milk dropped to tenth. Among young children 24–47.9 months, cow's milk was still the first source of energy but other milk sources were no longer on the list (Table 2).

Foods and other beverages consumed as the top 10 sources of energy among infants aged 6–11 months included soups and stews, cookies, yogurt, fruit, tortillas, eggs and egg dishes, and traditional beverages (Table 2). Food diversity increased with age, but these top sources of energy for 6–11.9-month-old remained in the top 10 sources of energy among toddlers and young children, except for yogurt (Table 2). Other foods added to the top 10 sources of energy in the two older groups were sweetened breads, which ranked fifth among toddlers and third among young children, dried beans, and sandwiches and tortas (Table 2). Among the top 10 sources of energy, cookies, sweetened breads, and traditional beverages collectively provided 7%, 14%, and 15% of total energy among 6–11.9-month-old infants, toddlers, and young children, respectively. These foods, together with other foods and beverages high in sugar, including sweetened tea and coffee, fruit-flavored drinks, carbonated sodas, and candy, provided 19% and 22% of daily energy intake among toddlers and young children, respectively.

Most of the top 10 milk and food sources of energy were also the top sources of protein and fat (Tables 3 and 4) and saturated fat (Supplementary Table S1) in all age groups. Breast milk, infant formula, and cow's milk were the top three sources of protein and fat among infants of 0–5.9 months and 6–11.9 months; cow's milk, soups and stews, and eggs and egg dishes were the top three sources of protein and fat among toddlers and young children (Table 3, Table 4 and Supplementary Table S1). Meats ranked fifth as a source of protein among both toddlers and young children. Tortillas ranked seventh and fourth as sources of protein among toddlers and young children, respectively. Overall, food sources of total fat and saturated fat were similar, with a slightly varied ranking (Table 4 and Supplementary Table S1).

Table 2. Food sources of energy among Mexican infants, toddlers, and young children aged 0–47.9 months by age group from ENSANUT 2012.

Rank	Age 0–5.9 Months		Age 6–11.9 Months		Age 12–23.9 Months		Age 24–47.9 Months	
	Food Group	% of Total	Food Group	% of Total	Food Group	% of Total	Food Group	% of Total
1	Breast milk	52.6	Breast milk	26.7	Cow's milk	13.2	Cow's milk	10.7
2	Infant formula	34.3	Infant formula	16.5	Soups & stews	7.8	Tortillas (plain)	8.3
3	Cow's milk	1.9	Cow's milk	10.2	Infant formula	6.9	Sweetened breads	7.0
4	Baby food (vegetables)	1.0	Soups & stews	6.5	Tortillas (plain)	5.4	Soups & stews	5.7
5	Infant Cereal	1.0	Cookies	4.3	Sweetened breads	4.9	Eggs & egg dishes	5.3
6			Yogurt	3.6	Traditional beverages	4.7	Cookies	4.2
7			Fresh or frozen fruit	3.2	Eggs & egg dishes	4.3	Dried beans	4.1
8			Tortillas (plain)	3.0	Fresh or frozen fruit	4.1	Sandwiches & tortas	4.1
9			Eggs & egg dishes	2.6	Cookies	3.9	Traditional beverages	3.3
10			Traditional beverages	1.7	Breast milk	3.2	Fresh or frozen fruit	3.2
11			Infant cereal	1.7	Yogurt	3.2	Breakfast cereals	2.9
12			Dried beans	1.4	Dried beans	2.8	Meats	2.9
13			Sweetened breads	1.0	Meats	2.7	Yogurt	2.9
14			100% fruit juice	1.0	Breakfast cereals	2.6	Salty snacks	2.8
15			Salty snacks	1.0	Sweetened tea and coffee	2.6	Sweetened tea and coffee	2.2
16					Salty snacks	2.2	Rice mixed dishes	2.1
17					Pasta mixed dishes	1.9	Carbonated sodas	1.7
18					Sandwiches & tortas	1.7	Candy	1.4
19					Rice mixed dishes	1.5	Vegetable & cheese tacos	1.2
20					100% fruit juice	1.5	Tamales	1.2
21					Fruit-flavored drinks	1.3	Fruit-flavored drinks	1.2
22					Tamales	1.2	Bread/rolls/biscuits/bagels	1.2
23							Beef or pork with vegetables and/or rice/pasta/potatoes	1.1
24							Pasta mixed dishes	1.1
25							100% fruit juice	1.1
26							Meat tacos	1.1
27							Chicken or turkey with vegetables and/or rice/pasta/potatoes	1.0
28							Enchiladas	1.0
29							White potatoes	1.0
All food groups		90.8		84.4		83.6		86.9

Table 3. Food sources of protein among Mexican infants, toddlers, and young children aged 0–47.9 months by age group from ENSANUT 2012.

Rank	Age 0–5.9 Months		Age 6–11.9 Months		Age 12–23.9 Months		Age 24–47.9 Months	
	Food Group	% of Total	Food Group	% of Total	Food Group	% of Total	Food Group	% of Total
1	Breast milk	48.0	Breast milk	21.5	Cow's milk	18.2	Cow's milk	14.8
2	Infant formula	40.1	Infant formula	15.9	Soups & stews	9.8	Eggs & egg dishes	10.2
3	Cow's milk	3.3	Cow's milk	13.2	Eggs & egg dishes	8.7	Soups & stews	7.2
4	Yogurt	1.5	Soups & stews	8.9	Infant formula	6.7	Tortillas (plain)	6.4
5	Baby food (vegetables)	1.4	Yogurt	5.3	Meats	6.4	Meats	6.0
6			Eggs & egg dishes	4.7	Dried beans	4.4	Dried beans	5.8
7			Tortillas (plain)	3.0	Tortillas (plain)	4.3	Sweetened breads	5.0
8			Dried beans	2.7	Yogurt	3.5	Sandwiches & tortas	4.9
9			Cookies	2.7	Sweetened breads	3.4	Yogurt	3.1
10			Meats	2.3	Traditional beverages	2.6	Breakfast cereals	2.5
11			Traditional beverages	1.9	Breakfast cereals	2.0	Cookies	2.2
12			Infant cereal	1.7	Cookies	1.9	Beef or pork with vegetables and/or rice/pasta/potatoes	1.7
13			Chicken or turkey with vegetables and/or rice/pasta/potatoes	1.4	Sandwiches & tortas	1.8	Chicken or turkey with vegetables and/or rice/pasta/potatoes	1.6
14					Sweetened tea and coffee	1.8	Traditional beverages	1.6
15					Breast milk	1.8	Sweetened tea and coffee	1.6
16					Chicken or turkey with vegetables and/or rice/pasta/potatoes	1.4	Rice mixed dishes	1.5
17					Pasta mixed dishes	1.1	Meat tacos	1.4
18					Salty snacks	1.1	Salty snacks	1.4
19					Rice mixed dishes	1.1	Fish/shellfish	1.1
20					Tamales	1.0	Bread/rolls/biscuits/bagels	1.1
21							Vegetable & cheese tacos	1.0
22							Tamales	1.0
23							Fresh or frozen fruit	1.0
24							Enchiladas	1.0
All food groups		94.3		85.2		83.0		85.1

Table 4. Food sources of fat among Mexican infants, toddlers, and young children aged 0–47.9 months by age group from ENSANUT 2012.

Rank	Age 0–5.9 Months		Age 6–11.9 Months		Age 12–23.9 Months		Age 24–47.9 Months	
	Food Group	% of Total	Food Group	% of Total	Food Group	% of Total	Food Group	% of Total
1	Breast milk	56.2	Breast milk	33.6	Cow's milk	16.8	Cow's milk	14.2
2	Infant formula	36.2	Infant formula	20.0	Infant formula	9.1	Eggs & egg dishes	9.8
3	Cow's milk	3.4	Cow's milk	13.2	Eggs & egg dishes	7.6	Sweetened breads	9.0
4			Soups & stews	4.8	Soups & stews	7.1	Meats	5.5
5			Cookies	3.7	Sweetened breads	6.1	Soups & stews	5.3
6			Eggs & egg dishes	3.5	Breast milk	4.8	Dried beans	5.1
7			Yogurt	3.2	Cookies	4.0	Sandwiches & tortas	5.0
8			Traditional beverages	1.5	Meats	4.0	Tortillas (plain)	4.2
9			Infant cereal	1.5	Dried beans	4.0	Salty snacks	4.1
10			Salty snacks	1.3	Salty snacks	3.0	Cookies	3.9
11			Dried beans	1.3	Sandwiches & tortas	2.5	Yogurt	2.7
12			Sweetened breads	1.0	Tortillas (plain)	2.4	Breakfast cereals	2.1
13			Tortillas (plain)	1.0	Traditional beverages	2.3	Beef or pork with vegetables and/or rice/pasta/potatoes	1.8
14					Breakfast cereals	2.2	Tamales	1.6
15					Pasta mixed dishes	2.0	Rice mixed dishes	1.6
16					Tamales	1.7	Chicken or turkey with vegetables and/or rice/pasta/potatoes	1.5
17					Yogurt	2.6	Vegetable & cheese tacos	1.4
18					Chicken or turkey with vegetables and/or rice/pasta/potatoes	1.2	Meat tacos	1.4
19					White potatoes	1.1	Pasta mixed dishes	1.3
20							Enchiladas	1.3
21							Traditional beverages	1.2
22							White potatoes	1.0
23							Sweetened tea and coffee	1.0
24							Infant formula	1.0
All food groups		95.8		89.6		84.5		87.0

The top contributors to energy were also the top sources of carbohydrate (Table 5). Tortillas ranked as the seventh source of carbohydrate among infants 6–11.9 months, then became the second and first source of carbohydrates among toddlers and young children, respectively. For added sugar, cookies, yogurt, fruit-flavored drinks, sweetened breads, and traditional beverages were the top sources across the age groups from 6–11.9 months onwards (Table 6). The contribution of carbonated sodas to added sugar was higher with increasing age, ranking fourteenth among infants 6–11.9 months, seventh among toddlers, and second among young children. Overall, the ranking of added sugar from traditional beverages was higher than carbonated sodas.

Fruit was the highest ranked source of dietary fiber among infants in both age categories. Among toddlers and young children, tortillas contributed the most fiber, followed by fruit (Table 7). From six months onwards, soups and stews were also an important source of fiber. Other top sources of fiber were vegetables, dried beans, pasta mixed dishes, and sweetened breads.

3.2. Vitamins

Breast milk, infant formula, cow's milk, and soups and stews were the main sources of vitamin A (Table 8), vitamin E (Table 9), folate (Table 10), and other B vitamins (Supplementary Tables 2–5), with a slightly varied order. Among toddlers and young children, in addition to different types of milk and soups and stews, eggs and egg dishes, dried beans, tortillas, breakfast cereals, and sweetened breads were also important sources of vitamin A, vitamin E, and B vitamins. Fruit ranked as the first source of vitamin C among toddlers and young children, followed by cow's milk, soups and stews, infant formula, and traditional beverages (Table 11). For folate, breast milk was the first source among infants; soups and stews were the first and second source among toddlers and young children, respectively, followed by dried beans and eggs and egg dishes (Table 10).

Table 5. Food sources of carbohydrates among Mexican infants, toddlers, and young children aged 0–47.9 months by age group from ENSANUT 2012.

Rank	Age 0–5.9 Months		Age 6–11.9 Months		Age 12–23.9 Months		Age 24–47.9 Months	
	Food Group	% of Total	Food Group	% of Total	Food Group	% of Total	Food Group	% of Total
1	Breast milk	50.3	Breast milk	22.5	Cow's milk	9.9	Tortillas (plain)	11.9
2	Infant formula	33.1	Infant formula	13.9	Tortillas (plain)	8.2	Cow's milk	8.2
3	Cow's milk	1.7	Cow's milk	7.2	Soups & stews	7.4	Sweetened breads	6.9
4	Baby food (vegetables)	1.3	Soups & stews	7.0	Fresh or frozen fruit	7.4	Soups & stews	5.5
5	100% fruit juice	1.3	Fresh or frozen fruit	5.5	Traditional beverages	6.4	Cookies	5.1
6	Fresh or frozen fruit	1.2	Cookies	5.3	Infant formula	5.9	Traditional beverages	4.6
7	Baby food (fruit)	1.1	Tortillas (plain)	4.9	Sweetened breads	4.9	Breakfast cereals	3.6
8	Infant cereal	1.1	Yogurt	3.9	Cookies	4.6	Sandwiches & tortas	3.3
9	Sweetened tea and coffee	1.0	Traditional beverages	3.0	Sweetened tea and coffee	3.6	Yogurt	3.3
10			Infant cereal	1.8	Yogurt	3.6	Fresh or frozen fruit	3.3
11			100% fruit juice	1.7	Breakfast cereals	3.0	Dried beans	3.0
12			Fruit-flavored drinks	1.6	100% fruit juice	2.6	Sweetened tea and coffee	2.9
13			Dried beans	1.5	Fruit-flavored drinks	2.6	Carbonated sodas	2.9
14			Infant cereal	1.2	Breast milk	2.2	Salty snacks	2.5
15			Rice mixed dishes	1.0	Pasta mixed dishes	2.2	Rice mixed dishes	2.5
16			Sweetened tea and coffee	1.0	Rice mixed dishes	2.0	Fruit-flavored drinks	2.3
17			Salty snacks	1.0	Dried beans	2.0	Candy	2.0
18			Sweetened breads	1.0	Salty snacks	2.0	100% fruit juice	1.8
19			Eggs & egg dishes	1.0	Tamales	1.1	Bread/rolls/biscuits/bagels	1.6
20			Vegetables	1.0	Sandwiches & tortas	1.1	Vegetable & cheese tacos	1.2
21					Candy	1.0	Pasta mixed dishes	1.2
22					Carbonated sodas	1.0	White potatoes	1.1
23							Tamales	1.1
All food groups		92.1		87.0		85.1		84.0

Table 6. Food sources of added sugar among Mexican infants, toddlers, and young children aged 0–47.9 months by age group from ENSANUT 2012.

Rank	Age 0–5.9 Months		Age 6–11.9 Months		Age 12–23.9 Months		Age 24–47.9 Months	
	Food Group	% of Total	Food Group	% of Total	Food Group	% of Total	Food Group	% of Total
1	Yogurt	30.9	Cookies	26.3	Yogurt	14.9	Traditional beverages	12.0
2	Sweetened tea and coffee	14.9	Yogurt	21.6	Cookies	11.8	Carbonated sodas	11.5
3	Traditional beverages	13.1	Fruit-flavored drinks	7.5	Sweetened breads	10.4	Sweetened breads	10.3
4	Bread/rolls/biscuits/bagels	11.6	Sweetened breads	6.4	Traditional beverages	10.3	Yogurt	10.3
5	Mexican desserts	6.0	Ice cream/frozen yogurt/puddings	6.3	Fruit-flavored drinks	8.2	Cookies	7.7
6	Cookies	5.8	Traditional beverages	6.4	Sweetened tea and coffee	7.6	Cow's milk	7.5
7	Fruit-flavored drinks	4.5	Candy	4.8	Carbonated sodas	5.6	Sweetened tea and coffee	6.8
8	Sweet breads	2.6	Bread/rolls/biscuits/bagels	2.3	Breakfast cereals	4.8	Fruit-flavored drinks	6.6
9	Carbonated sodas	2.6	Breakfast cereals	2.0	Candy	4.6	Candy	6.3
10	Canned fruit	1.8	Mexican desserts	1.9	100% fruit juice	3.6	Breakfast cereals	5.1
11	Preserves/jelly	1.8	Salty snacks	1.8	Cow's milk	3.0	Ice cream/frozen yogurt/puddings	2.4
12	Ice cream, frozen yogurt, puddings	1.0	100% fruit juice	1.7	Cakes	2.0	100% fruit juice	1.9
13			Sweetened tea and coffee	1.7	Ice cream/frozen yogurt/puddings	1.8	Bread/rolls/biscuits/bagels	1.6
14			Carbonated sodas	1.5	Mexican desserts	1.7	Cakes	1.5
15			Canned fruit	1.4	Salty snacks	1.6	Yakult	1.5
16			Yakult	1.3	Yakult	1.2	Mexican desserts	1.2
17			Sugars	1.1	Bread/rolls/biscuits/bagels	1.1	Sandwiches & tortas	1.1
18					Artificially sweetened powdered beverage	1.0	Artificially sweetened powdered beverage	1.0
All food groups		96.6		96.0		95.2		95.3

Table 7. Food sources of fiber among Mexican infants, toddlers and young children aged 0–47.9 months by age group from ENSANUT 2012.

Rank	Age 0–5.9 Months		Age 6–11.9 Months		Age 12–23.9 Months		Age 24–47.9 Months	
	Food Group	% of Total	Food Group	% of Total	Food Group	% of Total	Food Group	% of Total
1	Baby food (fruit)	22.1	Fresh or frozen fruit	18.8	Tortillas (plain)	17.8	Tortillas (plain)	19.9
2	Fresh or frozen fruit	15.0	Soups & stews	18.0	Fresh or frozen fruit	15.4	Fresh or frozen fruit	11.4
3	Vegetables	9.7	Tortillas (plain)	14.8	Soups & stews	12.5	Soups & stews	8.6
4	Baby food (vegetables)	9.3	Cookies	5.3	Dried beans	5.7	Dried beans	7.0
5	Infant formula	8.1	Vegetables	5.0	Pasta mixed dishes	5.0	Sweetened breads	4.7
6	Infant cereal	7.8	Dried beans	4.3	Sweetened breads	4.5	Sandwiches & tortas	4.3
7	Soups & stews	5.4	Traditional beverages	4.0	Cookies	3.4	Cookies	3.4
8	Pasta mixed dishes	4.3	Infant cereal	2.2	Traditional beverages	3.1	Salty snacks	2.9
9	Sweetened tea and coffee	3.1	Baby food (fruit)	2.1	Breakfast cereals	2.6	Traditional beverages	2.9
10	Tortillas (plain)	2.9	Pasta mixed dishes	2.0	Vegetables	2.4	Breakfast cereals	2.4
11	Yakult	1.6	Eggs & egg dishes	1.6	Salty snacks	2.2	Pasta mixed dishes	2.1
12	Canned fruit	1.5	White potatoes	1.6	Rice mixed dishes	2.1	Vegetables	1.9
13	100% Vegetable juice	1.0	Chicken or turkey with vegetables and/or rice/pasta/potatoes	1.5	Tamales	2.0	Rice mixed dishes	1.8
14	Cookies	1.0	Rice mixed dishes	1.4	Sandwiches & tortas	1.6	Meat tacos	1.8
15			Fruit-flavored drinks	1.3	100% fruit juice	1.4	Vegetable & cheese tacos	1.8
16			Sweetened breads	1.2	Eggs & egg dishes	1.2	Tamales	1.6
17			Salty snacks	1.2	Vegetable & cheese tacos	1.2	Enchiladas	1.6
18			Infant formula	1.0	Fruit-flavored drinks	1.2	Eggs & egg dishes	1.4
19					White potatoes	1.0	Cow's milk	1.3
20							Bread/rolls/biscuits/bagels	1.2
21							White potatoes	1.2
22							Fruit-flavored drinks	1.0
All food groups		92.8		87.3		86.3		86.2

Table 8. Food sources of vitamin A among Mexican infants, toddlers, and young children aged 0–47.9 months by age group from ENSANUT 2012.

Rank	Age 0–5.9 Months		Age 6–11.9 Months		Age 12–23.9 Months		Age 24–47.9 Months	
	Food Group	% of Total	Food Group	% of Total	Food Group	% of Total	Food Group	% of Total
1	Breast milk	55.2	Breast milk	34.2	Cow's milk	26.7	Cow's milk	26.3
2	Infant formula	35.3	Infant formula	20.3	Infant formula	10.5	Eggs & egg dishes	12.0
3	Baby food (vegetables)	3.0	Cow's milk	15.6	Soups & stews	9.7	Soups & stews	8.4
4	Cow's milk	1.1	Soups & stews	7.0	Eggs & egg dishes	8.7	Breakfast cereals	6.1
5	Infant cereal	1.0	Eggs & egg dishes	2.9	Breast milk	6.0	Traditional beverages	4.2
6			Infant cereal	1.8	Traditional beverages	4.2	Fresh or frozen fruit	3.5
7			Vegetables	1.5	Breakfast cereals	4.0	Dried beans	3.4
8			Traditional beverages	1.4	Dried beans	2.7	Sandwiches & tortas	3.3
9			Fresh or frozen fruit	1.0	Fresh or frozen fruit	2.7	Sweetened tea and coffee	2.0
10			Breakfast cereals	1.0	100% fruit juice	2.0	Rice mixed dishes	1.9
11					Vegetables	1.8	Infant formula	1.7
12					Rice mixed dishes	1.5	Yogurt	1.6
13					Meats	1.4	Vegetables	1.5
14					Cookies	1.2	100% fruit juice	1.4
15					Sweetened tea and coffee	1.1	Meats	1.2
16					Infant cereal	1.1	Cookies	1.2
17							Tamales	1.1
All food groups		95.6		86.7		85.3		80.8

Table 9. Food sources of vitamin E among Mexican infants, toddlers, and young children aged 0–47.9 months by age group from ENSANUT 2012.

Rank	Age 0–5.9 Months		Age 6–11.9 Months		Age 12–23.9 Months		Age 24–47.9 Months	
	Food Group	% of Total	Food Group	% of Total	Food Group	% of Total	Food Group	% of Total
1	Infant formula	48.0	Infant formula	24.1	Eggs & egg dishes	11.9	Eggs & egg dishes	14.7
2	Breast milk	41.9	Breast milk	21.2	Infant formula	11.3	Cow's milk	7.9
3	Pasta mixed dishes	1.1	Soups & stews	8.8	Cow's milk	10.1	Soups & stews	6.1
4	Baby food (vegetables)	1.1	Cow's milk	6.9	Soups & stews	9.0	Dried beans	5.5
5	Vegetables	1.0	Eggs & egg dishes	5.3	Fresh or frozen fruit	5.6	Tortillas (plain)	5.0
6			Fresh or frozen fruit	3.6	Pasta mixed dishes	5.0	Salty snacks	5.0
7			Cookies	2.7	Dried beans	4.0	Sandwiches & tortas	4.8
8			Tortillas (plain)	2.4	Salty snacks	3.9	Breakfast cereals	4.8
9			Pasta mixed dishes	1.9	Breakfast cereals	3.3	Fresh or frozen fruit	4.6
10			Infant cereal	1.9	Cookies	3.3	Sweetened breads	3.0
11			Vegetables	1.5	Tortillas (plain)	3.2	Pasta mixed dishes	2.6
12			Breakfast cereals	1.4	Meats	2.2	Cookies	2.3
13			Salty snacks	1.3	Sandwiches & tortas	2.1	Meat tacos	2.2
14			Dried beans	1.1	Traditional beverages	1.9	White potatoes	2.0
15			Traditional beverages	1.1	Sweetened breads	1.8	Rice mixed dishes	1.8
16			Baby food (fruit)	1.1	Breast milk	1.8	Beef or pork with vegetables and/or rice/pasta/potatoes	1.7
17					White potatoes	1.5	Infant formula	1.7
18					Chicken or turkey with vegetables and/or rice/pasta rice/potatoes	1.4	Chicken or turkey with vegetables and/or rice/pasta/potatoes	1.6
19					Tamales	1.3	Vegetable & cheese tacos	1.6
20					Rice mixed dishes	1.2	Enchiladas	1.6
21					100% fruit juice	1.1	Meats	1.5
22							Tamales	1.0
All food groups		93.1		86.3		86.9		83.0

Table 10. Food sources of folate among Mexican infants, toddlers, and young children aged 0–47.9 months by age group from ENSANUT 2012.

Rank	Age 0–5.9 Months		Age 6–11.9 Months		Age 12–23.9 Months		Age 24–47.9 Months	
	Food Group	% of Total	Food Group	% of Total	Food Group	% of Total	Food Group	% of Total
1	Breast milk	48.1	Breast milk	20.3	Soups & stews	14.4	Sweetened breads	10.9
2	Infant formula	39.0	Soups & stews	15.3	Dried beans	8.3	Soups & stews	10.7
3	Baby food (vegetables)	2.8	Infant formula	15.2	Fresh or frozen fruit	8.0	Dried beans	10.2
4	Vegetables	2.1	Dried beans	6.3	Eggs & egg dishes	7.5	Eggs & egg dishes	8.8
5	Soups & stews	1.3	Fresh or frozen fruit	5.6	Sweetened breads	7.0	Breakfast cereals	7.0
6	Fresh or frozen fruit	1.0	Vegetables	4.8	Cow's milk	6.8	Fresh or frozen fruit	6.4
7			Cow's milk	3.8	Infant formula	6.7	Cow's milk	4.7
8			Eggs & egg dishes	3.8	Breakfast cereals	5.6	Cookies	3.7
9			Cookies	3.4	Cookies	3.5	Sandwiches & tortas	3.2
10			Sweetened breads	1.6	Rice mixed dishes	2.6	Rice mixed dishes	3.2
11			Breakfast cereals	1.5	Vegetables	2.1	Tortillas (plain)	3.0
12			Rice mixed dishes	1.4	Tortillas (plain)	2.0	Salty snacks	1.6
13			Salty snacks	1.3	Breast milk	1.9	Vegetables	1.6
14			Infant cereal	1.3	100% fruit juice	1.8	100% fruit juice	1.5
15			Yogurt	1.0	Pasta mixed dishes	1.6	Traditional beverages	1.1
16					Salty snacks	1.5	Bread/rolls/biscuits/bagels	1.0
17					Traditional beverages	1.5	Enchiladas	1.0
18					Tamales	1.3	Pasta mixed dishes	1.0
19					Sandwiches & tortas	1.1	Infant formula	1.0
20							Yogurt	1.0
All food groups		94.3		86.6		86.2		82.6

Table 11. Food sources of vitamin C among Mexican infants, toddlers, and young children aged 0–47.9 months by age group from ENSANUT 2012.

Rank	Age 0–5.9 Months		Age 6–11.9 Months		Age 12–23.9 Months		Age 24–47.9 Months	
	Food Group	% of Total	Food Group	% of Total	Food Group	% of Total	Food Group	% of Total
1	Breast milk	50.5	Breast milk	28.7	Fresh or frozen fruit	17.8	Fresh or frozen fruit	15.1
2	Infant formula	36.5	Infant formula	16.5	Cow's milk	10.8	Cow's milk	11.7
3	100% fruit juice	2.3	Soups & stews	8.8	Soups & stews	9.9	Soups & stews	9.2
4	Vegetables	2.2	Fresh or frozen fruit	8.5	Infant formula	8.9	Traditional beverages	8.0
5	Baby food (vegetables)	1.6	Cow's milk	7.4	Fruit-flavored drinks	7.1	Fruit-flavored drinks	7.3
6	Baby food (fruit)	1.1	Fruit-flavored drinks	3.3	Traditional beverages	6.6	Dried beans	6.2
7			Infant cereal	3.3	100% fruit juice	5.8	Breakfast cereals	4.9
8			Vegetables	3.2	Dried beans	4.5	100% fruit juice	4.5
9			100% fruit juice	2.2	Breast milk	4.3	Rice mixed dishes	2.6
10			Dried beans	1.9	Breakfast cereals	2.9	White potatoes	1.8
11			Traditional beverages	1.6	Rice mixed dishes	2.2	Eggs & egg dishes	1.8
12			White potatoes	1.1	Vegetables	2.0	Sweetened breads	1.6
13			Baby food (fruit)	1.0	Eggs & egg dishes	1.5	Cookies	1.5
14					Pasta mixed dishes	1.4	Pasta mixed dishes	1.4
15					Cookies	1.2	Vegetables	1.4
16							Infant formula	1.3
17							Vegetable & cheese tacos	1.3
18							Beef or pork with vegetables and/or rice/pasta/potatoes	1.2
19							Enchiladas	1.1
20							Tamales	1.0
21							Sandwiches & tortas	1.0
All food groups		94.2		87.5		86.9		85.9

3.3. Minerals and Electrolytes

Among infants, in general, breast milk and infant formula were the top two sources of calcium (Table 12), iron (Table 13), zinc (Table 14), and potassium (Table 15). Among toddlers and young children, in addition to cow's milk, infant formula, yogurt, soups and stews, tortillas, eggs and egg dishes, and dried beans were also important sources of the above minerals.

Except for young children, infant formula ranked as the first source of iron among both infants 0–5.9 months and 6–11.9 months and toddlers, followed by breast milk, soups and stews, cow's milk, and eggs and egg dishes (Table 13). Tortillas ranked fifth as a source of iron among infant 6–11.9 months and toddlers. Cow's milk was the number one source of iron among young children, followed by eggs and egg dishes, tortillas, and sweetened breads. In addition to different types of milk, yogurt and soups and stews were the top sources of potassium. Fruit was another major source of potassium across all age groups, with the contribution higher with increasing age (Table 15). Soups and stews were the highest contributors of sodium among all age groups except infants 0–5.9 months, followed by cow's milk, eggs and egg dishes, and dried beans (Table 16).

Table 12. Food sources of calcium among Mexican infants, toddlers, and young children aged 0–47.9 months by age group from ENSANUT 2012.

Rank	Age 0–5.9 Months		Age 6–11.9 Months		Age 12–23.9 Months		Age 24–47.9 Months	
	Food Group	% of Total	Food Group	% of Total	Food Group	% of Total	Food Group	% of Total
1	Breast milk	47.2	Breast milk	25.8	Cow's milk	30.1	Cow's milk	28.3
2	Infant formula	40.5	Infant formula	20.1	Yogurt	11.7	Yogurt	9.8
3	Yogurt	2.9	Cow's milk	16.4	Infant formula	10.0	Tortillas (plain)	7.5
4	Cow's milk	2.6	Yogurt	12.2	Traditional beverages	4.9	Traditional beverages	5.6
5	Water	1.1	Soups & stews	3.3	Tortillas (plain)	4.3	Sandwiches & tortas	4.8
6			Infant cereal	3.0	Soups & stews	3.7	Breakfast cereals	4.5
7			Tortillas (plain)	2.2	Breast milk	3.5	Eggs & egg dishes	3.8
8			Traditional beverages	2.0	Eggs & egg dishes	3.1	Sweetened tea and coffee	3.3
9			Eggs & egg dishes	1.2	Breakfast cereals	3.0	Sweetened breads	3.3
10					Sweetened tea and coffee	2.8	Dried beans	3.2
11					Dried beans	1.9	Soups & stews	2.1
12					Sweetened breads	1.9	Fresh or frozen fruit	1.5
13					Sandwiches & tortas	1.9	Infant formula	1.4
14					Fresh or frozen fruit	1.7	Salty snacks	1.3
15					Infant cereal	1.3	Candy	1.0
16					Salty snacks	1.0	Vegetable & cheese tacos	1.0
17							Enchiladas	1.0
All food groups		94.3		86.2		86.8		83.4

Table 13. Food sources of iron among Mexican infants, toddlers, and young children aged 0–47.9 months by age group from ENSANUT 2012.

Rank	Age 0–5.9 Months		Age 6–11.9 Months		Age 12–23.9 Months		Age 24–47.9 Months	
	Food Group	% of Total	Food Group	% of Total	Food Group	% of Total	Food Group	% of Total
1	Infant formula	47.7	Infant formula	22.7	Infant formula	10.1	Cow's milk	9.8
2	Breast milk	34.1	Soups & stews	11.3	Soups & stews	9.7	Eggs & egg dishes	8.4
3	Cow's milk	2.1	Breast milk	7.1	Cow's milk	9.1	Tortillas (plain)	8.3
4	Soups & stews	1.8	Cow's milk	6.7	Eggs & egg dishes	7.0	Sweetened breads	7.8
5	Water	1.6	Tortillas (plain)	4.9	Tortillas (plain)	5.9	Soups & stews	6.7
6	Baby food (vegetables)	1.6	Cookies	4.4	Sweetened breads	5.8	Breakfast cereals	6.6
7	Vegetables	1.5	Infant cereal	4.3	Dried beans	5.3	Dried beans	5.9
8	Fresh or frozen fruit	1.2	Dried beans	4.3	Breakfast cereals	5.1	Cookies	4.6
9	Baby food (fruit)	1.1	Eggs & egg dishes	3.5	Cookies	4.1	Sandwiches & tortas	3.6
10			Baby food (fruit)	2.5	Traditional beverages	3.7	Meats	2.9
11			Traditional beverages	2.4	Meats	2.7	Traditional beverages	2.7
12			Salty snacks	1.9	Fresh or frozen fruit	2.6	Salty snacks	2.4
13			Rice mixed dishes	1.9	Sweetened tea and coffee	2.3	Rice mixed dishes	2.1
14			Vegetables	1.8	Salty snacks	2.0	Infant formula	1.7
15			Sweetened breads	1.6	100% fruit juice	1.7	Sweetened tea and coffee	1.6
16			Breakfast cereals	1.5	Tamales	1.7	100% fruit juice	1.2
17			Fresh or frozen fruit	1.4	Rice mixed dishes	1.7	Meat tacos	1.1
18			100% fruit juice	1.3	Sandwiches & tortas	1.3	Tamales	1.1
19			Sweetened tea and coffee	1.3	Pasta mixed dishes	1.3	Enchiladas	1.0
20					Infant cereal	1.2	Bread/rolls/biscuits/bagels	1.0
21							Fresh or frozen fruit	1.0
22							Beef or pork with vegetables and/or rice/pasta/potatoes	1.0
All food groups		92.7		87.4		84.3		82.5

Table 14. Food sources of zinc among Mexican infants, toddlers, and young children aged 0–47.9 months by age group from ENSANUT 2012.

Rank	Age 0–5.9 Months		Age 6–11.9 Months		Age 12–23.9 Months		Age 24–47.9 Months	
	Food Group	% of Total	Food Group	% of Total	Food Group	% of Total	Food Group	% of Total
1	Breast milk	44.3	Breast milk	21.1	Cow's milk	18.9	Cow's milk	16.0
2	Infant formula	43.3	Infant formula	19.6	Infant formula	9.4	Tortillas (plain)	8.8
3	Yogurt	2.2	Cow's milk	12.6	Soups & stews	7.7	Eggs & egg dishes	7.6
4	Cow's milk	1.9	Yogurt	7.0	Eggs & egg dishes	6.2	Soups & stews	5.9
5	Baby food (vegetables)	1.3	Soups & stews	6.8	Yogurt	6.1	Dried beans	5.7
6			Tortillas (plain)	3.8	Tortillas (plain)	5.8	Yogurt	5.0
7			Infant cereal	3.8	Dried beans	4.2	Breakfast cereals	4.8
8			Dried beans	2.9	Breakfast cereals	4.0	Sandwiches & tortas	4.6
9			Eggs & egg dishes	2.8	Meats	3.8	Meats	4.3
10			Traditional beverages	2.2	Traditional beverages	3.0	Sweetened breads	3.7
11			Vegetables	1.4	Sweetened breads	2.2	Salty snacks	1.8
12			Cookies	1.3	Breast milk	2.0	Cookies	1.7
13			Meats	1.1	Cookies	1.7	Beef or pork with vegetables and/or rice/pasta/potatoes	1.7
14			Breakfast cereals	1.0	Sandwiches & tortas	1.7	Traditional beverages	1.6
15					Pasta mixed dishes	1.4	Rice mixed dishes	1.5
16					Salty snacks	1.4	Meat tacos	1.4
17					Infant cereal	1.3	Sweetened tea and coffee	1.4
18					Sweetened tea and coffee	1.1	Infant formula	1.4
19					Rice mixed dishes	1.0	Vegetable & cheese tacos	1.2
20					Tamales	1.0	Enchiladas	1.1
21							Tamales	1.1
22							Chicken or turkey with vegetables and/or rice/pasta	1.0
All food groups		93.0		87.4		83.9		83.3

Table 15. Food sources of potassium among Mexican infants, toddlers, and young children aged 0–47.9 months by age group from ENSANUT 2012.

Rank	Age 0–5.9 Months		Age 6–11.9 Months		Age 12–23.9 Months		Age 24–47.9 Months	
	Food Group	% of Total	Food Group	% of Total	Food Group	% of Total	Food Group	% of Total
1	Breast milk	48.4	Breast milk	20.8	Cow's milk	15.1	Cow's milk	14.7
2	Infant formula	35.0	Infant formula	14.0	Soups & stews	10.9	Soups & stews	8.6
3	Baby food (vegetables)	2.2	Cow's milk	10.9	Fresh or frozen fruit	8.9	Fresh or frozen fruit	7.2
4	Cow's milk	1.9	Soups & stews	9.9	Infant formula	5.8	Dried beans	6.7
5	Vegetables	1.6	Fresh or frozen fruit	6.8	Dried beans	4.8	Tortillas (plain)	5.3
6	Fresh or frozen fruit	1.5	Eggs & egg dishes	3.6	Sweetened tea and coffee	4.2	Eggs & egg dishes	4.7
7	100% fruit juice	1.5	Yogurt	3.4	Traditional beverages	4.2	Sweetened tea and coffee	4.0
8	Sweetened tea and coffee	1.2	Dried beans	2.9	Tortillas (plain)	3.5	Yogurt	3.8
9	Baby food (fruit)	1.0	100% fruit juice	2.3	Eggs & egg dishes	3.4	Meats	3.1
10			Tortillas (plain)	2.2	100% fruit juice	3.4	Sandwiches & tortas	3.0
11			Vegetables	2.0	Yogurt	3.3	Traditional beverages	2.5
12			Traditional beverages	1.6	Meats	2.7	Breakfast cereals	2.3
13			Infant cereal	1.5	Fruit-flavored drinks	2.3	100% fruit juice	2.3
14			Sweetened tea and coffee	1.5	Vegetables	1.8	Salty snacks	2.0
15			Fruit-flavored drinks	1.3	Breakfast cereals	1.7	Fruit-flavored drinks	1.9
16			Chicken or turkey with vegetables and/or rice/pasta/potatoes	1.2			Sweetened breads	1.9
17					Pasta mixed dishes	1.4	Rice mixed dishes	1.6
18					Rice mixed dishes	1.4	White potatoes	1.6
19					White potatoes	1.2	Vegetables	1.4
20					Salty snacks	1.2	Beef or pork with vegetables and/or rice/pasta/potatoes	1.3
21					Sandwiches & tortas	1.2	Chicken or turkey with vegetables and/or rice/pasta/potatoes	1.2
22					Sweetened breads	1.0	Vegetable & cheese tacos	1.1
23							Meat tacos	1.1
24							Enchiladas	1.0
25							Tamales	1.0
All food groups		94.3		85.9		85.7		85.3

Table 16. Food sources of sodium among Mexican infants, toddlers, and young children aged 0–47.9 months by age group from ENSANUT 2012.

Rank	Age 0–5.9 Months		Age 6–11.9 Months		Age 12–23.9 Months		Age 24–47.9 Months	
	Food Group	% of Total	Food Group	% of Total	Food Group	% of Total	Food Group	% of Total
1	Breast milk	44.6	Soups & stews	16.8	Soups & stews	17.6	Soups & stews	12.2
2	Infant formula	37.4	Breast milk	15.9	Cow's milk	9.9	Eggs & egg dishes	10.6
3	Soups & stews	3.0	Infant formula	12.6	Eggs & egg dishes	8.4	Dried beans	7.3
4	Baby food (vegetables)	2.5	Cow's milk	8.7	Dried beans	7.2	Cow's milk	6.9
5	Vegetables	1.7	Eggs & egg dishes	6.0	Meats	4.2	Sandwiches & tortas	5.8
6	Cow's milk	2.6	Cookies	5.0	Infant formula	4.1	Meats	5.1
7	Water	1.3	Dried beans	3.6	Sweetened breads	3.4	Sweetened breads	4.6
8	Infant cereal	1.0	Yogurt	2.3	Cookies	3.2	Salty snacks	3.9
9			Salty snacks	1.9	Salty snacks	3.2	Rice mixed dishes	3.3
10			Chicken or turkey with vegetables and/or rice/pasta/potatoes	1.9	Traditional beverages	3.2	Tortillas (plain)	3.3
11			Infant cereal	1.7	Rice mixed dishes	2.9	Cookies	3.2
12			Traditional beverages	1.6	Pasta mixed dishes	2.8	Breakfast cereals	2.5
13			Meats	1.4	Breakfast cereals	2.7	Beef or pork with vegetables and/or rice/pasta/potatoes	2.1
14			Rice mixed dishes	1.4	Tortillas (plain)	2.1	White potatoes	1.6
15			Tortillas (plain)	1.1	Sandwiches & tortas	2.0	Bread/rolls/biscuits/bagels	1.6
16			Vegetables	1.1	White potatoes	1.6	Vegetable & cheese tacos	1.5
17			Pasta mixed dishes	1.1	Beef or pork with vegetables and/or rice/pasta/potatoes	1.5	Pasta mixed dishes	1.5
18					Breast milk	1.2	Tamales	1.4
19					Chicken or turkey with vegetables and/or rice/pasta/potatoes	1.1	Enchiladas	1.3
20					Sweetened tea and coffee	1.0	Chicken or turkey with vegetables and/or rice/pasta/potatoes	1.3
21					Bread/rolls/biscuits/bagels	1.0	Carbonated sodas	1.1
22							Meat tacos	1.0
All food groups		94.1		84.1		84.3		83.1

173

4. Discussion

The results of this study provide a comprehensive picture of food sources of energy and nutrients and show the shifts with age among Mexican children aged 0–47.9 months. Previous studies on nutrient intake in this population reported inadequate intakes of iron, calcium, vitamin D, vitamin E, folate, and fiber and excessive intakes of energy, added sugars, saturated fat, and sodium [14–18]. Our data have provided important insights on those findings.

4.1. Milk Sources

Overall, breast milk, infant formula, and cow's milk were the top sources of energy, protein, fat, carbohydrates, vitamins (vitamin A, vitamin E, vitamin C, and B vitamins), and minerals (calcium, iron, zinc, and potassium), especially in younger groups. This is similar to what we observed in studies in the USA [26,29] and in China [30]. However, one difference in this study is that cow's milk was one of the major sources of energy among infants 6–11.9 months. This is a concern because cow's milk is considered to be an inappropriate milk for children under the age of one year as early feeding of cow's milk is associated with an increased risk of developing iron-deficiency anemia [31]. The reasons include its low iron content, poor iron availability, and associated occult intestinal blood loss [32].

4.2. Low Nutrient-Dense Foods and Beverages

As infants and toddlers have a small stomach capacity but high nutrient needs to support their rapid growth, complementary foods should be nutrient-dense, i.e., relatively low in calories and high in vitamins and minerals [3]. However, low nutrient-dense and energy-rich cookies, sweetened breads, and traditional beverages were consumed as core foods in the diet of Mexican children.

These observations are very much aligned with previous findings that showed a high proportion of energy was provided by caloric beverages [12,33] and that added sugar consumption was high among Mexican children aged 1–4 years [16,18]. Our study provided further details as to what foods and beverages contributed to the high added sugar consumption and the relative role of each food. In addition, we found that consumption of sweetened foods and beverages started as early as the second six months of life and some food items shifted with increasing age. For example, the contribution of carbonated sodas to added sugar doubled in young children compared to toddlers. It is important that energy-rich foods, which provide little nutritional benefit, are limited [34]. Reduced consumption of cookies, sweetened breads, sugar sweetened beverages along with lower sugar content of traditional beverages would markedly decrease the total intake of added sugar in Mexican children.

4.3. Food Sources of Iron

Iron-rich foods are lacking in young Mexican children. Iron is of particular importance after six months of age as the infant's iron stores, which are laid down during gestation, are declining [35]. Thus, complementary foods need to provide iron, either from animal-source foods or from fortification, as recommended in the official Mexican guidelines on nutrition [36] and a recent Mexican complementary feeding consensus paper [37]. Given the detrimental consequences of iron deficiency disorders on cognitive and neurological development [38], a recent position paper on complementary feeding stressed the recommendation of iron-rich food consumption [34]. Previous studies in Mexico have shown that iron intake of infants did not meet recommendations [14], heme-iron intake was low [17], and iron-deficiency anemia was prevalent (23%) [10]. It has already been reported that complementary feeding practices in Mexico lack animal foods [39,40]. In our study, we found that meats provided less than 1% of energy among infants 6–11.9 month olds and were not among the top 10 food sources of energy in toddlers and young children. As a result, meats did not markedly contribute to the intake of iron or vitamins. Also of note, iron-fortified infant cereal made a minimal contribution to nutrient intake in this population. However, it is important to note that Mexican tortilla flour is fortified with iron [41], which might explain why tortillas appears as the third to fifth sources of iron after 12 months of age.

Surprisingly, cow's milk was found to be a top source of iron (ranked first among young children). This may be caused by two reasons. One is that a proportion of fortified cow's milk (19.6%) was grouped into cow's milk in this study and hence increased the iron contribution from the cow's milk category. The other reason might be that even though cow's milk is not high in iron, it is frequently consumed, making it a significant iron source.

4.4. Role of Local Foods

The ranking of a food as a source of energy or a nutrient reflects not only the concentration of a nutrient in a food but also the frequency of consumption of the food. Soups and stews were found to be top contributors to energy and almost all nutrients after milk including total fat, saturated fat, and sodium. Soups and stews are frequently consumed in this population [12,13]. Since soups and stews in Mexico typically contain meat (usually chicken), vegetables, and tortillas, it is understandable that these food mixtures can provide a wide range of nutrients.

Tortillas were a top source of energy, protein, carbohydrates, a number of B vitamins, calcium, iron, and zinc, and were the number one source of dietary fiber among toddlers and young children. Again, as a staple food in Mexico, high consumption of tortillas makes them a major contributor to macro- and micronutrients. On the contrary, although the contribution of vegetables (consumed as discrete items rather than as food mixtures) to nutrient intake was minimal, indicating low vegetable consumption, vegetables appeared to be in the top three or top five sources of fiber among infants. This is due to the high content of fiber in vegetables, even though they are infrequently consumed. On the other hand, the fact that tortillas were the number one source of fiber among toddlers and young children suggests that good food sources of fiber are really lacking and explains why fiber intake was low in 87% of children aged 1–4 years in Mexico [16]. In addition to the above, we also found that eggs and egg dishes and dried beans (both among the top 10 sources of energy), were top contributors to a number of key nutrients including protein, vitamin A, folate, iron, zinc, potassium, and fiber (dried beans only) in the diet of this population.

4.5. Limitations

This study was cross-sectional in design, so it is not possible to evaluate changes in food sources among the same children as they grow. We used a single day 24-h dietary recall, which may not reflect usual intake. The grouping of food items was designed to reflect local food culture and to help us understand the relative role of specific types of foods and beverages, but the choice of food groups could have had an influence on the rankings. If no detailed information was available, standard recipes were used for foods prepared at home, which could have led to either underestimation or overestimation of certain nutrients. Nevertheless, a major strength of this study is the use of small age categories and food groups to describe, in detail, the food sources of energy and nutrients and shifts with age in children aged 0–47.9 months using a nationally representative sample of Mexico.

5. Conclusions

This study provides important insights on food sources of energy and nutrients among Mexican children aged 0–47.9 months. The results show that, in addition to milk sources, other types of foods and beverages commonly consumed in Mexico had major contributions to the intakes of energy and nutrients. Foods and beverages high in sugar such as cookies, sweetened breads, and traditional beverages were among the food items commonly consumed from a very young age and contributed increasingly with age to the intake of energy and added sugar. Milk and soups and stews were top contributors to all nutrients. Tortillas and eggs and egg dishes were among the top contributors to iron and zinc. High-fiber foods like vegetables or dried beans were not the top sources of fiber in the diets of children in Mexico. The intake of more nutrient-dense foods such as vegetables, beans, lean meats, and fortified cereals should be encouraged to help address shortfalls in nutrients. Core foods like soups and stews and eggs and egg dishes were the top contributors to sodium, suggesting that they may be suitable targets for sodium reduction. The findings from this study can assist healthcare professionals to develop food-based recommendations to correct the inadequate or excessive intake of certain nutrients in the diets of infants and young children in Mexico.

Supplementary Materials: The following are available online at http://www.mdpi.com/2072-6643/9/5/494/s1, Table S1: Food sources of saturated fat, Table S2: Food sources of thiamine, Table S3: Food sources of riboflavin, Table S4: Food sources of niacin, Table S5: Food sources of vitamin B6.

Acknowledgments: We acknowledge the help of Barry Popkin in accessing and analyzing the ENSANUT data. We thank Phil Bardsley for his work in managing data and programming. Special thanks to Denise Deming, who wrote an initial version of the abstract for the 2016 Experimental Biology Conference and conducted preliminary analyses. We would like to thank the field workers who assisted with the data collection and also the mothers/infants who participated in the study.

Author Contributions: L.D. contributed to data analysis and was responsible for interpreting the data and writing the manuscript, and had final responsibility for this manuscript. M.C.A. contributed to formulating the research question and data analysis, and interpreted the data. A.L.E. and S.V.-C. contributed to data interpretation and the critical review and editing of the manuscript. All authors read and approved the final manuscript.

Conflicts of Interest: The authors declare no conflict of interest. L.D., M.C.A., and A.L.E. are employees of Nestec, S.A. (Nestlé Research Center), Lausanne, Switzerland and S.V.-C. is an employee of Nestlé Infant Nutrition, Mexico City, Mexico. The opinions expressed in the article are those of the authors alone and do not necessary reflect the views of recommendations of their affiliations.

References

1. Weng, S.F.; Redsell, S.A.; Swift, J.A.; Yang, M.; Glazebrook, C.P. Systematic review and meta-analyses of risk factors for childhood overweight identifiable during infancy. *Arch. Dis. Child.* **2012**, *97*, 1019–1026. [CrossRef] [PubMed]

2. Dyer, J.S.; Rosenfeld, C.R. Metabolic imprinting by prenatal, perinatal, and postnatal overnutrition: A review. *Semin. Reprod. Med.* **2011**, *29*, 266–276. [CrossRef] [PubMed]

3. Dewey, K.G. The challenge of meeting nutrient needs of infants and young children during the period of complementary feeding: An evolutionary perspective. *J. Nutr.* **2013**, *143*, 2050–2054. [CrossRef] [PubMed]

4. Word Health Organization. *Guiding Principles for Complementary Feeding of the Breastfed Child*; Pan American Health Organization: Washington, DC, USA, 2002.

5. Schwartz, C.; Scholtens, P.A.; Lalanne, A.; Weenen, H.; Nicklaus, S. Development of healthy eating habits early in life. Review of recent evidence and selected guidelines. *Appetite* **2011**, *57*, 796–807. [CrossRef] [PubMed]

6. Barquera, S.; Nonato, I.C.; Barrera, L.H.; Pedroza, A.; Rivera, J.Á. Prevalence of obesity in Mexican adults 2000–2012. *Salud Pública Mex.* **2013**, *55*, S151–S160. [PubMed]

7. Rivera, J.Á.; de Cosío, T.G.; Pedraza, L.S.; Aburto, T.C.; Sánchez, T.G.; Martorell, R. Childhood and adolescent overweight and obesity in Latin America: A systematic review. *Lancet Diabetes Endocrinol.* **2014**, *2*, 321–332. [CrossRef]

8. Rivera-Dommarco, J.Á.; Cuevas-Nasu, L.; González de Cosío, T.; Shamah-Levy, T.; García-Feregrino, R. Stunting in Mexico in the last quarter century: Analysis of four national surveys. *Salud Pública Mex.* **2013**, *55*, S161–S169. [PubMed]

9. Villalpando, S.; de la Cruz, V.; Levy, T.S.; Rebollar, R.; Contreras-Manzano, A. Nutritional status of iron, vitamin B12, folate, retinol and anemia in children 1 to 11 years old: Results of the ENSANUT 2012. *Salud Pública Mex.* **2015**, *57*, 372–384. [CrossRef] [PubMed]

10. De la Cruz-Góngora, V.; Villalpando, S.; Mundo-Rosas, V.; Shamah-Levy, T. Prevalence of anemia in Mexican children and adolescents: Results from three national surveys. *Salud Pública Mex.* **2013**, *55*, S180–S189. [PubMed]

11. Rivera, J.Á.; Pedraza, L.S.; Aburto, T.C.; Batis, C.; Sánchez-Pimienta, T.G.; González de Cosío, T.; López-Olmedo, N.; Pedroza-Tobías, A. Overview of the dietary intakes of the Mexican population: Results from the National Health and Nutrition Survey 2012. *J. Nutr.* **2016**, *146*, 1851S–1855S. [CrossRef] [PubMed]

12. Rodríguez-Ramírez, S.; Muñoz-Espinosa, A.; Rivera, J.Á.; González-Castell, D.; González de Cosío, T. Mexican children under 2 years of age consume food groups high in energy and low in micronutrients. *J. Nutr.* **2016**, *146*, 1916S–1923S. [CrossRef] [PubMed]

13. Deming, D.M.; Afeiche, M.C.; Reidy, K.C.; Eldridge, A.L.; Villalpando-Carrión, S. Early feeding patterns among Mexican babies: Findings from the 2012 National Health and Nutrition Survey and implications for health and obesity prevention. *BMC Nutr.* **2015**. [CrossRef]

14. Piernas, C.; Miles, D.R.; Deming, D.M.; Reidy, K.C.; Popkin, B.M. Estimating usual intakes mainly affects the micronutrient distribution among infants, toddlers and pre-schoolers from the 2012 Mexican National Health and Nutrition Survey. *Public Health Nutr.* **2016**, *19*, 1017–1026. [CrossRef] [PubMed]

15. Pedroza-Tobías, A.; Hernández-Barrera, L.; López-Olmedo, N.; García-Guerra, A.; Rodríguez-Ramírez, S.; Ramírez-Silva, I.; Villalpando, S.; Carriquiry, A.; Rivera, J.Á. Usual vitamin intakes by Mexican populations. *J. Nutr.* **2016**, *146*, 1866S–1873S. [CrossRef] [PubMed]

16. López-Olmedo, N.; Carriquiry, A.L.; Rodríguez-Ramírez, S.; Ramírez-Silva, I.; Espinosa-Montero, J.; Hernández-Barrera, L.; Campirano, F.; Martínez-Tapia, B.; Rivera, J.Á. Usual intake of added sugars and saturated fats is high while dietary fiber is low in the Mexican population. *J. Nutr.* **2016**, *146*, 1856S–1865S. [CrossRef] [PubMed]

17. Sánchez-Pimienta, T.G.; López-Olmedo, N.; Rodríguez-Ramírez, S.; García-Guerra, A.; Rivera, J.Á.; Carriquiry, A.L.; Villalpando, S. High prevalence of inadequate calcium and iron intakes by Mexican population groups as assessed by 24-hour recalls. *J. Nutr.* **2016**, *146*, 1874S–1880S. [CrossRef] [PubMed]

18. Sánchez-Pimienta, T.G.; Batis, C.; Lutter, C.K.; Rivera, J.A. Sugar-sweetened beverages are the main sources of added sugar intake in the Mexican population. *J. Nutr.* **2016**, *146*, 1888S–1896S. [CrossRef] [PubMed]

19. Romero-Martínez, M.; Shamah-Levy, T.; Franco-Núñez, A.; Villalpando, S.; Cuevas-Nasu, L.; Gutiérrez, J.P.; Rivera-Dommarco, J.Á. National Health and Nutrition Survey 2012: Design and coverage. *Salud Pública Mex.* **2013**, *55*, S332–S340.

20. Devaney, B.; Ziegler, P.; Pac, S.; Karwe, V.; Barr, S.I. Nutrient intakes of infants and toddlers. *J. Am. Diet. Assoc.* **2004**, *104*, S14–S21. [CrossRef] [PubMed]

21. Butte, N.F.; Fox, M.K.; Briefel, R.R.; Siega-Riz, A.M.; Dwyer, J.T.; Deming, D.M.; Reidy, K.C. Nutrient intakes of US infants, toddlers, and preschoolers meet or exceed dietary reference intakes. *J. Am. Diet. Assoc.* **2010**, *110*, S27–S37. [CrossRef] [PubMed]

22. Instituto Nacional de Salud Pública. *Bases de Datos de Valor Nutritivo de los Alimentos (National Institute of Public Health. Food Composition Table)*; National Institute of Public Health: Cuernavaca, Mexico, 2012.

23. United States Department of Agriculture, Agricultural Research Service. SR-27 Home Page. Available online: https://www.ars.usda.gov/northeast-area/beltsville-md/beltsville-human-nutrition-research-center/nutrient-data-laboratory/docs/sr27-home-page/ (accessed on 1 April 2015).

24. Brownman, S.A.; Friday, J.E.; Moshfegh, A.J. MyPyramid Equivalents Database, 2.0 for USDA Survey Foods, 2003–2004. Available online: https://www.ars.usda.gov/ARSUserFiles/80400530/pdf/mped/mped2_doc.pdf (accessed on 16 March 2017).

25. University of Minnesota. Nutrition Coordinating Center—NDSR 2016 User Manual. Appendix 11—Nutrient Information, page A11.5. Available online: http://www.ncc.umn.edu/products/ndsr-user-manual/ (accessed on 12 May 2017).

26. Fox, M.K.; Reidy, K.; Novak, T.; Ziegler, P. Sources of energy and nutrients in the diets of infants and toddlers. *J. Am. Diet. Assoc.* **2006**, *106*, S28–S42. [CrossRef] [PubMed]

27. Fox, M.K.; Condon, E.; Briefel, R.R.; Reidy, K.C.; Deming, D.M. Food consumption patterns of young preschoolers: Are they starting off on the right path? *J. Am. Diet. Assoc.* **2010**, *110*, S52–S59. [CrossRef] [PubMed]

28. Siega-Riz, A.M.; Deming, D.M.; Reidy, K.C.; Fox, M.K.; Condon, E.; Briefel, R.R. Food consumption patterns of infants and toddlers: Where are we now? *J. Am. Diet. Assoc.* **2010**, *110*, S38–S51. [CrossRef] [PubMed]

29. Grimes, C.A.; Szymlek-Gay, E.A.; Campbell, K.J.; Nicklas, T.A. Food sources of total energy and nutrients among U.S. Infants and toddlers: National Health and Nutrition Examination Survey 2005–2012. *Nutrients* **2015**, *7*, 6797–6836. [CrossRef] [PubMed]

30. Wang, H.; Denney, L.; Zheng, Y.; Vinyes Pares, G.; Reidy, K.; Wang, P.; Zhang, Y. Food sources of energy and nutrients in the diets of infants and toddlers in urban areas of China, based on one 24-hour dietary recall. *BMC Nutr.* **2015**. [CrossRef]

31. Griebler, U.; Bruckmuller, M.U.; Kien, C.; Dieminger, B.; Meidlinger, B.; Seper, K.; Hitthaller, A.; Emprechtinger, R.; Wolf, A.; Gartlehner, G. Health effects of cow's milk consumption in infants up to 3 years of age: A systematic review and meta-analysis. *Public Health Nutr.* **2016**, *19*, 293–307. [CrossRef] [PubMed]
32. Borgna-Pignatti, C.; Marsella, M. Iron deficiency in infancy and childhood. *Pediatr Ann.* **2008**, *37*, 329–337. [PubMed]
33. Barquera, S.; Campirano, F.; Bonvecchio, A.; Hernandez-Barrera, L.; Rivera, J.A.; Popkin, B.M. Caloric beverage consumption patterns in Mexican children. *Nutr. J.* **2010**, *9*, 47. [CrossRef] [PubMed]
34. Fewtrell, M.; Bronsky, J.; Campoy, C.; Domellof, M.; Embleton, N.; Fidler Mis, N.; Hojsak, I.; Hulst, J.M.; Indrio, F.; Lapillonne, A.; et al. Complementary feeding: A position paper by the European Society for Paediatric Gastroenterology, Hepatology, and Nutrition (ESPGHAN) committee on nutrition. *J. Pediatr. Gastroenterol. Nutr.* **2017**, *64*, 119–132. [CrossRef] [PubMed]
35. Baker, R.D.; Greer, F.R. Diagnosis and prevention of iron deficiency and iron-deficiency anemia in infants and young children (0–3 years of age). *Pediatrics* **2010**, *126*, 1040–1050. [CrossRef] [PubMed]
36. NORMA Oficial Mexicana NOM-043-SSA2–2012 Basic Health Services. Promotion and Health Education to Food. Criteria to Provide Guidance. Available online: http://dof.gob.mx/nota_detalle_popup.php?codigo=5285372 (accessed on 16 March 2017).
37. Romero-Velarde, E.; Villalpando-Carrión, S.; Pérez-Lizaur, A.B.; Iracheta-Gerez, M.; Alonso-Rivera, C.G.; López-Navarrete, G.E.; García-Contreras, A.; Ochoa-Ortiz, E.; Zarate-Mondragón, F.; López-Pérez, G.T.; et al. Consenso para las prácticas de alimentación complementaria en lactantes sanos. *Bol. Med. Hosp. Infant. Mex.* **2016**, *73*, 338–356.
38. Lozoff, B.; Beard, J.; Connor, J.; Barbara, F.; Georgieff, M.; Schallert, T. Long-lasting neural and behavioral effects of iron deficiency in infancy. *Nutr. Rev.* **2006**, *64*, S34–S43. [CrossRef] [PubMed]
39. González-Cosío, T.; Rivera-Dommarco, J.; Moreno-Macias, H.; Monterrubio, E.; Sepulveda, J. Poor compliance with appropriate feeding practices in children under 2 y in Mexico. *J. Nutr.* **2006**, *136*, 2928–2933.
40. Denney, L.; Reidy, C.K.; Eldridge, A.L. Differences in complementary feeding of 6 to 23 month olds in china, us and Mexico. *J. Nutr. Health Food Sci.* **2016**, *4*, 1–8.
41. Tovar, L.R.; Larios-Saldaña, A. Iron and zinc fortification of corn tortilla made either at the household or at industrial scale. *Int. J. Vitam. Nutr. Res.* **2005**, *75*, 142–148. [CrossRef] [PubMed]

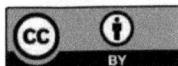

nutrients

MDPI

Article

Advising Consumption of Green Vegetables, Beef, and Full-Fat Dairy Products Has No Adverse Effects on the Lipid Profiles in Children

Ellen José van der Gaag [1,*], Romy Wieffer [2] and Judith van der Kraats [1]

[1] Ziekenhuisgroep Twente, Hengelo, Geerdinksweg 141, Hengelo 7555 DL, The Netherlands; e.gaagvander@zgt.nl (E.J.v.d.G.); judithvanderkraats@hotmail.com (J.v.d.K.)
[2] Isala Zwolle, Dokter van Heesweg 2, Zwolle 8025 AB, The Netherlands; romywieffer@gmail.com
* Correspondence: e.gaagvander@zgt.nl; Tel.: +31-088-708-5315

Received: 14 March 2017; Accepted: 16 May 2017; Published: 19 May 2017

Abstract: In children, little is known about lipid profiles and the influence of dietary habits. In the past, we developed a dietary advice for optimizing the immune system, which comprised green vegetables, beef, whole milk, and full-fat butter. However, there are concerns about a possible negative influence of the full-fat dairy products of the diet on the lipid profile. We investigated the effect of the developed dietary advice on the lipid profile and BMI (body mass index)/BMI-z-score of children. In this retrospective cohort study, we included children aged 1–16 years, of whom a lipid profile was determined in the period between June 2011 and November 2013 in our hospital. Children who adhered to the dietary advice were assigned to the exposed group and the remaining children were assigned to the unexposed group. After following the dietary advice for at least three months, there was a statistically significant reduction in the cholesterol/HDL (high-density lipoproteins) ratio ($p < 0.001$) and non-HDL-cholesterol ($p = 0.044$) and a statistically significant increase in the HDL-cholesterol ($p = 0.009$) in the exposed group, while there was no difference in the BMI and BMI z-scores. The dietary advice has no adverse effect on the lipid profile, BMI, and BMI z-scores in children, but has a significant beneficial effect on the cholesterol/HDL ratio, non-HDL-cholesterol, and the HDL-cholesterol.

Keywords: children; dietary advice; full-fat dairy products; green vegetables; beef; cholesterol; lipid profile; BMI; cardiovascular risk factors

1. Introduction

Little is known about cholesterol and lipid profiles in children, except from children known to have familiar dyslipidemia. However, concerns about the cholesterol levels are troubling parents when doctors advise to give full-fat dairy products to their children. Are these concerns realistic or not? At this moment, adult recommendations are also used for children.

There are circumstances when full-fat dairy products are investigated for their possible positive contribution to different health aspects in children. One aspect is the functioning of the immune system, which is partly dependent on the nutritional status. Nutrients, such as vitamins and minerals, play an important role in the strengthening of the immune system. As a consequence, an adequate nutritional status, and thereby a strong immune system, might prevent infections [1–7].

In a previous study, we compared the dietary intake of children with recurrent respiratory infection (without immunological disorders) and healthy children [8]. These children usually have respiratory complaints without an adequate explanation, like immunological deficiencies. The outcomes showed that the group of children with recurrent infections eats less beef, natural milk, and green vegetables compared to the healthy children.

Following this study, a nutrient-rich diet has been developed as a possible intervention for recurrent infections using the NEVO (Nederlands Voedingsstoffenbestand) tables, a Dutch nutrient database containing information about the nutrients of each food [9]. There are more international databases containing macro and micronutrients. We choose this database because this database contains the most information about the regular food that is eaten and sold in The Netherlands.

The diet is based on foods high in nutrients that could support the immune system, namely green vegetables, beef, whole milk, and butter (Table 1). This are also the food groups that are not frequently consumed by children with recurrent infections. Compared to other vegetables, green vegetables contain more zinc, vitamin A, and vitamin C. Beef contains more iron, zinc, vitamin A and vitamin E compared with other types of meat [9]. These nutrients have immune supporting effects and play a role in the antiviral mechanisms, which could positively affect recurrent upper respiratory tract infections [2–7]. Looking at the full-fat dairy products, whole milk, and butter are a source of lipids, vitamins, and essential fatty acids, such as linoleic acid and alpha-linolenic acid [9]. The lipids can act as a carrier for vitamins A, D, E, and K, [10] which can have a positive effect on the immune system [9,10]. In addition, the extra fats in whole milk have anti-microbial properties and can act as bacteriostatics [9,11].

Table 1. Nutrients in food products of the dietary advice compared to other food products (according to the NEVO tables [9]).

Food Product	Nutrients per 100 Grams									
	Vitamin A (ug)	Vitamin D (ug)	Vitamin E (mg)	Iron (mg)	Zinc (mg)	Calorie (kcal)	Saturated Fats (g)	Total Unsaturated Fats (g)	N-3 Fats (g)	Linoleic Acid (N-6 fat) (g)
Spinach cooked	652	-	3.5	2.4	1.20	25	0.1	0.7	0.5	0.1
Broccoli cooked	116	-	2.5	0.9	0.62	27	0.1	0.2	0.1	-
Cauliflower cooked	0	-	0.1	0.3	0.26	23	0.1	0.2	0.2	-
Chicory cooked	1	-	0.2	0.2	0.17	17	-	0.1	-	0.1
Beef > 10% fat	68	0.5	2.4	2.8	5.84	277	6.2	10.5	0.2	2.9
Chicken breast	18	0.1	1.1	0.7	0.74	158	1.4	1.8	0.1	0.8
Pork 10%–19% fat	25	0.6	1.1	1.0	2.65	378	5.4	10.1	0.2	3.2
Butter	903	1.2	2.5	0.1	0.09	737	52.9	19.9	0.5	1.3
Margarine	800	7.5	9.5	0.1	-	349	8.5	34.5	5.9	19
Whole milk	36	-	0.1	-	0.46	62	2.2	0.8	-	0.1
Skimmed milk	1	-	-	-	0.46	35	0.1	-	-	-
Adequate intake or recommended dietary allowance/day for children [12,13]	♂/♀ 2–5 years: 350 ug	♂/♀ 4–8 years: 10 ug	♂/♀ 2–5 years: 5 mg	♂/♀ 2–5 years: 8 mg	♂/♀ 2–5 years: 6 mg	4–8 years: ♂1720 kcal ♀1552 kcal	♂/♀ 4–8 years: 10 En%	♂/♀ all ages: 8–38 En%	4–8 years: 0.15–0.2 g	♂/♀ 4–8 years: 2 En%

This previous study showed that the dietary advice had significant positive effects on the length and gravity of respiratory tract infections in children [14]. Furthermore, another study showed that the same dietary advice decreases some symptoms of medically unresolved fatigue in children [1,15].

Strengthening the immune system just by changing food habits might be a solution for many patients with recurrent infections but without an immunological disorder or for patients with medically unresolved fatigue. However, there are thoughts that the saturated fats in the recommended whole milk and butter could have a negative influence on the lipid profile and/or the risk of cardiovascular disease. The National Heart Foundation of Australia states that the intake of saturated fatty acids is highly associated with an increased risk of coronary heart disease due to elevated LDL-cholesterol (low-density lipoproteins cholesterol) and serum cholesterol levels [16]. The American Heart Association (AHA) and American Academy of Pediatrics advise the use of dairy products that are fat-free or low in fat, in order to minimize the intake of saturated fat. They mention that a decline in saturated fat and cholesterol intake has been associated with a reduction in cardiovascular disease [17]. The Dutch Centre of Food recommends replacing saturated fats with unsaturated fats, which should lower the risk of cardiovascular disease [18].

Recently, conflicting findings have been reported regarding the association of saturated fats and the risk of cardiovascular disease. Several studies show no evidence for the assumed association and some even describe an inverse association [19–21].

The aim of our study was to determine whether the developed dietary advice—relatively high in saturated fats—has an influence on the BMI (body mass index) of children and on risk factors of cardiovascular disease. The total cholesterol/HDL (high-density lipoproteins) ratio is an important predictor of later risk of cardiovascular disease [22,23]. Additionally, the American Academy of Pediatrics recommends non-HDL concentration as an important benchmark for the screening of cardiovascular risk in children [24]. Therefore, we used the lipid profile of children in order to determine whether the dietary advice with its beneficial effect on at least respiratory tract infections in children can be safely used.

2. Materials and Methods

The present study is a non-randomized retrospective cohort study. The determination of the lipid profile of the children was executed by blinded laboratory workers. The measurements of weight and height were not blindly executed.

We performed a laboratory search in our laboratory database for patient blood samples. Included in the search were children aged from 1 to 16 years with at least two measurements of a lipid profile in the period between June 2011 and November 2013 at hospital ZGT (Hospital Group Twente) Hengelo/Almelo in the Netherlands. Patient charts were hand-searched for dietary habits/advice. If no details were given in the patient charts, dietary habits were addressed as unknown. When no abnormalities were noted, we assumed it was according to the Dutch dietary guidelines [12]. Children who had followed the dietary advice were assigned to the exposed group and the remaining children were assigned to the unexposed group. A schematic overview of the data collection is shown in Figure 1.

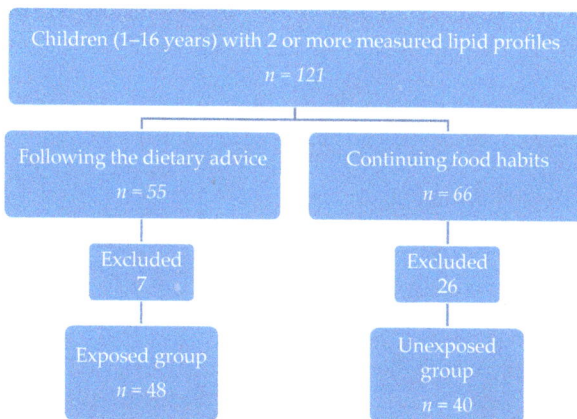

Figure 1. Schematic overview of the data collection.

We excluded all children with a disorder that might influence the lipid profile, such as familiar hypercholesterolemia, hypothyroidism, diabetes mellitus type I and II, obesity, metabolic disorders, and medication which influences the lipid profile (according to [25]). As shown in Table 2, in the exposed group six patients were excluded based on the exclusion criteria described above, and one patient withdrew informed consent. Following the exclusion criteria, 26 patients were excluded in the unexposed group.

Table 2. Overview of the excluded patients.

Exposed Group	(*n* = 55)	Unexposed Group	(*n* = 66)
Incomplete lipid profile	2	Incomplete lipid profile	5
Familiar hypercholesterolemia	2	Familiar hypercholesterolemia	3
Obesity	1	Obesity	13
Age < 1 year or > 16 years	1	Age < 1 year or > 16 years	1
Diabetes mellitus	0	Diabetes mellitus	3
Metabolic disorder	0	Metabolic disorder	1
Medication	0	Medication	0
Dropouts	1	Dropouts	0
Exposed group	(*n* = 48)	Unexposed group	(*n* = 40)

The children visited the pediatric outpatient clinic for several complaints. In the exposed group, most of them suffered from recurrent infections, subclinical hypothyroidism or tiredness. The unexposed group consisted of children with recurrent infections, abdominal complaints, epilepsy, failure to thrive, behavioral disorders.

The dietary advice, based on the NEVO tables [9], consists of eating beef three times a week, green vegetables five times a week (both age-related portions, according to the Dutch Center of Food), at least one glass (200 mL) of full-fat milk (3.4% fat) each day, and the use of five grams per slice of bread of natural butter (80% fat) for at least three months. Each item of the advice counted for 25% and children had to score at least 75% to meet the criteria of the exposed group. All other dietary habits remained unchanged. The children who did not follow the dietary advice were included in the unexposed group. For ethical reasons we were not allowed to approach them and had to assume that there were no large changes in their food habits during the period of follow-up.

We recorded information of all children from both groups: gender, age, weight, height, duration, and degree of following the dietary advice, lipid profile at the time of presentation, and follow-up.

The height of the children was measured with a vertical ruler. The children were weighed in underwear and all measurements were performed by a pediatrician. The children's BMI was calculated by dividing their weight in kilograms by the square of their height in meters. The BMI *z*-score is calculated on the basis of gender, age, height, and weight [26]. The BMI *z*-score can be calculated only from the age of 24 months. This means that no BMI *z*-score was calculated in children younger than two years. These data were calculated, but not added in the tables, due to lacking data in the younger children.

Both for the start of the dietary advice, and at the end of the follow-up, the lipid profile was determined in all children. At the time of blood collection by venapuncture the children had an empty stomach, as nutrition can affect LDL and triglyceride concentrations [27]. The lipids from the lipid profile are total cholesterol, high-density lipoprotein cholesterol (HDL-C), cholesterol/HDL ratio, low-density lipoprotein cholesterol (LDL-C), triglycerides (TG), and non-HDL. The lipid profile was measured by enzymatic colorimetric techniques with the COBAS 6000 (Roche Diagnostics, Almere, The Netherlands). The LDL was calculated with Friedewald's formula: LDL = total cholesterol − HDL − (0.45 × TG). The primary outcome of this study, the cholesterol/HDL ratio, was calculated by dividing the total cholesterol by HDL cholesterol [23]. The non-HDL can be calculated by the following formula: total cholesterol − HDL cholesterol = non-HDL cholesterol (non-HDL).

We used SPSS Statistics 20 (SPSS Inc., Chicago, IL, USA) to execute our data analysis. Normality was checked by visual expectation of histograms and Shapiro-Wilk test. Continuous variables were expressed as the mean with the standard deviation (SD) or the median with the interquartile range (IQR); categorical variables were expressed as counts with corresponding percentages. Differences in baseline characteristics between groups was tested using an independent *t*-test or Mann-Whitney (continuous variables) or Pearson's chi-square (categorical). To test changes of the lipid profile between measurements within each group a paired *T*-test or Wilcoxon was used. Concerning the BMI and

BMI z-score, several data were lacking. Therefore, the BMI and BMI z-scores were tested using mixed models analysis. For all comparisons, a *p*-value ≤ 0.05 was regarded as significant.

3. Results

3.1. Baseline Data

The baseline data of the unexposed and exposed group are presented in Table 3. The demographic characteristics, period of follow-up, the lipid profiles, and the BMI characteristics did not differ significantly at the start of this study.

Table 3. Baseline characteristics of the unexposed and exposed group.

Characteristic	Unexposed Group *n* = 40	Exposed Group *n* = 48	*p*-Value
Gender (n, %)MenWomen	24 (60%) 16 (40%)	25 (52%) 23 (48%)	0.457
Age (years) (median, IQR)	4.7 (2.3–9.0)	2.6 (1.6–8.0)	0.102
Follow-up (months)(median, IQR)	5.0 (4.0–8.0)	4.5 (4.0–8.8)	0.744
BMI (median, IQR)	15.9 (15.1–17.5)	16.7 (15.4–18.5)	0.408

IQR (interquartile range); SD (standard deviation).

3.2. Changes within Groups

The baseline, follow up and differences in lipid profile within the two groups between the start and follow-up are shown in Table 4. In the exposed group, the HDL-cholesterol increased significantly with 0.14 mmol/L (*p* = 0.009), 95% CI (−0.24 to −0.04) (confidence interval). The cholesterol/HDL ratio was significantly reduced (*p* < 0.001), 95% CI (0.35–0.84), as was the non-HDL (*p* = 0.044), 95% CI (0.01–0.34). The decrease in the cholesterol/HDL is caused by the significant increase in the HDL-cholesterol. The total cholesterol did not change significantly and barely affects the cholesterol/HDL ratio. No significant changes occurred in the BMI and BMI z-score (a change of −0.06) in the exposed group. There were no significant changes of the lipid profile or BMI and BMI z-score (change of 0.09) in the unexposed group.

Table 4. Changes in lipid profile and BMI of both groups between the start and end of follow-up.

Measurements	Unexposed Group *n* = 40				Exposed Group *n* = 48			
	Baseline	Follow-up	Change (95%-CI/IQR))	*p*-Value	Baseline	Follow-up	Change (95%-CI)	*p*-Value
Total cholesterol (mmol/L) (median, IQR)	4.05 (3.83–4.70)	4.20 (3.70–4.68)	−0.06 [a] (−0.11–0.22)	0.581 [d]	4.20 (3.5–5.0)	4.35 (3.7–4.7)	−0.03 [a] (−0.25–0.18)	0.738 [c]
HDL-cholesterol (mmol/L) (median, IQR)	1.35 (0.93–1.59)	1.30 (0.95–1.57)	−0.01 [b] (−0.19–0.12)	0.842 [c]	1.17 (0.88–1.48)	1.35 (1.12–1.53)	0.14 [a] (0.04–0.24)	0.009 [d]
Cholesterol/HDL (mmol/L) (median, IQR)	3.45 (2.57–4.70)	3.40 (2.53–4.45)	0,00 [b] (−0.35–0.38)	0.883 [d]	3.75 (3.00–4.95)	3.15 (2.80–4.95)	−0.30 [b] (−1.2–0.17)	< 0.001 [c]
Triglycerides (mmol/L) (median, IQR)	0.96 (0.70–1.93)	1.00 (0.80–1.47)	0.05 [b] (−0.38–0.30)	0.821 [d]	1.10 (0.80–1.67)	1.05 (0.80–1.50)	−0.07 [a] (−0.31–0.16)	0.469 [d]
LDL-cholesterol (mmol/L) (median, IQR)	2.30 (2.00–2.80)	2.30 (1.90–2.88)	0.00 [a] (−0.15–0.13)	0.852 [c]	2.55 (1.70–3.00)	2.40 (1.93–2.80)	−0.10 [b] (−0.60–0.30)	0.384 [c]
Non-HDL cholesterol (mmol/L) (median, IQR)	3.01 (2.54–3.49)	2.83 (2.40–3.39)	−0.06 [a] (−0.21–0.08)	0.384 [c]	3.14 (2.56–3.61)	2.98 (2.45–3.28)	−0.17 [a] (−0.34—0.01)	0.044 [d]
BMI (median, IQR)	15.9 (15.1–17.5)	15.8 (15.1–17.5)	0.24 [a] (-0.05–0.54)	0.178 [d]	16.7 (15.4–18.5)	16.0 (14.9–18.0)	0.00 [b] (−0.63–0.30)	0.719 [d]

[a] Normally distributed (mean, 95% CI); [b] non-normally distributed (median, IQR); [c] paired *t*-test; [d] Wilcoxon signed rank test.

4. Discussion

Our research shows that consumption of green vegetables, beef, whole milk, and butter has no adverse effect on the lipid profile in children. The dietary advice, no advice with respect to carbohydrate intake, but relatively high in saturated fats is even shown to have a favorable effect on the lipid profile: it gave a significant increase in HDL cholesterol, and a decrease in non-HDL cholesterol and the cholesterol/HDL ratio.

In a previous study the dietary advice has been shown to have a significant improving effect on the incidence and duration of recurrent respiratory tract infections [15]. This nutritional advice will probably be discouraged by major national and international organizations since the idea exists that saturated fats have a negative effect on the lipid profile and/or the cholesterol/HDL ratio and, thus, increases the risk of cardiovascular disease.

The American Heart Association and the American Academy of Pediatrics recommend not offering any whole-milk products to children, because of the higher concentrations of saturated fats and, therefore, the increased risk of later cardiovascular disease [17]. The Dutch Nutrition Centre recommends that children should not eat full-fat products at all, due to the relatively high concentration of saturated fats. According to the nutrition center the intake of saturated fats has a negative impact on the cholesterol/HDL ratio and, therefore, increases the risk of cardiovascular disease [18].

Over the years, various studies have been published discussing the relationship between saturated fatty acids and cardiovascular disease. The idea that consuming saturated fats can lead to death from cardiovascular disease has certainly not been confirmed by all studies. A meta-analysis of randomized trials showed that saturated fat has an increasing effect on HDL cholesterol. The increase in the HDL-cholesterol is greater when consuming saturated fats, compared to consuming unsaturated fats [28], which can contribute to a decrease in total cholesterol/HDL cholesterol ratio [29]. *The Lancet* published a systematic review of 61 prospective studies, which showed that higher HDL cholesterol levels reduce the risk of death from cardiovascular disease [30].

Contrary to expectations, a large meta-analysis by Siri-Tarino and colleagues shows that there is no significant link between the consumption of saturated fats and an increased risk of cardiovascular disease in general and coronary heart disease in particular [20]. In line with this, a meta-analysis by Skeaf and Miller commissioned by the World Health Organization concluded that the amount of saturated fats in a diet does not have an impact on the risk of coronary heart disease [31]. The American Heart Association claims that replacing saturated fat with carbohydrates lowers the risk of cardiovascular disease. In contrast, a meta-analysis of prospective studies shows that replacing saturated fat with carbohydrates leads to a significantly increased risk of cardiovascular disease [32]. This is supported by Musunuru, who concluded that it is not the saturated fats, but the carbohydrates in a diet that cause atherogenic dyslipidemia [33].

Next to the inconsistent data about dairy fats and cardiovascular risk factors, there are also inconsistent data about the risk of dairy fat on developing diabetes mellitus. A recent study from the Nurses' Health Study and the Health Professionals Follow-Up Study show a protective effect of high plasma dairy fatty acid concentrations and lower incidence of diabetes mellitus [34].

As an alternative to butter with its saturated fats, margarine was developed. This "skinny" dairy product is enriched with "healthy" omega-6 fatty acids. However, the replacement of saturated fatty acids and trans-fatty acids by omega-6 fatty acids is associated with an increased risk of coronary heart disease and overall mortality [35]. We now know that omega-6 fatty acids have pro-inflammatory characteristics while omega-3 fatty acids have anti-inflammatory ones. A diet with a large amount of omega-6 fatty acids and a high omega-6/omega-3 ratio enhances the development of diseases such as cancer, cardiovascular disease, inflammatory and autoimmune diseases. In contrast, high levels of omega-3 fatty acids have suppressive effects on those diseases [36]. The investigated dietary advice contributes to a good fatty-acid balance due to its green vegetables, which contain a relatively high amount of omega-3 fatty acids and are low in omega-6 fatty acids [9]. Recently, a study showed that people who eat a lot of green leafy vegetables have a 32% lower risk of myocardial infarction [37]. In addition, green vegetables have other positive effects concerning health, such as reducing the risk of many forms of cancer [38,39]. Additionally, the dietary advice contributes to the inhibition of oxidation of LDL cholesterol, a crucial step in atherosclerosis, with its relatively high levels of Vitamin A and E in beef, compared to other types of meat [40].

The BMI and BMI z-scores in the exposed group did not significantly change during the months of follow-up. If we calculate the caloric intake of the dietary advice, using age-adequate quantities advised by the Dutch Food Center [12], the diet contains 94 more calories compared to a diet with identical quantities of low-fat milk and margarine [9]. By contrast, beef contains 1.5 times fewer calories compared to, for example, pork, which has 82 calories per serving [9,41]. This almost neutralizes the extra calories ingested by a child with the intake of whole milk and butter. Additionally, whole milk has a favorable glycemic control and, thereby, possibly an inhibitory effect on appetite and food intake [42]. Several investigations show that a higher intake of dairy products does not increase body weight, results that are consistent with the results of our study [43,44].

This study suggests that diet quality can have some benefits for children. However, one of the limitations of this study is the retrospective design. Adherence to the dietary advice was retrospectively controlled through evaluative questions during the consultation with the pediatrician. A more reliable way of checking the nutritional advice is to let patients fill out a daily food questionnaire.

Due to the retrospective design the food habits of the unexposed group could not all be traced. In this case we had to assume that they did not consume full fat dairy (in The Netherlands semi-skimmed milk and low-fat butter are advised) and no changes in diet occurred during follow-up. In a research design such as a randomized controlled trial, the unexposed group could also fill out a food questionnaire so that any changes in diet can be detected.

Following the retrospective design of this study the unexposed and exposed group could not be randomized. A probable advantage is that the patients (and/or their parents) in the exposed group were possibly more motivated to follow the diet given the fact that they chose to follow the diet themselves.

There were missing values in the BMI and, thereby, the BMI z-scores of the children, so that the conclusions of BMI and BMI z-score are based on a smaller number of patients than we included. Furthermore, the mean period of follow-up was 4.4 months, which means that we cannot draw conclusions about these outcomes in the long term. We require long-term follow-up studies to evaluate the course of the lipid profile.

5. Conclusions

This retrospective study shows diet quality in childhood can have some useful benefits. Earlier, it was shown that a dietary advice of green vegetables, beef, whole milk, and full-fat butter reduces the number of days with a respiratory tract infection in children. In this study we have shown that the dietary advice has no adverse effect on the lipid profile, BMI, and BMI z-score in children. Conversely, the dietary advice has a significant beneficial effect on the HDL-cholesterol, cholesterol/HDL ratio, and non-HDL-cholesterol. The dietary advice can, therefore, be safely recommended and might be beneficial for children with recurrent respiratory tract infections. However, the findings of this retrospective study should be further investigated in randomized controlled trials.

Acknowledgments: The authors would like to thank van der Palen (epidemiologist) and Josien Timmerman with their help with the statistical analysis.

Author Contributions: Ellen van der Gaag was responsible for the study design, implementation of the study and writing. Romy Wieffer conducted the data interpretation, literature research, and writing. Judith van der Kraats collected and analyzed the data and performed the literature research. All authors designed the approach, commented, edited, and approved the paper, and are responsible for the final version of the paper.

Conflicts of Interest: The authors declare no conflict of interest.

References

1. Field, C.J.; Johnson, I.R.; Schley, P.D. Nutrients and their role in host resistance to infection. *J. Leukocyte Biol.* **2002**, *71*, 16–32. [PubMed]
2. Jimenez, C.; Leets, I.; Puche, R.; Anzola, E.; Montilla, R.; Parra, C.; Aguilera, A.; Garcia-Casal, M.N. A single dose of vitamin A improves haemoglobin concentration, retinol status and phagocytic function of neutrophils in preschool children. *Brit. J. Nutr.* **2010**, *103*, 798–802. [CrossRef] [PubMed]
3. Maggini, S.; Wenzlaff, S.; Hornig, D. Essential role of vitamin C and zinc in child immunity and health. *J. Int. Med. Res.* **2010**, *38*, 386–414. [CrossRef] [PubMed]
4. Prasad, A.S. Zinc: Role in immunity, oxidative stress and chronic inflammation. *Curr. Opin. Clin. Nutr.* **2009**, *12*, 646–652. [CrossRef] [PubMed]
5. Wintergerst, E.S.; Maggini, S.; Hornig, D.H. Immune-enhancing role of vitamin C and zinc and effect on clinical conditions. *Ann. Nutr. Metab.* **2006**, *50*, 85–94. [CrossRef] [PubMed]
6. Cherayil, B.J. Iron and immunity: Immunological consequences of iron deficiency and overload. *Arch. Immunol. Ther. Exp.* **2010**, *58*, 407–415. [CrossRef] [PubMed]
7. Ekiz, C.; Agaoglu, L.; Karakas, Z.; Gurel, N.; Yalcin, I. The effect of iron deficiency anemia on the function of the immune system. *Hematol. J.* **2005**, *5*, 579–583. [CrossRef] [PubMed]
8. Munow, M.; van der Gaag, E.J. Ailing Toddlers: Is There a Relation between Behavior and Health? Book of Abstracts 27th Annual Meeting of the European Society for Pediatric Infectious Diseases; 2009; p. 764. Available online: http://www.scirp.org/%28S%28351jmbntvnsjt1aadkposzje%29%29/reference/ReferencesPapers.aspx?ReferenceID=962833 (accessed on 18 May 2017).
9. National Institute for Public Health and the Environment (RIVM)/the Kingdom of the Netherlands. Dutch Food Composition Database 2014. Available online: http://nevo-online.rivm.nl/ (accessed on 12 May 2014).
10. German, J.B. Dietary lipids from an evolutionary perspective: Sources, structures and functions. *Matern. Child Nutr.* **2011**, *7*, 2–16. [CrossRef] [PubMed]
11. Batovska, D.; Todorova, I.; Tsvetkova, I.; Najdenski, H. Antibacterial study of the medium chain fatty acids and their 1-monoglycerides: Individual effects and synergistic relationships. *Pol. J. Microbiol.* **2009**, *58*, 43–47. [PubMed]
12. Dietary Reference Intakes: Energy, Proteins, Fats and Digestible Carbohydrates. Health Council Neth. Available online: https://www.narcis.nl/publication/RecordID/oai:cris.maastrichtuniversity.nl:publications%2Fdc7e056b-a54d-471d-a496-ec334fd5ad1e (accessed on 13 June 2013).
13. Brink, E.J.; Breedveld, B.C.; Peters, J.A.C. Aanbevelingen Voor Vitamines, Mineralen en Spoorelementen. Factsheet The Netherlands Nutrition Centre. Available online: http://www.voedingscentrum.nl/Assets/Uploads/voedingscentrum/Documents/Professionals/Pers/Factsheets/Factsheet%20Aanbevelingen%20voor%20vitamines,%20mineralen%20en%20spoorelementen.pdf (accessed on 15 December 2016).
14. Ten Velde, L.G.H.; Leegsma, J.; van der Gaag, E.J. Recurrent upper respiratory tract infections in children;the influence of green vegetables, beef, whole milk and butter. *Food Nutr. Sci.* **2013**, *4*, 71–77. [CrossRef]
15. Steenbruggen, T.G.; Hoekstra, S.J.; van der Gaag, E.J. Could a change in diet revitalize children who suffer from unresolved fatigue? *Nutrients* **2015**, *7*, 1965–1977. [CrossRef] [PubMed]
16. Shrapnel, W.S.; Calvert, G.D.; Nestle, P.J.; Truswell, A.S. Diet and coronary heart disease. *Natl. Heart Found. Aust. Med. J. Aust.* **1992**, *156*, S9–S16.
17. Gidding, S.S.; Dennison, B.A.; Birch, L.L.; Daniels, S.R.; Gillman, M.W.; Lichtenstein, A.H.; Rattay, K.T.; Steinberger, J.; Stettler, N.; van Horn, L. Dietary recommendations for children and adolescents: A guide for practitioners. *Pediatrics* **2006**, *117*, 544–559. [CrossRef] [PubMed]
18. The Netherlands Nutrition Centre. Verzadigd vet. Available online: http://www.voedingscentrum.nl/encyclopedie/verzadigd-vet.aspx (accessed on 15 May 2016).
19. Muskiet, F.A.J.; Muskiet, M.H.A.; Kuipers, R.S. Het faillissement van de verzadigd vethypothese van cardiovasculaire ziektes. *Ned. Tijdschr. Klin. Chem. Labgeneesk* **2012**, *37*, 192–211. (In Dutch).
20. Siri-Tarino, P.W.; Sun, Q.; Hu, F.B.; Krauss, R.M. Meta-analysis of prospective cohort studies evaluating the association of saturated fat with cardiovascular disease. *Am. J. Clin. Nutr.* **2010**, *91*, 535–546. [CrossRef] [PubMed]

21. Kratz, M.; Baars, T.; Guyenet, S. The relationship between high-fat dairy consumption and obesity, cardiovascular, and metabolic disease. *Eur. J. Nutr.* **2013**, *52*, 1–24. [CrossRef] [PubMed]

22. Kinosian, B.; Glick, H.; Garland, G. Cholesterol and coronary heart disease predicting risks by levels and ratios. *Ann. Intern. Med.* **1994**, *121*, 641–647. [CrossRef] [PubMed]

23. The Netherlands Nutrition Centre. Cholesterol. Available online: http://www.voedingscentrum.nl/encyclopedie/cholesterol.aspx (accessed on 16 May 2016).

24. Department of Health and Human Services. National Heart Lung and Blood Institute. Expert Panel on Integrated Guidelines for Cardiovascular Health and Risk Reduction in Children and Adolescents. Available online: https://www.nhlbi.nih.gov/files/docs/guidelines/peds_guidelines_full.pdf (accessed on 15 January 2017).

25. The Netherlands National Health Care Institute. Farmacotherapeutisch kompas. Available online: https://www.farmacotherapeutischkompas.nl/ (accessed on 5 January 2014).

26. U.S. Department of Health and Human Services. National Center for Health Statistics, Z-Score Data Files. Available online: https://www.cdc.gov/growthcharts/zscore.htm (accessed on 14 February 2014).

27. Kubo, T.; Takahashi, K.; Furujo, M.; Hyodo, Y.; Tsuchiya, H.; Hattori, M.; Fujinaga, S.; Urayama, K. Usefulness of non-fasting lipid parameters in children. *J. Pediatr. Endocr. Metab.* **2017**, *30*, 77–83. [CrossRef] [PubMed]

28. Mensink, R.P.; Zock, P.L.; Kester, A.D.; Katan, M.B. Effects of dietary fatty acids and carbohydrates on the ratio of serum total to HDL cholesterol and on serum lipids and apolipoproteins: A meta-analysis of 60 controlled trials. *Am. J. Clin. Nutr.* **2003**, *77*, 1146–1155. [PubMed]

29. Huth, P.J.; Park, K.M. Influence of dairy product and milk fat consumption on cardiovascular disease risk: A review of the evidence. *Adv. Nutr.* **2012**, *3*, 266–285. [CrossRef] [PubMed]

30. Lewington, S.; Whitlock, G.; Clarke, R.; Sherliker, P.; Emberson, J.; Halsey, J.; Qizilbash, N.; Peto, R.; Collins, R. Blood cholesterol and vascular mortality by age, sex, and blood pressure: A meta-analysis of individual data from 61 prospective studies with 55,000 vascular deaths. *Lancet* **2007**, *370*, 1829–1839. [CrossRef] [PubMed]

31. Skeaf, C.M.; Miller, J. Dietary fat and coronary heart disease: Summary of evidence from prospective cohort and randomized controlled trails. *Ann. Nutr. Metab.* **2009**, *55*, 173–201. [CrossRef] [PubMed]

32. Jakobsen, M.U.; O'Reilly, E.J.; Heitmann, B.L.; Pereira, M.A.; Bälter, K.; Fraser, G.E.; Goldbourt, U.; Hallmans, G.; Knekt, P.; Liu, S. Major types of dietary fat and risk of coronary heart disease: A pooled analysis of 11 cohort studies. *Am. J. Clin. Nutr.* **2009**, *89*, 1425–1432. [CrossRef] [PubMed]

33. Musunuru, K. Atherogenic dyslipidemia: Cardiovascular risk and dietary intervention. *Lipids* **2010**, *45*, 907–914. [CrossRef] [PubMed]

34. Yakoob, M.Y.; Shi, P.; Willet, W.C.; Rexrode, K.M.; Campos, H.; Orav, E.J.; Hu, F.B.; Mozaffarian, D. Circulating Biomarkers of dairy fat and risk of incident diabetes mellitus among men and women in the United States in two large prospective cohorts. *Circulation* **2016**, *133*, 1645–1654. [CrossRef] [PubMed]

35. Ramsden, C.E.; Hibbeln, J.R.; Majchrzak, S.F.; Davis, J.M. N-6 fatty acid-specific and mixed polyunsaturate dietary interventions have different effects on CHD risk: A meta-analysis of randomised controlled trials. *Brit. J. Nutr.* **2010**, *104*, 1586–1600. [CrossRef] [PubMed]

36. Simopoulos, A.P. The importance of the Omega-6/Omega-3 fatty-acid ratio in cardiovascular disease and other chronic diseases. *Exp. Biol. Med.* **2008**, *233*, 674–688. [CrossRef] [PubMed]

37. Ahmed, F. Health: Edible advice. *Nature* **2010**, *468*, S10–S12. [CrossRef] [PubMed]

38. Cohen, J.H.; Kristal, A.R.; Standford, J.L. Fruit and vegetable intakes and prostate cancer risk. *J. Natl. Cancer Inst.* **2000**, *92*, 61–68. [CrossRef]

39. Ambrosone, C.B.; McCann, S.E.; Freudenheim, J.L.; Marshall, J.R.; Zhang, Y.; Shields, P.G. Breast cancer risk in premenopausal women is inversely associated with consumption of broccoli, a source of isothiocyanates, but is not modified by GST genotype. *J. Nutr.* **2004**, *134*, 1134–1138. [PubMed]

40. Zhang, P.Y.; Xu, X.; Li, X.C. Cardiovascular diseases: Oxidative damage and antioxidant protection. *Eur. Rev. Med. Pharmacol. Sci.* **2014**, *18*, 3091–3096. [PubMed]

41. The Netherlands Nutrition Centre. Hoeveel en wat kan ik per dag eten? Available online: http://www.voedingscentrum.nl/nl/schijf-van-vijf/eet-niet-teveel-en-beweeg/hoe-eet-ik-niet-te-veel.aspx (accessed on 21 March 2014).

42. Haug, A.; Høstmark, A.T.; Harstad, O.M. Bovine milk in human nutrition—A review. *Lipids Health Dis.* **2007**, *6*, 25. [CrossRef] [PubMed]
43. Snijder, M.B.; van der Heijden, A.A.W.A.; van Dam, R.M.; Stehouwer, C.D.A.; Hiddink, G.J.; Nijpels, G.; Heine, R.J.; Bouter, L.M.; Dekker, J.M. Is higher dairy consumption associated with lower body weight and fewer metabolic disturbances? *Am. J. Clin. Nutr.* **2007**, *85*, 989–995. [PubMed]
44. Rautiainen, S.; Wang, L.; Lee, I.M.; Manson, J.E.; Buring, J.E.; Sesso, H.D. Dairy consumption in association with weight change and risk of becoming overweight or obese in middle-aged and older woman: A prospective cohort study. *Am. J. Clin. Nutr.* **2016**, *103*, 979–988. [CrossRef] [PubMed]

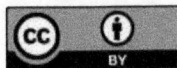

nutrients

MDPI

Article

A Polish Study on the Influence of Food Neophobia in Children (10–12 Years Old) on the Intake of Vegetables and Fruits

Dominika Guzek [1,*], Dominika Głąbska [2], Ewa Lange [2] and Marzena Jezewska-Zychowicz [1]

[1] Department of Organization and Consumption Economics, Faculty of Human Nutrition and Consumer Sciences, Warsaw University of Life Sciences (SGGW-WULS), 159C Nowoursynowska Street, 02-787 Warsaw, Poland; marzena_jezewska_zychowicz@sggw.pl

[2] Department of Dietetics, Faculty of Human Nutrition and Consumer Sciences, Warsaw University of Life Sciences (SGGW-WULS), 159C Nowoursynowska Street, 02-787 Warsaw, Poland; dominika_glabska@sggw.pl (D.G.); ewa_lange@sggw.pl (E.L.)

* Correspondence: dominika_guzek@sggw.pl

Received: 31 March 2017; Accepted: 27 May 2017; Published: 2 June 2017

Abstract: Adhering to the recommended intake of fruits and vegetables is an important habit that should be inculcated in children, whereas food neophobia is indicated as one of the most important factors creating food preferences that may interfere. The aim of the presented study was to analyze the association between the food neophobia level and the intake of fruits and vegetables in children aged 10–12 years. The study was conducted among a group of 163 children (78 girls and 85 boys). The assessment of the food neophobia level was based on the Food Neophobia Scale (FNS) questionnaire and the assessment of the fruit and vegetable intake was based on the food frequency questionnaire. A negative correlation between the food neophobia level and the vegetable intake was observed both for girls ($p = 0.032$; R = -0.2432) and for boys ($p = 0.004$; R = -0.3071), whereas for girls differences in vegetable intake were observed also between various food neophobia categories ($p = 0.0144$). It may be concluded that children with higher food neophobia level are characterized by lower vegetable intake than children with lower food neophobia level. For fruits and juices of fruits and vegetables, associations with food neophobia level were not observed.

Keywords: food neophobia; Food Neophobia Scale (FNS); children; fruits; vegetables; juices

1. Introduction

Inadequate intake of fruits and vegetables is indicated as a reason for 6.7 million deaths worldwide each year, which was estimated for the year 2010 [1]. The World Health Organization indicated in a report [2] that, if consumed in the recommended amounts, fruits and vegetables reduce the risk of noncommunicable diseases, including coronary heart disease, stroke, and some types of cancers.

Especially in the case of children, vegetable intake is perceived as beneficial, and consuming them in every meal is a positive behavior that may contribute to healthier dietary patterns [3]. Moreover, it was confirmed in a Polish study on a group of girls that the pattern associated with high fruit and vegetable intake was connected with greater restrictions in the intake of products high in sugar, fat, and starch [4].

In spite of the beneficial effects of fruits and vegetables, in a study of 52 countries taking part in the World Health Survey (2002–2003), the intake was stated to be lower than the lowest recommended number of five servings per day (80 g of fruits/vegetables per serving) for 77.6% of men and 78.4% of women from all the countries [5]. Similarly, in the Child and Adolescent Health Surveys (KiGGS wave 1), it was found that in the age group of 3–17 years, girls consumed 2.7 and boys consumed 2.4 servings of fruits and vegetables per day, whereas only 12.2% of girls and 9.4% of boys consumed five servings per day [6].

It is emphasized that even higher fruit and vegetable intake must be considered, as the World Health Organization recommends 600 g (7.5 servings) per day in adults and 480 g (6 servings) per day in children aged 5–14 years [7]. Achieving the recommended intake of fruits and vegetables in children is a challenge. On the one hand, established children's dietary patterns predict adulthood dietary patterns, but on the other, compared with adults, there are additional factors influencing children's fruit and vegetable intake [2]. Considering both factors, parental role modeling is important, as it is a significant predictor of children's dietary patterns [8]. In general, it may be indicated that the two determining factors, not observed in the case of adults, are parental intake and home accessibility, while the other most prominent determinants indicated for children are gender, age, socioeconomic position of the family, and preferences [9].

Among all the determinants of food choices indicated for children, only their preferences are directly dependent on them. However, children typically prefer familiar, bland, and sweet products, whereas in the case of unknown food products, aversion may occur [10]. Food neophobia is indicated as the most important factor creating food preferences in the case of younger children [11], but also, in the case of children aged 10–11 years, it is emphasized that they should be introduced to unfamiliar fruits and vegetables in order to increase their taste preferences [12].

The aim of the presented study was to analyze the association between the food neophobia level and the intake of fruits and vegetables in children aged 10–12 years.

2. Materials and Methods

2.1. Ethics Approval

The study was conducted according to the guidelines laid down in the Declaration of Helsinki, and all the procedures involving human subjects were approved by the Ethics Committee of the Faculty of Human Nutrition and Consumer Sciences of the Warsaw University of Life Sciences (SGGW-WULS) in Warsaw, Poland (No. 10/2016; 12.12.2016).

2.2. Study Participants

The study group was recruited in the group of children aged 10–12 years from Warsaw, who participated in the scientific nutrition workshops for children conducted in the Dietary Outpatient Clinic of the Faculty of Human Nutrition and Consumer Sciences of the SGGW-WULS. Inclusion criteria were children aged 10–12 years, not suffering from any developmental disorder affecting intellectual abilities, including various intellectual or cognitive deficits. The information about nutritional workshops for children aged 10–12 years was placed on the web page, and 258 children were signed up for the workshops by their parents. The workshops' participants were proposed to take part in the study for analyzing the association between food neophobia level and fruit and vegetable intake. One hundred and seventy-five children agreed to participate, and their parents or legal guardians also provided written consent to participate. The exclusion criterion was nonprovision of written consent to participate.

The participants were asked to fill in two questionnaires: the Food Neophobia Scale (FNS) questionnaire by Pliner and Hobden [13] and the food frequency questionnaire consisting of 31 questions about various groups of products. Because not all participants filled in both questionnaires and due to some missing data, 163 participants (78 girls and 85 boys) were included in the final analysis. The study design and number of participants are presented in Figure 1.

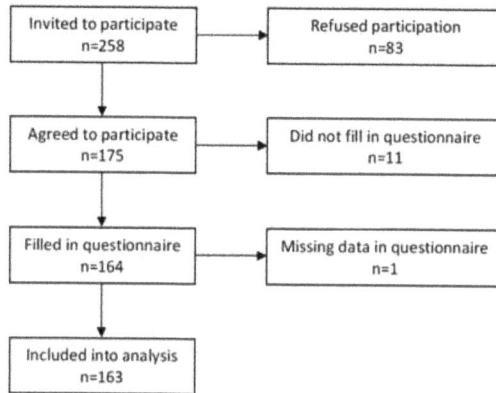

Figure 1. Study design and number of participants.

2.3. Assessment of the Food Neophobia Level

The FNS questionnaire was applied in order to assess the food neophobia level in the analyzed individuals. Each individual received the list of sentences and was asked to rate his or her level of agreement with each sentence, using one of the seven categories of answer (scale from strongly disagree to strongly agree). Because the 10-item FNS questionnaire of Pliner and Hobden [13] includes five positive items (indicating neophilic individuals) and five negative items (indicating neophobic individuals), negative responses were reversed during the analysis of data [14]. In the present group, Cronbach's alpha was at a respectable level (0.78; $n = 163$), and the same respectable level was observed for the group of boys (0.78; $n = 78$), whereas for the group of girls, it was stated to be very good (0.85; $n = 85$), indicating good internal consistency [15].

The calculated food neophobia level ranged from 10 to 70 and, on the basis of the level, the participants were divided into three tertiles characterized by various food neophobia levels: low values (first tertile) are attributed to a low neophobia level (neophilic), medium values (second tertile) are attributed to a medium neophobia level, and high values (third tertile) are attributed to a high neophobia level (neophobic) [16].

2.4. Assessment of the Fruit and Vegetable Intake

The food frequency questionnaire was applied in order to assess the typical intake of fruits and vegetables as well as fruit and vegetable juices among the analyzed individuals. In order to reduce overestimation due to high self-appraisal, the respondents were asked not only about fruits and vegetables, and fruit and vegetable juices, but also about all the most important food products groups, without giving any information as to which items would be assessed. Potatoes were also categorized as a separate group to avoid misinterpreting them as vegetables. The applied questionnaire was previously positively validated on the basis of a Bland-Altman plot in a group of 172 children.

Each individual received the list of food products groups with specified serving size and was asked about the exact number of servings (calculated not only in integers, but also decimal parts) of the products specified in the questionnaire consumed per day/week/month (depending on the product), according the methodology described previously [17]. In the case of fruits and vegetables, participants were asked to specify the number of servings consumed per day, whereas in the case of fruit and vegetable juices, they were asked to specify the number of servings consumed per week. In the case of fruits and vegetables, the described serving size was 100 g, so the numbers of servings were multiplied by 100 g to obtain the typical intake value per day. In the case of fruit and vegetable juices, the described serving size was 250 g, so the number of servings was multiplied by 250 g and divided by seven (days) to obtain a typical intake value per day. The serving sizes were not only expressed in terms of grams, but also described using typical household measures.

2.5. Statistical Analysis

The obtained data are presented as means ± standard deviation (SD) with minimum, maximum, and median values. The distributions of the analyzed factors were verified by using the Shapiro-Wilk test. Internal reliability of the FNS for the group was tested using the Cronbach's alpha coefficient. Differences between groups were identified by using the U Mann-Whitney test and Kruskal-Wallis ANOVA test (applied for nonparametric distribution). Analyses of the correlations were verified by using Spearman's rank correlation coefficient (applied for nonparametric distribution).

The accepted level of significance was set at $p \leq 0.05$. Statistical analysis was conducted using Statistica software version 8.0 (StatSoft Inc., Tulsa, OK, USA).

3. Results

The assessment of fruit intake observed for the analyzed groups of girls and boys in various food neophobia categories is presented in Table 1. No differences in fruit intake in the groups of children characterized by various neophobia levels were stated for both girls and boys. Also, no differences in fruit intake between girls and boys from the same neophobia level were observed.

Table 1. Fruit intake (g/day) for boys and girls in Food Neophobia Scale categories—mean ± SD, as well as median, minimum, and maximum values are presented, and compared between genders and between food neophobia categories.

Food Neophobia Category (Tertile of Food Neophobia Scale)	Girls; n = 78		Boys; n = 85		p-Value
	Mean ± SD	Median (Minimum–Maximum)	Mean ± SD	Median (Minimum–Maximum)	
Low (first)	198.1 ± 122.0	200.0 * (0.0–500.0)	202.1 ± 156.2	200.0 * (10.0–600.0)	0.7077
Medium (second)	180.8 ± 99.1	175.0 * (50.0–400.0)	187.9 ± 108.3	200.0 * (50.0–400.0)	0.7594
High (third)	163.5 ± 126.9	100.0 * (50.0–600.0)	175.9 ± 116.2	150.0 * (0.0–500.0)	0.4121
p-Value		0.8890		0.2736	

* distribution different than normal (verified using Shapiro-Wilk test—$p \leq 0.05$).

The assessment of vegetable intake observed for the analyzed groups of girls and boys in various food neophobia categories is presented in Table 2. No differences in vegetable intake in the group of boys characterized by various neophobia levels were found. In the group of girls, it was found that the differences in vegetable intake observed between various food neophobia categories were statistically significant (p = 0.0144). At the same time, no differences in vegetable intake between girls and boys from the same neophobia level were observed.

Table 2. Vegetable intake (g/day) for boys and girls in Food Neophobia Scale categories—mean ± SD, as well as median, minimum, and maximum values are presented, and compared between genders and between food neophobia categories.

Food Neophobia Category (Tertile of Food Neophobia Scale)	Girls; n = 78		Boys; n = 85		p-Value
	Mean ± SD	Median (Minimum–Maximum)	Mean ± SD	Median (Minimum–Maximum)	
Low (first)	165.4 ± 119.0	100.0 * (0.0–400.0)	158.2 ± 107.3	100.0 * (50.0–500.0)	0.9635
Medium (second)	167.3 ± 103.9	200.0 * (0.0–400.0)	161.2 ± 144.8	100.0 * (50.0–800.0)	0.3796
High (third)	118.8 ± 105.2	100.0 * (0.0–500.0)	97.5 ± 76.4	100.0 * (0.0–300.0)	0.4988
p-Value		0.0144		0.0983	

* distribution different than normal (verified using Shapiro-Wilk test—$p \leq 0.05$).

The assessment of fruit and vegetable juice intake observed for the analyzed groups of girls and boys in various food neophobia categories is presented in Table 3. No differences in fruit and vegetable juice intake in the groups of children characterized by various neophobia levels were stated for both girls and boys. Also, no differences in fruit and vegetable juice intake between girls and boys from the same neophobia level were observed.

Table 3. Fruit and vegetable juice intake (g/day) for boys and girls in Food Neophobia Scale categories—mean ± SD, as well as median, minimum, and maximum values are presented, and compared between genders and between food neophobia categories.

Food Neophobia Category (Tertile of Food Neophobia Scale)	Girls; n = 78		Boys; n = 85		p-Value
	Mean ± SD	Median (Minimum–Maximum)	Mean ± SD	Median (Minimum–Maximum)	
Low (first)	115.4 ± 106.6	89.3 * (0.0–428.6)	195.8 ± 225.0	107.1 * (0.0–1000.0)	0.3245
Medium (second)	140.1 ± 119.0	107.1 * (0.0–357.1)	153.9 ± 147.9	107.1 * (0.0–535.7)	0.7998
High (third)	136.7 ± 185.2	71.4 * (0.0–642.9)	154.3 ± 127.5	142.9 * (0.0–500.0)	0.1496
p-Value		0.9602		0.5550	

* distribution different than normal (verified using Shapiro-Wilk test—$p \leq 0.05$).

To verify the differences in fruit and vegetable intake observed between girls of various food neophobia categories, analysis of correlation between the food neophobia level and the intake of fruits, vegetables, and fruit and vegetable juices was conducted (Table 4). It was confirmed that neither for fruits nor for fruit and vegetable juices, the association between food neophobia level and intake exists, for both girls and boys. Simultaneously, the previously indicated association for vegetables was proven. It was stated that the negative correlation between the food neophobia level and vegetable intake exists in both girls ($p = 0.032$; $R = -0.2432$) and boys ($p = 0.004$; $R = -0.3071$); thus, it may be indicated that children with a higher neophobia level are characterized by lower vegetable intake than children with a lower neophobia level.

Table 4. Analysis of correlation between food neophobia level and fruit intake, vegetable intake, as well as fruit and vegetable juice intake.

	Girls; n = 78		Boys; n = 85	
	p	R	p	R
Fruits	0.069	−0.2071 *	0.842	−0.0219 *
Vegetables	0.032	−0.2432 *	0.004	−0.3071*
Fruit and vegetable juices	0.416	−0.0933 *	0.490	−0.0759 *

* Spearman's rank coefficient.

4. Discussion

Considering the low fruit and vegetable intake in children, indicating the factors that may influence it as well as suggesting the possible ways to overcome the observed trend may be crucial to improve the nutritional value of diet by increasing its variety [18]. Food neophobia (defined as reluctance or avoidance of unknown food products) and pickiness (defined as consuming an inadequate variety of food products, due to the rejection of substantial number of them) are indicated as the most important factors that may cause low vegetable intake [19]. Pickiness is not always reasoned by food neophobia [20] but, in the case of food neophobia, pickiness of unknown food products is common [21].

Food neophobia in children may be associated not only with pickiness, but also with unwillingness to even try unfamiliar food products, which might result in following an improperly balanced diet [18]. Because of food neophobia in adolescence, neophobic behaviors may be transferred to adulthood [22], as it was indicated that such behaviors often remain stable from the age of 13 years to adulthood [23]. At the same time, the age of 9 years is indicated as critical because before that age, the development of food behaviors takes place [24]. Taking this into account, the analysis of food neophobia, its determinants, and consequences among the group of children aged 10–12 years is of a great value, as at such an age there is still a possibility of creating preferences and to trying to reduce the level of neophobic behaviors.

It needs to be emphasized that, in spite of the fact that in preschool children (early childhood) parents can influence dietary patterns [25], in the late childhood, parental influence is reduced in comparison with early childhood, which is associated inter alia with not participating in family dinners [26]. However, the influence of peers is also an important factor, which was proven in the case of vegetable choices, as it was observed that eating vegetables with peers was associated not only with choosing nonpreferred ones, while peers did so, but also with changing preferences [27].

Fruit and vegetable choices in general are associated with children preferences and accessibility [14], which are related to the factors associated not only with the family but also with the country. In the Polish population, it is indicated that national traditions and customs may influence vegetable intake, as they may, for example, cause higher cabbage intake, which is associated with a number of traditional recipes of cabbage dishes that are commonly consumed [28]. However, among the most preferred and most frequently consumed vegetables in Poland in the group of school children are carrots, cucumbers, radishes, and tomatoes; among the most preferred fruits are strawberries, tangerines, oranges, and blueberries, whereas among the most frequently consumed fruits are apples, tangerines, bananas, and oranges [29]. At the same time, in a group of Spanish children and young people, among the most preferred fruits and vegetables are similar products such as apples, bananas, carrots, tomatoes, and lettuce [30].

Vegetable intake is important in the context of food neophobia, as it concerns mainly fruits and vegetables [31]. Moreover, it is indicated that in general, for children, vegetables are characterized by a lower acceptance level than fruits [32], and is even observed to be the lowest among the acceptance levels for all the food product groups [33]. This may partly explain the results of the present study, and the fact that vegetable intake was more prone than fruit intake to be reduced in the case of children characterized by a high food neophobia level. This may result from the fact that vegetables are not as sweet as fruits, and sometimes even have a bitter taste [34], and thus may be subjected to natural rejection evolved as an adaptive safeguard reaction to the potential toxicity of food products [35]. However, in the case of the analyzed group, who have had more experiences with a variety of food products compared to younger children, factors other than naturally evolved reactions must be rather taken into account.

Among the factors influencing vegetable intake, food neophobia and pickiness have been indicated as the important ones. In the study of Galloway et al. [36], it was indicated that girls characterized by high food neophobia and pickiness had higher vegetable intake than those characterized by low food neophobia and pickiness. However, in the mentioned study, in a comparison between the groups of girls with high food neophobia accompanied by low pickiness and those with low food neophobia accompanied by high pickiness, no differences between groups were indicated [36]. In the case of the present study, a similar association was observed; however, new conclusions may be formulated. It may be supposed that food neophobia not only influences vegetable intake when combined with pickiness but, in the population of Polish children, may also be the strong independent factor that may influence it alone. However, to draw more general conclusions, further studies should be conducted also in countries other than Poland.

Another new insight into the area of food neophobia is associated with the fact that, in the study of Galloway et al. [36], only a group of girls was analyzed. It is well known that among girls and boys, food preferences may differ, wherein girls are characterized by a higher general preference of fruits and vegetables compared to boys [33]. Moreover, it is indicated that not only boys are characterized by a higher food neophobia level than girls, but also adult males than females [37]. However, concerning food neophobia, in the majority of studies on the association between food neophobia level and intake of fruits and vegetables in children, the authors analyze data for the combined groups of boys and girls [38–42], whereas only a few studies present data for boys and girls separately or for only one gender [33,36,43].

Although the attitude toward food products may differ between boys and girls, analyzing them as one combined group may result in changing observed associations. For example, a study by Falciglia et al. [18] reported that no relationship between food neophobia level and vegetable intake was observed, however, this finding may have resulted from analyzing boys and girls together.

At the same time, in the study of Tsuji et al. [43], a high food neophobia level in Japanese boys was associated with low vegetable intake, which was not observed in the group of girls. On the one hand, it is in agreement with the results of Galloway et al. [36], as in the mentioned study not a high food neophobia level alone, but only that combined with a high level of pickiness was associated with low vegetable intake in girls. However, on the other hand, it should be mentioned that vegetable intake in the Japanese diet is different from that in the Western diet, while, for example, a higher level of soya intake must be considered [43].

The results of the conducted study indicated that both girls and boys, aged 10–12 years, with a higher food neophobia level may be characterized by lower vegetable intake than children with a lower food neophobia level. It must also be emphasized that, in the case of girls, the association was stronger than that found in boys, as was observed in both the analysis of correlations and comparison between the groups of various food neophobia levels.

Such an observation may be useful for public health purposes. In order to obtain the recommended vegetable intake in children, the reduction of the food neophobia levels may be essential. It may be achieved by taste education and food exposures, which may lead to creating new dietary habits [44,45]. However, it is also observed that implementing taste education and food exposures has produced contradictory results; for vegetables, either a successful education [27] or lack of success was observed [45] in various studies. Taking this into account, not only the association between food neophobia level and vegetable intake must be assessed, but also the most efficient ways of education must be analyzed in order to achieve the reduction of food neophobia levels.

In spite of the promising results of this study, some limitations exist. On the one hand, the general heterogeneity of the analyzed group is positive, as it represents a group representative of the Polish population of children aged 10–12 years more realistically than a homogeneous group. However, on the other hand, it may be argued that in a heterogeneous group, the observed associations may be influenced by the existing variations between individuals. Moreover, in spite of the fact that the food frequency questionnaire is one the most commonly applied methods in dietary research, this tool is also limited by specific error associated with fact that it is a retrospective method, based on the memory of respondents [46]. However, the applied food frequency questionnaire was a previously validated and comprehensive questionnaire, in which respondents were asked not only about fruit and vegetable intake, but also about all food products groups, without specifying which items would be assessed. Applying a self-administrated questionnaire is also a well-known method to reduce a social desirability bias, and is thus considered better than other methods of questionnaire administration. Such an approach may reduce the effect of desirable bias, but it is still not completely eliminated [47]. Taking into account the aim of this study, it may be indicated that the systematic errors resulting from the applied method did not influence the association between the food neophobia level and the observed intake of fruits and vegetables in children aged 10–12 years.

Simultaneously, it must be emphasized that the varying results of the studies conducted worldwide may result from differences in the applied methodology, as well as from cultural differences between children from analyzed countries. The previously indicated differences of the most commonly chosen fruits and vegetables between Asian and European countries, as well as the indicated similarities of the most commonly chosen fruits and vegetables between European countries, are confirmed by the broad data from international comparisons. Taking into account the data from 2013, it must be indicated that fruit intake in Poland was similar to those in countries in the geographical proximity, such as Czech Republic, Slovakia, Hungary, Latvia, Ukraine, Republic of Moldavia, Romania, and the Russian Federation [48], and vegetable intake in Poland was also similar to those in countries such as Hungary, Lithuania, Slovenia, Serbia, Croatia, Republic of Moldavia, as well as Germany and Austria [48].

Given the abovementioned data, it must be emphasized that the obtained results could be useful to compare with results from other countries characterized by similar intake. Still, further studies are also recommended in order to confirm these observations in other European or non-European countries.

5. Conclusions

1. Children, aged 10–12 years, with a higher food neophobia level may be characterized by lower vegetable intake than children with a lower neophobia level.
2. The association between food neophobia level and vegetable intake in the case of girls aged 10–12 years seems to be stronger than that in the case of boys.
3. In the case of children aged 10–12 years, in order to increase the vegetable intake, education must be conducted to achieve a reduction in the food neophobia level. However, further studies are also needed.

Author Contributions: D.Gu. made study conception and design; D.Gu., D.Gł., E.L. performed the research; D.Gł., analyzed the data; D.Gu., D.Gł., E.L., M.J.-Z. wrote the paper. All the authors read and approved the final manuscript.

Conflicts of Interest: The authors declare no conflict of interest

References

1. Lim, S.S.; Vos, T.; Flaxman, A.D.; Danaei, G.; Shibuya, K.; Adair-Rohani, H.A.; AlMazroa, M.A.; Amann, M.; Anderson, R.; Andrews, K.G.; et al. A comparative risk assessment of burden of disease and injury attributable to 67 risk factors and risk factor clusters in 21 regions, 1990–2010: A systematic analysis for the Global Burden of Disease Study 2010. *Lancet* **2012**, *380*, 2224–2260. [CrossRef]
2. Increasing Fruit and Vegetable Consumption to Reduce the Risk of Noncommunicable Diseases Biological, Behavioural and Contextual Rationale. WHO, 2014. Available online: http://www.who.int/elena/titles/bbc/fruit_vegetables_ncds/en/ (accessed on 27 March 2017).
3. Lee, H.A.; Hwang, H.J.; Oh, S.Y.; Park, E.A.; Cho, S.J.; Kim, H.S.; Park, H. Which Diet-Related Behaviors in Childhood Influence a Healthier Dietary Pattern? From the Ewha Birth and Growth Cohort. *Nutrients* **2017**, *9*, 4. [CrossRef] [PubMed]
4. Galinski, G.; Lonnie, M.; Kowalkowska, J.; Wadolowska, L.; Czarnocinska, J.; Jezewska-Zychowicz, M.; Babicz-Zielinska, E. Self-Reported Dietary Restrictions and Dietary Patterns in Polish Girls: A Short Research Report (GEBaHealth Study). *Nutrients* **2016**, *8*, 796. [CrossRef] [PubMed]
5. Hall, J.N.; Moore, S.; Harper, S.B.; Lynch, J.W. Global variability in fruit and vegetable consumption. *Am. J. Prev. Med.* **2009**, *36*, 402–409. [CrossRef] [PubMed]
6. Borrmann, A.; Mensink, G.B.; KiGGS Study Group. Fruit and vegetable consumption by children and adolescents in Germany: Results of KiGGS wave 1. *Bundesgesundheitsblatt Gesundheitsforschung Gesundheitsschutz* **2015**, *58*, 1005–1014. (In German) [CrossRef] [PubMed]
7. Lock, K.; Pomerleau, J.; Causer, L.; McKee, M. Low fruit and vegetable consumption. In *Comparative Quantification of Health Risks. Global and Regional Burden of Disease Attribution to Selected Major Risk Factors*; Ezzati, M., Lopez, A.D., Rodgers, A., Murray, C.J.L., Eds.; Nonserial Publication; World Health Organization: Geneva, Switzerland; pp. 597–728.
8. Hebestreit, A.; Intemann, T.; Siani, A.; De Henauw, S.; Eiben, G.; Kourides, Y.A.; Kovacs, E.; Moreno, L.A.; Veidebaum, T.; Krogh, V.; et al. Dietary patterns of European children and their parents in association with family food environment: Results from the I. Family Study. *Nutrients* **2017**, *10*, 126. [CrossRef] [PubMed]
9. Rasmussen, M.; Krølner, R.; Klepp, K.-I.; Lytle, L.; Brug, J.; Bere, E.; Due, P. Determinants of fruit and vegetable consumption among children and adolescents: A review of the literature. Part I: Quantitative studies. *Int. J. Behav. Nutr. Phys. Act.* **2006**, *2*, 1–19.
10. Wardle, J.; Cooke, L. Genetic and environmental determinants of children's food preferences. *Br. J. Nutr.* **2008**, *99*, 15–21. [CrossRef] [PubMed]
11. Russell, C.G.; Worsley, A. A population-based study of preschoolers' food neophobia and its associations with food preferences. *J. Nutr. Educ. Behav.* **2008**, *40*, 11–19. [CrossRef] [PubMed]

12. Chu, Y.L.; Farmer, A.; Fung, C.; Kuhle, S.; Veugelers, P. Fruit and vegetable preferences and intake among children in Alberta. *Can. J. Diet. Pract. Res.* **2013**, *74*, 21–27. [CrossRef] [PubMed]

13. Pliner, P.; Hobden, K. Development of a scale to measure the trait of food neophobia in humans. *Appetite* **1992**, *19*, 105–120. [CrossRef]

14. Knaapila, A.; Tuorila, H.; Silventoinen, K.; Keskitalo, K.; Kallela, M.; Wessma, M.; Peltonen, L.; Cherkas, L.C.; Spector, T.D.; Perola, M. Food neophobia shows heritable variation in humans. *Physiol. Behav.* **2007**, *91*, 573–578. [CrossRef] [PubMed]

15. DeVellis, R.F. *Scale Development*; Sage Publications: Newbury Park, NJ, USA, 1991.

16. Tuorila, H.; Mustonen, S. Reluctant trying of an unfamiliar food induces negative affection for the food. *Appetite* **2010**, *43*, 418–421. [CrossRef] [PubMed]

17. Głąbska, D.; Guzek, D.; Sidor, P.; Włodarek, D. Vitamin D dietary intake questionnaire validation conducted among young Polish women. *Nutrients* **2016**, *5*, 36. [CrossRef] [PubMed]

18. Falciglia, G.A.; Couch, S.C.; Gribble, L.S.; Pabst, S.M.; Frank, R. Food neophobia in childhood affects dietary variety. *J. Am. Diet. Assoc.* **2000**, *100*, 1474–1481. [CrossRef]

19. Dovey, T.; Staples, P.; Gibson, E.; Halford, J. Food neophobia and 'picky/fussy' eating in children: A review. *Appetite* **2008**, *50*, 181–193. [CrossRef] [PubMed]

20. Ong, C.; Phuah, K.Y.; Salazar, E.; How, C.H. Managing the "picky eater" dilemma. *Singap. Med. J.* **2014**, *55*, 184–190. [CrossRef]

21. Mennella, J.A.; Nicklaus, S.; Jagolino, A.L.; Yourshaw, L.M. Variety is the spice of life: Strategies for promoting fruit and vegetable acceptance during infancy. *Physiol. Behav.* **2008**, *22*, 29–38. [CrossRef] [PubMed]

22. Lytle, L.A.; Seifert, S.; Greenstein, J.; McGovern, F. How do children's eating patterns and food choices change over time? Results from a cohort study. *Am. J. Health Promot.* **2000**, *14*, 222–228. [CrossRef] [PubMed]

23. Nicklaus, S.; Boggio, V.; Chabanet, C.; Issanchou, S. A prospective study of food variety seeking in childhood, adolescence and early adult life. *Appetite* **2005**, *44*, 289–297. [CrossRef] [PubMed]

24. Laureati, M.; Bergamaschi, V.; Pagliarini, E. School-based intervention with children. Peer-modeling, reward and repeated exposure reduce food neophobia and increase liking of fruits and vegetables. *Appetite* **2014**, *83*, 26–32. [CrossRef] [PubMed]

25. Nicklas, T.A.; Baranowski, T.; Baranowski, J.C.; Cullen, K.; Rittenberry, L.; Olvera, N. Family and child-care provider influences on preschool children's fruit, juice, and vegetable consumption. *Nutr. Rev.* **2001**, *59*, 224–235. [CrossRef] [PubMed]

26. Gillman, M.W.; Rifas-Shiman, S.L.; Frazier, A.L.; Rockett, H.R.; Camargo, C.A., Jr.; Field, A.E.; Berkey, C.S.; Colditz, G.A. Family dinner and diet quality among older children and adolescents. *Arch. Fam. Med.* **2000**, *9*, 235–240. [CrossRef] [PubMed]

27. Birch, L.L. Effects of peer models' food choices and eating behaviors on preschoolers' food preferences. *Child Dev.* **1980**, *51*, 489–496. [CrossRef]

28. Czarnocińska, J.; Anioła, J.; Grabowska, J.; Galiński, G.; Wądołowska, L. Food preferences, frequency and intake by schoolgirls. *Pol. J. Food Nutr. Sci.* **2009**, *59*, 251–254.

29. Babicz-Zielińska, E. Preference and consumption of vegetables and fruit among schoolchildren. *Pol. J. Food Nutr. Sci.* **1999**, *8*, 109–116.

30. Pérez-Rodrigo, C.; Ribas, L.; Serra-Majem, L.; Aranceta, J. Food preferences of Spanish children and young people: The enKid study. *Eur. J. Clin. Nutr.* **2003**, *57*, 45–48. [CrossRef] [PubMed]

31. Lafraire, J.; Rioux, C.; Giboreau, A.; Picard, D. Food rejections in children: Cognitive and social/environmental factors involved in food neophobiaand picky/fussy eating behavior. *Appetite* **2016**, *96*, 347–357. [CrossRef] [PubMed]

32. Coulthard, H.; Palfreyman, Z.; Morizet, D. Sensory evaluation of a novel vegetable in school age children. *Appetite* **2016**, *1*, 64–69. [CrossRef] [PubMed]

33. Cooke, L.J.; Wardle, J. Age and gender differences in children's food Preferences. *Br. J. Nutr.* **2005**, *93*, 741–746. [CrossRef] [PubMed]

34. Forestell, C.A.; Mennella, J.A. Early Determinants of Fruit and Vegetable Acceptance. *Pediatrics* **2007**, *120*, 1247–1254. [CrossRef] [PubMed]

35. Glendinning, J.I. Is the bitter rejection response always adaptive? *Physiol. Behav.* **1994**, *56*, 1217–1227. [CrossRef]

36. Galloway, A.; Lee, Y.; Birch, L.L. Predictors and consequences of food neophobia and pickiness in young girls. *J. Am. Diet. Assoc.* **2003**, *103*, 692–698. [CrossRef] [PubMed]

37. Hursti, U.; Sjödén, P. Food and general neophobia and their relationship with self-reported food choice: Familial resemblance in Swedish families with children of ages 7–17 years. *Appetite* **1997**, *29*, 89–103. [CrossRef] [PubMed]

38. Cooke, L.; Wardle, J.; Gibson, E. Relationship between parental report of food neophobia and everyday food consumption in 2–6-year-old children. *Appetite* **2003**, *41*, 205–206. [CrossRef]

39. Cooke, L.; Wardle, J.; Gibson, E.; Sapochnik, M.; Sheiham, A.; Lawson, M. Demographic, familial and trait predictors of fruit and vegetable consumption by pre-school children. *Public Health Nutr.* **2004**, *7*, 295–302. [CrossRef] [PubMed]

40. Cooke, L.; Carnell, S.; Wardle, J. Food neophobia and mealtime food consumption in 4–5 year old children. *Int. J. Behav. Nutr. Phys.* **2006**, *3*, 14. [CrossRef] [PubMed]

41. Wardle, J.; Carnell, S.; Cooke, L. Parental control over feeding and children's fruit and vegetable intake: How are they related? *J. Am. Diet. Assoc.* **2005**, *105*, 227–232. [CrossRef] [PubMed]

42. Coulthard, H.; Blissett, J. Fruit and vegetable consumption in children and their mothers. Moderating effects of child sensory sensitivity. *Appetite* **2009**, *52*, 410–415. [CrossRef] [PubMed]

43. Tsuji, M.; Nakamura, K.; Tamai, Y.; Wada, K.; Sahashi, Y.; Watanabe, K.; Ohtsuchi, S.; Ando, K.; Nagata, C. Relationship of intake of plant-based foods with 6-n-propylthiouracil sensitivity and food neophobia in Japanese preschool children. *Eur. J. Clin. Nutr.* **2012**, *66*, 47–52. [CrossRef] [PubMed]

44. Stein, L.J.; Nagai, H.; Nakagawa, M.; Beauchamp, G.K. Effects of repeated exposure and health-related information on hedonic evaluation and acceptance of a bitter beverage. *Appetite* **2003**, *40*, 119–129. [CrossRef]

45. Park, B.K.; Cho, M.S. Taste education reduces food neophobia and increases willingness to try novel foods in school children. *Nutr. Res. Pract.* **2016**, *10*, 221–228. [CrossRef] [PubMed]

46. Gibson, R.S. *Principles of Nutritional Assessment*, 2nd ed.; Oxford University Press: New York, NY, USA, 2005.

47. Nederhof, A.J. Methods of coping with social desirability bias: A review. *Eur. J. Soc. Psychol.* **1985**, *15*, 263–280. [CrossRef]

48. Data and Statistics—Food Supply—Statistics by Country. Available online: https://knoema.com/atlas/topics/Agriculture (accessed on 25 May 2017).

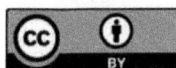

nutrients

MDPI

Article

Parents' Qualitative Perspectives on Child Asking for Fruit and Vegetables

Alicia Beltran, Teresia M. O'Connor, Sheryl O. Hughes, Debbe Thompson, Janice Baranowski, Theresa A. Nicklas and Tom Baranowski *

USDA/ARS Children's Nutrition Research Center, Department of Pediatrics, Baylor College of Medicine, Houston, TX 77030, USA; abeltran@bcm.edu (A.B.); teresiao@bcm.edu (T.M.O.); shughes@bcm.edu (S.O.H.); dit@bcm.edu (D.T.); jbaranow@bcm.edu (J.B.); tnicklas@bcm.edu (T.A.N.)
* Correspondence: tbaranow@bcm.edu; Tel.: +1-713-798-6762

Received: 14 March 2017; Accepted: 31 May 2017; Published: 5 June 2017

Abstract: Children can influence the foods available at home, but some ways of approaching a parent may be better than others; and the best way may vary by type of parent. This study explored how parents with different parenting styles would best receive their 10 to 14 years old child asking for fruits and vegetables (FV). An online parenting style questionnaire was completed and follow-up qualitative telephone interviews assessed home food rules, child influence on home food availability, parents' preferences for being asked for food, and common barriers and reactions to their child's FV requests. Parents (*n* = 73) with a 10 to 14 years old child were grouped into authoritative, authoritarian, permissive, or uninvolved parenting style categories based on responses to questionnaires, and interviewed. Almost no differences in responses were detected by parenting style or ethnicity. Parents reported their children had a voice in what foods were purchased and available at home and were receptive to their child's asking for FV. The most important child asking characteristic was politeness, especially among authoritarian parents. Other important factors were asking in person, helping in the grocery store, writing requests on the grocery shopping list, and showing information they saw in the media. The barrier raising the most concern was FV cost, but FV quality and safety outside the home environment were also considerations.

Keywords: fruit; vegetables; asking skills; parenting style; children

1. Introduction

Fruit and vegetable consumption has been inversely correlated with all-cause mortality, especially cardiovascular disease mortality [1], and with hypertension, coronary heart disease, and stroke [2]. Despite these health benefits, children's FV consumption is below recommended levels [3]. Focusing on children is important because establishing healthy eating behaviors at any child age tracks into adulthood [4]. A determinant of child FV consumption is home availability [5], i.e., having the item in the home (e.g., carrots in the refrigerator) [6].

Parents influence their children's dietary intake [7]. Keeping healthy foods in the home and unhealthy foods out of the home (i.e., home availability) were consistently the most important parental influences on child intake [8]. In addition, parents influence children's eating behavior through their parenting style [9], i.e., the emotional tone set by the parent for the parent–child relationship. Four general types of parenting style have been identified: authoritarian (highly demanding, and controlling; low emotional warmth), authoritative (highly demanding and controlling; high emotional support and responsiveness), permissive/indulgent (low control and non-demanding, high emotional support and responsiveness), and uninvolved (low demanding, low responsiveness) [10,11]. Parenting style was related to the healthfulness of joint parent–child food shopping selections [12]. Uninvolved parenting style moderated the relationship of child emotional eating and BMIz scores [13]. Maternal indulgent feeding style (i.e., parenting style specific to food) and restrictive parenting practices were related to BMIz score increase over an 18 month interval [14]. Ethnic group differences have been detected in parenting style [15].

Parent–child relationships, however, are a two-way interaction [16]. Children have influenced home food availability by expressing their preferences [17,18] and making requests [19]. Children have developed knowledge, skills, and values for decision making to influence purchases for the home [20,21]. One strategy to increase home FV availability is to teach children to effectively ask parents for their favorite FV. Early adolescence (e.g., 10–14 years old) is a time when children are beginning to establish independence [22], and thus an ideal time to learn new ways to relate to parents. A role-playing intervention improved child asking and negotiation skills and showed a positive effect on home FV availability [23], while another reported that a school based intervention increased parent report of child asking for FV [24]. Asking behaviors at baseline among fourth or fifth grade children predicted home FV availability, but small increases in asking behaviors did not increase home FV availability [25]. Children 12–15 years of age expressed reluctance to ask for FV due to the anticipated negative reaction of their parents [26], which may affect how they ask for FV, and depress impact. Furthermore, parents with the alternative parenting styles may respond differently to various ways of child asking.

Given child reluctance to ask parents to increase FV at home [26], more effective asking interventions may be created if nutrition education interventionists understood how parents might respond to their child's FV asking behaviors and whether these responses vary by parenting style. Given ethnic group differences in parenting style [15], it would also be valuable to understand differences in parent responses by ethnic group.

This study explored how parents from different ethnic groups with different parenting styles would best receive asking for FV from their 10–14-year-old child, and thereby provide the basis for an intervention teaching children asking skills to enhance home FV availability.

2. Materials and Methods

2.1. Study Design

This study was conducted in two phases in 2006. Phase I was a cross sectional online survey that assessed parenting styles. Parents were categorized by parenting style (i.e., authoritative, authoritarian, permissive, or uninvolved). Phase II was an intensive telephone interview with the parent primarily responsible for home food purchase and preparation. Participants were stratified by parenting style and ethnic group based on survey responses. While the project was based in Houston, TX, USA, and the more intensive recruitment activities were located in Houston, respondents from across the USA could participate since inclusion required only completing a web-based questionnaire and responding to a telephone interview. Participants were asked in the survey to select the state and city in which they were located.

2.2. Sample and Recruitment

Eligible participants were parents or guardians with a 10–14-year-old child, had Internet access, were English or Spanish speaking, and were the person in the household responsible for home food purchase, preparation, and serving. Participants were excluded if their 10–14-year-old child had a health condition that affected their dietary intake.

Participants were recruited via a national Children's Nutrition Research Center newsletter, the Children's Nutrition Research Center volunteer list and webpage, health related electronic mailing lists; flyers, a health fair, and radio advertisements targeted to the African American population. Since African American children tend to eat fewer FV [27] and are less likely to participate in research [28], an attempt was made to increase participation from this group. This convenience approach to recruitment and enrollment lasted nine months. A total of 537 participants entered the website and consented to participate, 8 participants declined to participate; of these, 198 parent/guardian and child pairs (36.3%) completed the online survey. Twenty-two participants did not qualify because they were not the parent or guardian of the child and one participant did not qualify because the child did not live with the parent. We have no data for why the 316 participants who consented electronically did not complete the survey.

2.3. Procedures

The study website informed parents about the purpose of the study, assured confidentiality and obtained online consent to participate for self and child. The parent then completed a screening and demographic questionnaire, the Children's Report of Parental Behavior Inventory (CRPBI-30) (Schludermann EH & Schludermann SM, 1988, unpublished results) adapted to parents (English or Spanish). After the parent completed the questionnaires, their 10–14-year-old child completed online assent, and answered the CRPBI-30 for children and youth [29].

The parent/guardian–child pairs who met the inclusion criteria were then categorized on parenting style calculated from the child CRPBI-30 responses. The goal was to enroll 100 participants: 40 authoritative and 40 authoritarian participants with 10 African American, White, Hispanic, and Other in each of these categories; and 10 participants each in the permissive and uninvolved cells. In our experience with research on parenting, theoretical saturation is usually attained with 10 or fewer participants, thereby providing an adequate sample for ethnicity differences within parenting style groups. Theoretically, we expected the permissive and uninvolved parenting style parents would be less likely to be responsive to child asking behaviors. For example, permissive parents would be expected to allow any food (healthy or not) the child wanted into the home; and uninvolved parents would not be expected to respond to any entreaty. Also, based on previous experience we knew there would be fewer permissive and uninvolved respondents, likely reflecting their indifference to participating in such projects. We continued enrollment for as long as participants were agreeing to be interviewed. The parent was then contacted for the 45-min telephone interview. Interviews were pilot tested. All interviewed parents were compensated $25. The Institutional Review Board of the Baylor College of Medicine approved the protocol and procedures.

2.4. Measures

The demographic and screening questionnaire included questions about ethnicity, parent education and parent household role. The revised children and youth report of parental behavior inventory questionnaire (CRPBI-30) is a short (30 item) version of the 108-item questionnaire (Schludermann EH & Schludermann SM, 1988, unpublished results), which measures three dimensions: acceptance/rejection, psychological control/autonomy, and firm/lax control. Each item was answered on a three-point scale (1 = not like my parent or guardian, 2 = a little like my parent or guardian, and 3 = a lot like my parent or guardian). In a sample of older adolescents reporting on their mothers, Cronbach's alphas and test–retest correlations were 0.75 and 0.84 for acceptance (10 items), 0.72 and 0.84 for psychological control (10 items), and 0.65 and 0.79 for firm control (10 items), respectively (Schludermann EH & Schludermann SM, 1988, unpublished results) and dimensions were associated with Family Satisfaction as measured by Olson's Family Satisfaction Scale [29].

2.5. Qualitative Interview

A semi-structured interview script was designed by researchers with expertise in child feeding behavior and qualitative interview techniques. The script guided the interview; prompts were used to assess different aspects of the questions while probes were used to expand or clarify the responses (see Table 1). The script explored the family rules about foods eaten at home, participation, and influence of the child in the decision making of the foods available at home, times when parents were willing to talk with the child about foods, ways in which the child could best ask the parent for foods, parent reactions towards specific child FV requests, and barriers to comply with their child's request.

Table 1. Questions used to guide the semi-structured interview

1. How much say, if any, does your child have about the foods and beverages you buy for home?
2. If your child wanted to talk with you about the foods they like or don't like, when are the best times or situations for them to talk with you?
3. If your child wanted to have specific foods available at home, describe the best way for them to ask you.
a. What other ways, other than asking, could they use to let you know about specific foods they wanted at home?
4. How likely would you be to buy fruit or vegetables if your child asked for them?
a. How would your response to your child change: • If no one else in your home would eat the fruit or vegetable? • If you've bought this fruit or vegetable in the past but had to throw it away? • If you personally do not like this fruit or vegetable? • If the fruit or vegetable is expensive? • If the fruit or vegetable cannot be prepared quickly? • If you don't know how to prepare this fruit or vegetable?
5. How likely would you be to do the following, if your child asked you to: • Buy 100% fruit juice for breakfast? • Buy fruit for an after-school snack? • Buy vegetables and dip for a snack (e.g., carrots and low fat ranch dip)? • Buy a salad for home? • Make a salad for home? • Make their favorite vegetable for dinner? • Add a fruit or vegetable to the grocery list? • Buy fruit at a restaurant? • Buy a salad at a restaurant? • Buy a vegetable at a restaurant?

2.6. Data Analysis

As prescribed by the originators, children's reports on two of the dimensions: acceptance and firm control were used to categorize their parents on the parenting style category based on median splits from the validation studies (Schludermann EH & Schludermann SM, 1988, unpublished results): authoritarian (high control, low acceptance), authoritative (high control, high acceptance), permissive (low control, high acceptance), and uninvolved (low control, low acceptance). Child responses were used to avoid the possible confounding of common response bias of parent report of parenting style with parent responses to the interview.

Audio-recordings were transcribed verbatim and transcriptions checked against audio-recordings prior to analysis to ensure accuracy. Analysis was conducted in phases: first, separate responses were identified on the transcripts, and entered into Excel (version 12, 2007 Microsoft Office Excel, Microsoft Corp, Redmond, WA, USA); coding was performed manually with thematic codes [30,31] reflecting the questions asked. Within questions, codes were derived as the classification proceeded. Interview response codes were grouped by parenting style and ethnicity to assess possible differences. Given the large number of interviews, coding was conducted independently by six staff members and a coordinator. All transcripts were coded by two coders. The coordinator discussed discrepancies with the independent coders until consensus was established; codings were revised based on the consensus opinion. Comparison summary tables were created to assess differences by ethnicity and then by parenting style.

3. Results

Seventy-three participants (36.9% of the 193 completing the web-based questionnaire) were interviewed: 36 authoritative, 30 authoritarian, 5 permissive, and 2 uninvolved parents (Table 2). The majority were mothers (98.6%) with an average 40.0 ± 5.0 years of age. More parents of girls were interviewed (60.3%). Participants were heavily sourced from Houston (55%), but came from across the

US (Table 2). Since no or only slight differences in responses were detected by parenting style, or by ethnicity in the authoritarian and authoritative categories, findings are presented by questions in the script. The few differences by parenting style and ethnicity are noted.

Table 2. Parent–child demographic characteristics.

Characteristic	*n* (%)	M (SD)
Total parent–child interviews	73 (100.0)	
Age of 10–14 yo child (years)		
10	13 (17.8)	
11	13 (17.8)	
12	17 (23.3)	
13	17 (23.3)	
14	13 (17.8)	
Parent Age		39.97 (5.89)
Child gender		
Male	29 (39.7)	
Female	44 (60.3)	
Parent gender		
Male	1 (1.4)	
Female	72 (98.6)	
Child Race/Ethnicity		
White	22 (30.1)	
AA	19 (26.0)	
Hispanic	23 (31.5)	
Other	9 (12.3)	
Parent Race/Ethnicity		
White	27 (37)	
AA	20 (27.4)	
Hispanic	20 (27.4)	
Other	6 (8.2)	
Parenting style		
Authoritative	36 (49.3)	
Authoritarian	30 (41.1)	
Permissive	5 (6.8)	
Uninvolved	2 (2.7)	
Highest Parent Education		
HS Graduate or less	10 (13.7)	
Some college/technical school	22 (30.1)	
College graduate	23 (31.5)	
Post graduate study	18 (24.7)	
Highest Household Education		
HS Graduate or less	11 (15.1)	
Some college/technical school	21 (28.8)	
College graduate	19 (26.0)	
Post graduate study	22 (30.1)	
State of participants		
California	2 (2.7)	
Colorado	1 (1.4)	
Maine	1 (1.4)	
Minnesota	2 (2.7)	
North Carolina	1 (1.4)	
New Mexico	4 (5.4)	
Oklahoma	1 (1.4)	
Oregon	1 (1.4)	
Texas Houston	40 (55)	
Other Cities	18 (24.6)	
Tennessee	1 (1.4)	
Wyoming	1 (1.4)	

Percentages that do not sum to 100% are due to rounding. Legend: AA = African-American; HS = High School.

3.1. Influence of the Child on the Food and Beverages Bought for Home

When asking parents how much influence their child had on the foods and beverages purchased for home, most of the parents (88%) said their child had a lot of, or some, influence. Three ways in which the child influenced the parent included: the child decided the type of food; the parent controlled the situation, but allowed the child some input upon request; and the parent asked what the child wanted to eat. "...somewhat my child has a say, because if he's not going to eat it, it's no use for me buying it. I have to buy something that I know he's going to eat, or he wants." (Interview 380, Authoritarian–African American)

Some parents (23%) said the child influenced them to buy what the child liked, implying they do not have to ask the child. A few parents (11%) reported the child had a say in food purchases depending on the type of food. If the parent considered the food healthy the parent would buy the requested food, but if the parent considered the food unhealthy, the parent would not purchase it. Some parents (37%) said their child had some say by adding food items to the shopping list, while others (52%) said their child went grocery shopping with them.

3.2. Types of Food Requested by the Child and the Parents' Reaction

Children requested a variety of foods; whether parents bought the requested food depended on the type of food. If the food requested was chips or cookies, a small group (11%) would not buy it. Another factor influencing the purchase was budget. A minority (7%) suggested buying a healthier version of the requested food, or buying the food for limited occasions or quantities. Only 14% of parents reported buying the food without any restrictions, in order to please the child. "...if they're saying, ...can we get green grapes and red grapes, ...if it is something healthy and they ask for it, and granted it is affordable, ...and in the budget ...they can have it, because I encourage them to eat good foods." (Interview 286, Authoritarian–White)

3.3. Times or Channels for the Parent and Child to Talk about Foods

Most parents (73%) reported that a good time to discuss purchasing a food was in the car, because they had time to talk, and the family was together as a captive audience. However, a small number of parents (18%) reported talking in the car was not a good time. Most parents (89%) reported mealtimes as a good time, preferring dinnertime, because they are together as a family, and talk about the day with food present. Another good time was while making the grocery list (53% of parents). "Usually ...at dinner, or ...because we spend a lot of time in the car driving to different activities and that's always a very good time for us to talk." (Interview 650, Authoritative–Other Ethnicity)

Some parents (30%) reported anytime was good to talk about food. The grocery store (18%), while cooking (10%), and before or after school (15%) were other times mentioned by small numbers of parents.

3.4. How Parents Liked Their Child to Ask for Food

Some parents (44%) reported a good way was just asking them in person. About 40% thought their child should ask in a polite manner. This was mentioned more often by the authoritarian parents (18/30) than authoritative (7/36) or permissive (2/5) parents. Across all groups, some of the parents (37%) indicated a good way was asking or selecting the food at the grocery store. "... if they ... asked me, "Mom, could you get me something today?" and they said it in a nice tone with a good attitude and they were happy about it". (Interview 722, Uninvolved–White)

Another good way was writing the food on the grocery list (52% of parents). "I keep a list that they can add to. But they pretty much know, ...what's okay to put on there." (Interview 310, Authoritative–White) Some parents (26%) reported another way to ask was showing them information from the TV or child magazine ads.

When asked whether a child could ask too often, a small group (8% of parents) reported they would prefer not having the child ask too often (not further specified). However, other parents (32%) indicated they would get what the child asked for, depending on the type of food and the attitude of the child.

3.5. Common Barriers to Comply with Child Requests

Most parents (84%) said they would buy FV if their child asked; further, they reported that buying only the FV their child ate was not a barrier. However, a small number (15%) indicated they would be careful with the amount of FV purchased, if no one else at home ate that particular FV. " ... if one liked it and the rest did not, I would just buy less of it, but I would still buy it." (Interview 311, Permissive-White)

Across all groups, some parents (58%) reported being willing to buy the FV even if it had to be thrown away in the past. However, if this was the case they would purchase less of it or less frequently in the future and a few authoritarian parents would remind the child this would be the last time. A small number of parents (26%) reported they were not likely to purchase the FV if it had been thrown away in the past.

Parents' FV preferences were not a barrier to buying FV for their child. Some parents (42% would buy an expensive FV if the child asked. Others (52%) would buy the requested FV depending on their budget and only if the FV were in season. A small number of parents (19%) would limit the quantity purchased. "If it's expensive but still a little reasonable I will buy it as long as it's something healthy and I know they will eat it..." (Interview 436, Authoritative–Hispanic)

Time for FV preparation and lack of knowledge about preparation were not considered barriers for most parents (66%). Some parents (19%) would purchase the FV and prepare them only when they had time to do so. Only a few parents (16%) reported the lack of time and knowledge to prepare FV to be a barrier and therefore not likely to buy them.

3.6. Reactions to Specific FV Requested by Their Child

Most parents (78%) had a positive reaction toward buying 100% fruit juice for breakfast, and F and V and dip for a snack for their child. A few parents (11%) reported not likely buying 100% fruit juice because of the high sugar content and price. A few parents (10%) would not buy V and dip for a snack because they believed their child would not eat it or was not in their budget. Most parents (59%) already bought salad for home, while some parents (11%) would not buy salad for home because of the quality of salad and beliefs their child would not eat it. "Maybe a fruit salad but a vegetable leaf salad, she will not touch it with a ten-foot pole." (Interview 439, Authoritarian–Hispanic)

Many (84%) reported they would make their child's favorite V for dinner when available. Most parents (75%) would add a F or V to the grocery list, if asked, and buy F at a restaurant (59%), even though a few (5%) thought it was expensive. However, some parents (36%) were not likely to buy F at a restaurant because of perceived low quality, high price, and preference to eat F at home. "No, I don't buy fruit or vegetables ...you don't know what they put inside, ...what kind of seasoning. ...how they prepare it." (Interview 146, Authoritative–African American)

Most, but not all, parents (79%) said they would very likely buy salad or a V at a restaurant for their child.

4. Discussion

Availability of FV at home has consistently been shown to be related to child vegetable intake [32], but reticence in child asking to increase FV has been reported [26]. This study explored how parents would best respond to their 10–14-year-old child asking for FV. In general, parents appeared to be receptive, but the receptiveness of some appeared to be tempered by whether the food requested was considered healthy, and the parent retained control over the situation by limiting the quantity purchased. Although differences in parental acceptance of child asking was expected by parenting style and ethnicity, only slight differences were found in parent responses across authoritative and authoritarian styles and ethnicities. Thus, tailoring an intervention to parenting style or ethnicity does not appear to be needed. Alternatively, an intervention should take steps to appeal to all ethnicities or to be ethnic neutral [33].

Most of this literature has emphasized how parents do or can influence children, and so few references exist for comparison on how children can influence parents and the home food environment [26]. Children directly and indirectly had an influence on what foods were available at home. This is the first report of parent receptiveness to child asking. Parents expressed some control over the food available at home, but kept in mind the child's preferences when buying food, or allowing the child to select the food. Similar observations have been reported about how child preferences influence food availability at home [17]. Furthermore, children's influence on food purchases has been fully recognized and successfully used by marketers [19,20]. A community-based gardening intervention showed children influenced the families' decision making [34]. Marketers have identified influence tactics used by the children to persuade their parents to fulfill their needs e.g., consultation, where the child involves a parent in making a decision [19] or ingratiation where the child gets the parent in a good mood, before asking the parent to comply with their request. Thus, teaching a child to state their FV preferences and ask for FV appear to be promising techniques for helping increase availability of FV in the home and thereby its consumption. Future research should investigate these four pathways of child influence in the context of FV asking.

Parents were aware of the importance of having "healthy food" available at home, and limiting availability of unhealthy food. Concern of parents to have healthy food available in the home has been shown in other studies [35]. Thus, since FV are generally considered healthy, most parents would appear to be receptive to FV requests.

The most important child asking characteristic was politeness, especially among authoritarian parents. Another important factor was the channel for asking, whether in person or by helping in the grocery store, writing it on the grocery list or showing parents the information in the media. These factors have been effective at influencing parents' purchases in other settings [19,20]. Any intervention encouraging stating preference or asking for FV should emphasize politeness on the child's part in each of the channels of asking irrespective of parenting style.

Although some parents reported situational barriers, most offered to still purchase FV requested, but in limited quantities or at different times. The barriers that raised more concern were FV costs and the quality and safety of the FV obtained at restaurants. The intervention might teach children to have realistic expectations for parent responses to their asking. Alternatively, this could be an opportunity to combine math training, microeconomics, and nutrition by teaching somewhat older children relative pricing, amounts purchased, and household budgeting.

A limitation of this study was our inability to recruit substantial numbers of parents who practiced permissive and uninvolved parenting, which restricts the comparisons and the generalizability of the findings. Only 36.3% of mothers who completed the online consent also completed the online survey. Mothers lived in diverse locations across the US, and we do not know their reason(s) for participating, or others for not participating, which may bias the results. Thus, the sample may not be representative of all mothers of children this age, thereby limiting generalizability. Since family structure influences food choices in households [36], further research is needed on how the composition of the household affects family negotiations towards foods available at home.

5. Conclusions

Parent–child communication is bidirectional. Parents showed openness to complying with their child FV requests, as long as certain minimal criteria were met. Children need to learn to ask parents for FV in a polite manner. The training should specifically address alternative channels, e.g., during meals, while preparing the grocery list, in the kitchen when the parent is cooking, in the car, or at the grocery store. Strategies should improve the asking skills to overcome some of the parents' perceived barriers like the lack of time to prepare FV, cost of FV, and FV food safety out of the home environment. Tailoring an intervention to parenting style or ethnicity does not appear to be necessary.

Acknowledgments: This work was funded by grant R21 HD058175 from the National Institute of Child Health and Human Development (NICHHD). This work is also a publication of the United States Department of Agriculture (USDA/ARS) Children's Nutrition Research Center, Department of Pediatrics, Baylor College of Medicine, Houston, Texas, and had been funded in part with federal funds from the USDA/ARS under Cooperative Agreement No. 58-6250-0-008.

Author Contributions: Tom Baranowski, Teresia M. O'Connor, Sheryl O. Hughes, Debbe Thompson, Janice Baranowski, and Theresa A. Nicklas conceived and designed the study. Alicia Beltran was involved in the design and planning of the research, conducted the data collection and analysis, and wrote a preliminary draft of the paper. All authors critically reviewed the manuscript and approved the final version submitted for publication.

Conflicts of Interest: The authors declare no conflict of interest.

References

1. Leenders, M.; Sluijs, I.; Ros, M.M.; Boshuizen, H.C.; Siersema, P.D.; Ferrari, P.; Weikert, C.; Tjønneland, A.; Olsen, A.; Boutron-Ruault, M.C.; et al. Fruit and vegetable consumption and mortality: European prospective investigation into cancer and nutrition. *Am. J. Epidemiol.* **2013**, *178*, 590–602. [CrossRef] [PubMed]
2. Boeing, H.; Bechthold, A.; Bub, A.; Ellinger, S.; Haller, D.; Kroke, A.; Leschik-Bonnet, E.; Müller, M.J.; Oberritter, H.; Schulze, M.; et al. Critical review: Vegetables and fruit in the prevention of chronic diseases. *Eur. J. Nutr.* **2012**, *51*, 637–663. [CrossRef] [PubMed]
3. Grimm, K.A.; Kim, S.A.; Yaroch, A.L.; Scanlon, K.S. Fruit and vegetable intake during infancy and early childhood. *Pediatrics* **2014**, *134*, S63–S69. [CrossRef] [PubMed]
4. Craigie, A.M.; Lake, A.A.; Kelly, S.A.; Adamson, A.J.; Mathers, J.C. Tracking of obesity-related behaviours from childhood to adulthood: A systematic review. *Maturitas* **2011**, *70*, 266–284. [CrossRef] [PubMed]
5. Kristiansen, A.L.; Bjelland, M.; Himberg-Sundet, A.; Lien, N.; Andersen, L.F. Associations between physical home environmental factors and vegetable consumption among Norwegian 3–5-year-olds: The BRA-study. *Public Health Nutr.* **2016**, *20*, 1173–1183. [CrossRef] [PubMed]
6. Cullen, K.W.; Baranowski, T.; Owens, E.; Marsh, T.; Rittenberry, L.; de Moor, C. Availability, accessibility and preferences for fruit, 100% juice and vegetables influence children's dietary behavior. *Health Educ. Behav.* **2003**, *30*, 615–626. [CrossRef] [PubMed]
7. Pearson, N.; Biddle, S.J.; Gorely, T. Family correlates of fruit and vegetable consumption in children and adolescents: a systematic review. *Public Health Nutr.* **2009**, *12*, 267–283. [CrossRef] [PubMed]
8. Yee, A.Z.; Lwin, M.O.; Ho, S.S. The influence of parental practices on child promotive and preventive food consumption behaviors: A systematic review and meta-analysis. *Int. J. Behav. Nutr. Phys. Act.* **2017**, *14*, 47. [CrossRef] [PubMed]
9. Gerards, S.M.; Sleddens, E.F.; Dagnelie, P.C.; de Vries, N.K.; Kremers, S.P. Interventions addressing general parenting to prevent or treat childhood obesity. *Int. J. Pediatr. Obes.* **2011**, *6*, e28–e45. [CrossRef] [PubMed]
10. Maccoby, E.; Martin, J. Socialization in the context of the family: Parent–child interaction. In *Handbook of Child Psychology: Socialization, Personality and Social Development*; Hetherington, E.M., Ed.; Wiley: New York, NY, USA, 1983; pp. 1–101.
11. Baumrind, D. Current patterns of parental authority. *Dev. Psychol.* **1971**, *4 1 Pt 2*, 1–103. [CrossRef] [PubMed]
12. Lucas-Thompson, R.G.; Graham, D.J.; Ullrich, E.; MacPhee, D. General and food-selection specific parenting style in relation to the healthfulness of parent–child choices while grocery shopping. *Appetite* **2017**, *108*, 353–360. [CrossRef] [PubMed]
13. Hankey, M.; Williams, N.A.; Dev, D. Uninvolved maternal feeding style moderates the association of emotional overeating to preschoolers' body mass index z-scores. *J. Nutr. Educ. Behav.* **2016**, *48*, 530–537. [CrossRef] [PubMed]
14. Hughes, S.O.; Power, T.G.; O'Connor, T.M.; Fisher, J.O.; Chen, T.A. Maternal feeding styles and food parenting practices as predictors of longitudinal changes in weight status in Hispanic preschoolers from low-income families. *J. Obes.* **2016**, *2016*. [CrossRef] [PubMed]

15. Clark, T.T.; Yang, C.; McClernon, F.J.; Fuemmeler, B.F. Racial differences in parenting style typologies and heavy episodic drinking trajectories. *Health Psychol.* **2015**, *34*, 697–708. [CrossRef] [PubMed]

16. Baranowski, T.; O'Connor, T.; Hughes, S.; Sleddens, E.; Beltran, A.; Frankel, L.; Mendoza, J.A.; Baranowski, J. Houston...We have a problem! Measurement of parenting. *Child Obes.* **2013**, *9*, 1–4. [CrossRef] [PubMed]

17. James, A.; Curtis, P.; Ellis, K. Negotiating family, negotiating food: Children as family participants? In *Children, Food and Identity in Everyday Life*; James, A., Kjørholt, A.T., Tingstad, V., Eds.; Palgrave Macmillan: Hampshire, UK, 2009; pp. 35–51.

18. Story, M.; Neumark-Sztainer, D.; French, S. Individual and environmental influences on adolescent eating behaviors. *J. Am. Diet. Assoc.* **2002**, *102*, S40–S51. [CrossRef]

19. Wimalasiri, J. A cross-national study on children's purchasing behavior and parental response. *J. Consum. Mark.* **2004**, *21*, 274–284. [CrossRef]

20. Kraak, V.; Pelletier, D.L. The influence of commercialism on the food purchasing behavior of children and teenage youth. *Fam. Econ. Nutr. Rev.* **1998**, *11*, 15–24.

21. John, D.R. Consumer socialization of children: A retrospective look at twenty-five years of research. *J. Consum. Res.* **1999**, *26*, 183–213. [CrossRef]

22. Thornburg, H.D. Is early adolescence really a stage of development? *Theory Pract.* **1983**, *22*, 79–84. [CrossRef]

23. Baranowski, T.; Davis, M.; Resnicow, K.; Baranowski, J.; Doyle, C.; Lin, L.S.; Smith, M.; Wang, D.T. Gimme 5 fruit, juice and vegetables for fun and health: Outcome evaluation. *Health Educ. Behav.* **2000**, *27*, 96–111. [CrossRef] [PubMed]

24. Sharma, S.; Helfman, L.; Albus, K.; Pomeroy, M.; Chuang, R.J.; Markham, C. Feasibility and acceptability of Brighter Bites: A food co-op in schools to increase access, continuity and education of fruits and vegetables among low-income populations. *J. Prim. Prev.* **2015**, *36*, 281–286. [CrossRef] [PubMed]

25. DeSmet, A.; Liu, Y.; De Bourdeaudhuij, I.; Baranowski, T.; Thompson, D. The effectiveness of asking behaviors among 9–11 year-old children in increasing home availability and children's intake of fruit and vegetables: Results from the Squire's Quest II self-regulation game intervention. *Int. J. Behav. Nutr. Phys. Act.* **2017**, *14*, 51. [CrossRef] [PubMed]

26. Middlestadt, S.E.; Lederer, A.M.; Smith, N.K.; Doss, D.; Hung, C.L.; Stevenson, L.D.; Fly, A.D. Determinants of middle-school students asking parents for fruits and vegetables: A theory-based salient belief elicitation. *Public Health Nutr.* **2013**, *16*, 1971–1978. [CrossRef] [PubMed]

27. Storey, M.; Anderson, P. Income and race/ethnicity influence dietary fiber intake and vegetable consumption. *Nutr. Res.* **2014**, *34*, 844–850. [CrossRef] [PubMed]

28. Erves, J.C.; Mayo-Gamble, T.L.; Malin-Fair, A.; Boyer, A.; Joosten, Y.; Vaughn, Y.C.; Sherden, L.; Luther, P.; Miller, S.; Wilkins, C.H. Needs, priorities, and recommendations for engaging underrepresented populations in clinical research: A community perspective. *J. Community Health* **2016**, *42*, 472–480. [CrossRef] [PubMed]

29. Olson, D.H.; Wilson, M. Family satisfaction. In *Families: What Makes Them Work*; Olson, D.H., McCubbin, H.I., Barnes, H., Larsen, A., Muxen, M., Wilson, M., Eds.; Sage Publications: Beverly Hills, CA, USA, 1983.

30. Bernard, H.R.; Ryan, G.W. *Analyzing Qualitative Data: Systematic Approaches*; Sage Publications: Thousand Oaks, CA, USA, 2010.

31. Braun, V.; Clarke, V. Using thematic analysis in psychology. *Qual. Res. Psychol.* **2006**, *3*, 77–101. [CrossRef]

32. Johnson, S.L. Developmental and environmental influences on young children's vegetable preferences and consumption. *Adv. Nutr.* **2016**, *7*, 220S–231S. [CrossRef] [PubMed]

33. Resnicow, K.; Baranowski, T.; Ahluwalia, J.S.; Braithwaite, R.L. Cultural sensitivity in public health: Defined and demystified. *Ethn. Dis.* **1999**, *9*, 10–21. [PubMed]

34. Heim, S.; Bauer, K.W.; Stang, J.; Ireland, M. Can a community-based intervention improve the home food environment? Parental perspectives of the influence of the delicious and nutritious garden. *J. Nutr. Educ. Behav.* **2011**, *43*, 130–134. [CrossRef] [PubMed]

Nutrients **2017**, *9*, 575

35. Nørgaard, M.K.; Brunsø, K. Family conflicts and conflict resolutions regarding food choices. *J. Consum. Behav.* **2011**, *10*, 141–151. [CrossRef]

36. Coveney, J. What does research on families and food tell us? Implications for nutrition and dietetic practice. *Nutr. Diet.* **2002**, *59*, 113–119.

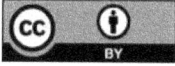

nutrients

MDPI

Article

Weight Status Is Related with Gender and Sleep Duration but Not with Dietary Habits and Physical Activity in Primary School Italian Children

Alice Rosi [1], Maria Vittoria Calestani [1], Liborio Parrino [2], Giulia Milioli [2], Luigi Palla [3], Elio Volta [4], Furio Brighenti [1] and Francesca Scazzina [1,*]

[1] Human Nutrition Unit, Department of Food and Drug, University of Parma, 43125 Parma, Italy; alice.rosi.g@gmail.com (A.R.); vittoria.calestani@hotmail.com (M.V.C.); furio.brighenti@unipr.it (F.B.)
[2] Sleep Disorders Center, Department of Medicine and Surgery, University of Parma, 43126 Parma, Italy; liborio.parrino@unipr.it (L.P.); giulia.milioli@gmail.com (G.M.)
[3] Department of Medical Statistics, Faculty of Epidemiology and Population Health, London School of Hygiene and Tropical Medicine, London WC1E 7HT, UK; luigi.palla@lshtm.ac.uk
[4] Giocampus Steering Committee, 43124 Parma, Italy; voltaelio@giocampus.it
*   Correspondence: francesca.scazzina@unipr.it; Tel.: +39-0521-903-841; Fax: +39-0521-903-832

Received: 30 April 2017; Accepted: 2 June 2017; Published: 6 June 2017

Abstract: The prevalence of overweight and obesity in children has risen greatly worldwide. Diet and poor physical activity are the two risk factors usually examined, but epidemiological evidence exists suggesting a link between sleep duration and overweight/obesity in children. The aim of this study was to describe the relationship among body mass index (BMI), diet quality, physical activity level, and sleep duration in 690 children attending the 5th grade in primary schools (9–11 years old) in the city of Parma (Italy) involved in the Giocampus educational program. This was achieved through (i) measuring anthropometric data to compute body mass index; (ii) administering a food questionnaire to evaluate adherence to the Mediterranean Diet (KIDMED score); and (iii) administering a lifestyle questionnaire to classify children physical activity level (PAL), sleep duration, and school achievement. A highly significant negative association was found between BMI and sleep hours. Moreover, there was a significant positive association between PAL and KIDMED scores. No evidence was found of association between BMI and PAL, nor between BMI and KIDMED score. Data from this study established that BMI is correlated to gender and sleep duration, defining sleep habits as one of the factors linked to overweight and obesity.

Keywords: Mediterranean diet; KIDMED; sleep; physical activity; children; school; BMI; lifestyle; Giocampus

1. Introduction

The incidence of overweight and obesity is increasing in all age groups worldwide. In Italy, overweight or obesity prevalence in children reach 35% in some regions, an extremely high level considering that obesity is high risk exposure for future health conditions [1,2]. In particular, overweight/obesity during childhood and adolescence is associated to a higher risk of developing chronic diseases during adulthood, such as several types of cancer, cardiovascular diseases, and metabolic syndrome [3]. The main determinants of overweight and obesity during childhood are an excessive energy intake, the lack of physical activity, and an inadequate sleep duration [4]. In the last few years, the time spent by children in outdoor activities or sports has considerably decreased, while time spent in screen activities, such as watching TV, playing videogames, or using electronic devices in their spare time has increased [5]. Even dietary habits have radically changed in recent years.

The consumption of high energy density and processed foods has risen significantly at the expense of fruit, vegetables, legumes, and whole cereals, the latter being those food groups the Mediterranean diet is based upon [6]. This fact is even more alarming as a high adherence to the Mediterranean diet has been related to a lower risk of developing chronic diseases and mortality in adults [7]. Different studies have also shown that a short sleep duration is often related to a non-balanced food intake and to unhealthy lifestyle habits, such as a reduction of physical activity [8–10]. Nevertheless, only a few studies have analyzed the relationship among dietary habits, physical activity, and sleep duration in school-aged children [11].

For all these reasons, it is paramount to create a surveillance system for monitoring the actual incidence of overweight and obesity in children and for defining the relative contribution of lifestyle habits (dietary, physical activity and sleep related). Moreover, it is important to educate children about a healthy lifestyle, explaining the importance of a balanced diet, regular physical activity, and adequate sleep duration [12]. In this framework, schools seem to be the optimal context for promoting programs aimed at improving lifestyle habits in children [13].

In the state primary schools in the city of Parma (Italy), an educational school program named "Giocampus" has been created for improving the wellbeing of future generations through healthy eating education and promotion of physical activity. An integrated "learning through playing" approach for delivering nutritional education has been successful in improving children's knowledge about healthy foods and a healthy lifestyle [14]. Professionally guided programs of physical education may also lead to significant progress in the development of conditional and coordinative abilities [15].

The aim of this study was to describe the relationship among body mass index (BMI), adherence to the Mediterranean diet (MD), physical activity level (PAL), and sleep duration in school-aged children attending the Giocampus program.

2. Materials and Methods

2.1. Participants and Study Design

The study was carried out during the 2015–2016 school years in the city of Parma (North Italy), in primary schools participating to the Giocampus program. All the students enrolled in the fifth grade (9–11 years old) were asked to participate in this observational study, through letters sent to the schools. Before acceptance, school principals, teachers, and parents were fully informed about the study protocol and the methods of assessment.

Data for each child were collected on the same day during school hours by two trained researchers through (i) measuring anthropometric data; (ii) administering a diet questionnaire aimed at defining the adherence to the MD; and (iii) administering a lifestyle questionnaire allowing classification of children PAL, sleep duration, and school achievement. The two questionnaires were administered directly to children.

The study was performed according to the Declaration of Helsinki and was approved by the Ethical Committee of the University of Parma (n5348-15/02/16).

2.2. Anthropometric Measurements

Anthropometric measurements were collected in the morning, during the physical activity class, ensuring privacy for each child, and following the WHO guidelines [16]. Body weight was measured to the nearest 100 g by using an electronic scale (MQ919, Maniquick, Niederkassel, Germany) with the child wearing only T-shirt and shorts, and was then corrected according to a simplified method validated within the Italian national surveillance system Okkio alla SALUTE [17]. Height was measured to the nearest 100 mm using a portable stadiometer (Leicester Tanita HR 001, Tanita, IL, USA). BMI was calculated as weight in kilograms divided by the square of the height in meters. Weight status was defined through the International Obesity Task Force gender- and age-related cut-offs for children BMI [18].

2.3. Dietary Habits

Adherence to the MD was assessed through the Mediterranean Diet Quality Index for children and adolescents (KIDMED) [19]. The KIDMED questionnaire comprises 16 dichotomous yes/no questions related to 12 positive and 4 negative dietary habits. Based on their correspondence with the principles of the MD, questions with a positive connotation were scored +1 point and questions with a negative connotation −1 point. A total KIDMED score ranging from 0 to 12 points was calculated for each child. The adherence to the MD was considered low, medium, or high if the KIDMED score was ≤3, between 4 and 7, and ≥8, respectively.

2.4. Physical Activity Level

According to the Italian national survey on children lifestyle [20], the PAL of children was defined by asking children about four types of activity they may be practicing during a usual week: transport-related activity, leisure time, screen-related activity, and sport. For each question, children chose one out of four possible answers, to which a score between 1 (sedentary habit) and 4 (high physical activity) was assigned. The mean score of the questions corresponded to the final activity level of the child, in keeping with the PAQ-C questionnaire [21]. Based on their final score, children were classified into one of four PAL categories as sedentary, low active, active, and very active [22,23].

2.5. Sleep Behaviors

Sleep habits were explored in terms of sleep duration and sleep pattern by asking about the wake up time in the morning and the time children went to sleep, for both weekdays and weekend days. Total sleep time was calculated in hours as the difference between bedtime and wake up time for weekdays and weekend days, and as the average weighted duration using the equation: (weekday time × 5 + weekend day time × 2)/7.

On the basis of the National Sleep Foundation recommendations for school-age children [24], sleep duration was classified as low if less than 9 h per night, recommended if between 9 and 11 h per night or high if more than 11 h per night.

In addition, sleep pattern was defined using the median value of the total week average sleep-wake schedule and classified as early bed/early rise (EE) (before 22:04 and before 07:38), early bed/late rise (EL) (before 22:04 and after 07:38), late bed/early rise (LE) (after 22:04 and before 07:38), or late bed/late rise (LL) (after 22:04 and after 07:38) [25,26].

2.6. School Achievement

School performance was assessed by asking the average grade (across subjects) of the current school year as a number, since in Italy school grades could range between 0 (very poor) and 10 (outstanding). In addition, child response was classified in three categories: mostly 10 and 9 (excellent-very good level), mostly 8 and 7 (good-very satisfactory level), and mostly 6 or less (satisfactory-poor level).

2.7. Statistical Analysis

All data were analyzed using descriptive statistics. Continuous variables were expressed as mean ± standard deviation (SD) of the total samples and by gender groups, BMI groups, or adherence to the MD groups. Categorical variables are presented as absolute frequencies and percentages of the total in the sample of respondents and by BMI groups or adherence to the MD groups.

The Kolmogorov–Smirnov test was applied to assess the normality of data distribution. The Student *t*-test was used to compare continuous variables between gender or BMI groups, while one-way ANOVA with Bonferroni post hoc test was used to compare among adherence to the MD groups, once the equality of variance was assessed by using the Levene's test. A Pearson chi-square test was performed to compare categorical variables between genders, BMI groups, and adherence to the MD groups.

The statistical analysis was completed through the Statistical Package for the Social Sciences (SPSS®, version 24.0, IBM, Chicago, IL, USA), with the significance set at $p < 0.05$.

3. Results

From a total of 1062 potentially eligible children, written consent to participate from parents was collected for 711 students (response rate 67%). In addition, 21 pupils did not give their verbal consent to participate or were absent during the assessment day. A total of 690 children, 357 females (52%) and 333 males (48%), with a mean age of 10.8 ± 0.4 years old, correctly completed all study requests. Children characteristics for the total sample and by gender are presented in Table 1.

Table 1. Participant characteristics (total sample and by gender).

Characteristic	Total Sample (*n* = 690)	Female (*n* = 357)	Male (*n* = 333)	*p* Value
Age (years)	10.8 ± 0.4	10.8 ± 0.3	10.8 ± 0.4	0.175
Weight (kg)	39.6 ± 8.7	39.2 ± 8.6	40.1 ± 8.8	0.152
Height (cm)	144.7 ± 6.8	145.0 ± 7.2	144.5 ± 6.5	0.357
BMI (kg/cm^2)	18.8 ± 3.2	18.5 ± 3.1	19.1 ± 3.3	0.019
KIDMED Score	6.5 ± 2.2	6.7 ± 2.1	6.4 ± 2.3	0.034
Physical Activity Level				<0.001
Low	92 (13.3)	57 (8.3)	35 (5.1)	
Medium	129 (18.7)	82 (11.9)	47 (6.8)	
High	372 (53.9)	177 (25.7)	195 (28.3)	
Very high	97 (14.1)	41 (5.9)	56 (8.1)	
Sleep Duration				
Total Sleep (hh)	9.5 ± 0.8	9.6 ± 0.7	9.4 ± 0.8	0.010
Week days (hh)	9.3 ± 0.8	9.4 ± 0.7	9.2 ± 0.8	<0.001
Weekend days (hh)	10.0 ± 1.4	10.3 ± 1.3	9.7 ± 1.5	<0.001
School Achievement	8.5 ± 1.0	8.5 ± 1.0	8.4 ± 1.0	0.467

Data are presented as mean $\pm$ SD of 690 (total sample), 357 (female) and 333 (male) independent measurements or as frequency (% of the total sample). A Pearson chi-square test was used to test the association of physical activity level with gender, while a *t*-test was used to compare all the other variables by gender.

No differences were found for weight and height between genders. The mean BMI corresponded to a normal weight status defined through the IOTF gender- and age-related cut-offs for both genders, despite its being higher in males ($p = 0.019$). In general, children had a medium adherence to the MD even by gender, with females being more adherent to the principles of the MD ($p = 0.034$). On the other hand, gender frequencies appear to differ by PAL ($x^2 = 17.1$, $df = 3$, $p < 0.001$), which was representative of a medium/high active lifestyle for both genders. According to the school-age children recommendations, children slept the recommended hours per night (9–11 h), and the sleep duration was found to be higher in females ($p = 0.010$ for the average total sleep and $p < 0.001$ for both weekdays and weekend days). School achievement was similar between genders, showing a good school performance of participants.

Irrespective of gender, 500 children (72.5%) had a low or normal weight, while 190 children were overweight-obese (Table 2). The two BMI groups frequencies appear to differ by gender ($x^2 = 8.7$, $df = 1$, $p = 0.003$), sleep duration ($x^2 = 9.7$, $df = 2$, $p = 0.008$), and school achievement categories ($x^2 = 12.0$, $df = 2$, $p = 0.002$), while they were similar for adherence to the MD, physical activity level, and sleep pattern. In addition, children in the under-normal weight group slept on average more hours per night ($p = 0.005$), and similar results were observed considering only weekdays or weekend days ($p = 0.017$ and $p = 0.033$, respectively).

Table 2. Dietary habits, lifestyle, school achievement, and sleeping behaviors by BMI.

Variable	Total Sample (*n* = 690)	Under-Normal Weight (*n* = 500)	Overweight—Obese (*n* = 190)	*p* Value
Gender				0.003
Female	357 (51.7)	276 (40.0)	81 (11.7)	
Male	333 (48.3)	224 (32.5)	109 (15.8)	
KIDMED Score				0.881
Low	64 (9.3)	46 (6.7)	18 (2.6)	
Medium	381 (55.2)	279 (40.4)	102 (14.8)	
High	245 (35.5)	175 (25.4)	70 (10.1)	
Physical Activity Level				0.729
Low	92 (13.3)	66 (9.6)	26 (3.8)	
Medium	129 (18.7)	96 (13.9)	33 (4.8)	
High	372 (53.9)	272 (39.4)	100 (14.5)	
Very high	97 (14.1)	66 (9.6)	31 (4.5)	
Sleep Duration				0.008
Low	149 (21.6)	94 (13.6)	55 (8.0)	
Recommended	525 (76.1)	392 (56.8)	133 (19.3)	
High	16 (2.3)	14 (2.0)	2 (0.3)	
Sleep Pattern				0.518
EE	211 (30.6)	149 (21.6)	62 (9.0)	
EL	123 (17.8)	93 (13.5)	30 (4.3)	
LE	125 (18.1)	86 (12.5)	39 (5.7)	
LL	231 (33.5)	172 (24.9)	59 (8.6)	
Sleep Time Quantity				
Mean sleep (hh)	9.5 ± 0.8	9.6 ± 0.8	9.4 ± 0.8	0.005
Week days (hh)	9.3 ± 0.8	9.4 ± 0.8	9.2 ± 0.8	0.017
Weekend days (hh)	10.0 ± 1.4	10.1 ± 1.4	9.8 ± 1.4	0.033
School Achievement				0.002
Mostly 10 and 9	360 (52.2)	279 (40.4)	81 (11.7)	
Mostly 8 and 7	314 (45.5)	213 (30.9)	101 (14.6)	
Mostly 6 or less	16 (2.3)	8 (1.2)	8 (1.2)	

Data are presented as frequency (% of the total sample) or as mean ± SD out of 690 (total sample), 500 (under weight and normal weight children), and 190 (overweight and obese children) independent measurements. A Pearson chi-square test was used to test the association of all categorical variables with BMI groups, while a *t*-Test was used to compare Sleep Time Quantity between BMI groups.

In relation to dietary habits, as shown in Table 3, only 9% of children showed a low adherence to the MD, while 55% showed a medium adherence, and 36% a high adherence. Associations were observed between adherence to MD and gender (χ^2 = 8.5, *df* = 2, *p* = 0.015), MD and physical activity level (χ^2 = 23.3, *df* = 6, *p* = 0.001), MD and school achievement categories (χ^2 = 10.9, *df* = 4, *p* = 0.028). Children with a low adherence to the MD had also a lower mean sleep duration (*p* = 0.010) and a lower sleep time during weekdays (*p* = 0.002).

Consistently with their adherence to the MD, children showed positive eating habits, with only small variations registered by gender. The KIDMED questionnaire responses to each single question for the total sample and by gender are presented in Figure 1.

Fruit and fruit juices were consumed daily by 83% of children, 48% had a second portion every day, and 35% ate nuts regularly. In addition, 73% of children had fresh or cooked vegetables regularly once a day, and 44% ate more than one portion of vegetables each day. In relation to protein-based food, 47% of participants ate fish regularly and 53% had pulses more than once a week. Pasta or rice was consumed almost every day by 84% of children. Almost 90% of children had breakfast regularly, 62% consumed cereals or grains for breakfast, 74% milk or dairy products, and 60% commercially baked goods or pastries. In addition, 36% ate two yoghurts and/or some cheese daily, and 88% used olive oil as a condiment when eating at home. Considering unhealthy habits, only 7% of students went more than once per week to a fast food restaurant, and 26% had sweets and/or candy several times every day.

Table 3. Dietary habits, lifestyle, school achievement, and sleeping behaviors by adherence to the Mediterranean diet (MD).

Variable	Total Sample (n = 690)	Low Adherence (n = 64)	Medium Adherence (n = 381)	High Adherence (n = 245)	p Value
Gender					0.015
Female	357 (51.7)	25 (3.6)	190 (27.5)	142 (20.6)	
Male	333 (48.3)	39 (5.7)	191 (27.7)	103 (14.9)	
BMI category					0.087
Underweight	51 (7.4)	4 (0.6)	27 (3.9)	20 (2.9)	
Normal weight	449 (65.1)	42 (6.1)	252 (36.5)	155 (22.5)	
Overweight	157 (22.8)	15 (2.2)	92 (13.3)	50 (7.2)	
Obese	33 (4.8)	3 (0.4)	10 (1.4)	20 (2.9)	
Physical Activity Level					0.001
Low	92 (13.3)	12 (1.7)	54 (7.8)	26 (3.8)	
Medium	129 (18.7)	17 (2.5)	81 (11.7)	31 (4.5)	
High	372 (53.9)	29 (4.2)	205 (29.7)	138 (20.0)	
Very high	97 (14.1)	6 (0.9)	41 (5.9)	50 (7.2)	
Sleep Duration					0.315
Low	149 (21.6)	19 (2.8)	81 (11.7)	49 (7.1)	
Recommended	525 (76.1)	45 (6.5)	289 (41.9)	191 (27.7)	
High	16 (2.3)	0 (0.0)	11 (1.6)	5 (0.7)	
Sleep Pattern					0.101
EE	211 (30.6)	17 (2.5)	111 (16.1)	83 (12.0)	
EL	123 (17.8)	6 (0.9)	65 (9.4)	52 (7.5)	
LE	125 (18.1)	15 (2.2)	69 (10.0)	41 (5.9)	
LL	231 (33.5)	26 (3.8)	136 (19.7)	69 (10.0)	
Sleep Time Quantity					
Mean sleep (hh)	9.5 ± 0.8	9.2 ± 0.8 [a]	9.5 ± 0.8 [b]	9.6 ± 0.8 [b]	0.010
Week days (hh)	9.3 ± 0.8	9.0 ± 0.7 [a]	9.3 ± 0.8 [b]	9.4 ± 0.7 [b]	0.002
Weekend days (hh)	10.0 ± 1.4	9.7 ± 1.9	10.0 ± 1.4	10.1 ± 1.3	0.182
School Achievement					0.028
Mostly 10 and 9	360 (52.2)	22 (3.2)	205 (29.7)	133 (19.3)	
Mostly 8 and 7	314 (45.5)	39 (5.7)	170 (24.6)	105 (15.2)	
Mostly 6 or less	16 (2.3)	3 (0.4)	6 (0.9)	7 (1.0)	

Data are presented as frequency (% of the total sample) or as mean ± SD out of 690 (total sample), 64 (children with a low adherence to the Mediterranean Diet (MD)), 381 (children with a medium adherence to the Mediterranean Diet), and 245 (children with a high adherence to the Mediterranean Diet) independent measurements. A Pearson chi-square test was used to test the association of all categorical variables with adherence to Mediterranean Diet, while an ANOVA with a Bonferroni post hoc test was used to compare Sleep Time Quantity among adherence to MD groups ("a,b": different letters in the same raw indicate significant differences among adherence groups).

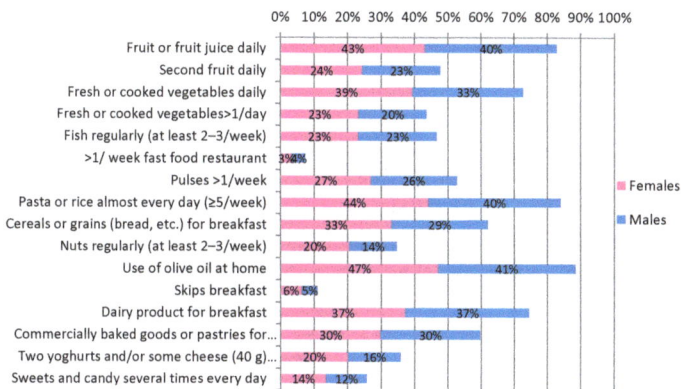

Figure 1. Responses to the KIDMED questionnaire of all children and by gender (percentage in respect to the total sample).

4. Discussion

This study describes the relationship among body mass index, diet quality, physical activity level, and sleep duration in a sample of healthy children (aged 9–11 years) attending an educational school program in Parma, Italy.

The amount of children classified as overweight or obese was 28%, a slightly lower percentage than the value (29%) observed in the region, where the city of Parma is located (Emilia-Romagna) [20]. In turn, the regional prevalence of overweight and obesity is lower when compared to the national situation (31%) [20]. The present study involved about 700 children and the prevalence of overweight and obesity is confirmed to be lower that observed in the data from another study, with a very similar sample size, conducted in Italy [27]. Our results showed a significantly higher overweight and obesity prevalence in boys than in girls, which is consistent with recent investigations [1].

In our study, children showed a medium adherence to the MD, with females significantly more faithful to the principles of the MD, showing a higher attention towards healthy behaviors. However, among 33 studies analyzing gender differences in MD adherence, only 7 studies were able to significantly spot it, and 6 out of 7 reported a higher adherence in girls [28]. In the studied population, the mean MD score (6.5) was higher than that observed in the most recent studies carried out in Italy [28]. Ferranti and colleagues [25] found a mean MD adherence of 4.3 in a population of more than 1500 adolescents. In another study, conducted on a Sicilian adolescent population, the mean MD score was 5.8 in rural areas and 4.8 in urban areas [29].

The detailed analysis obtained from each single question of the KIDMED questionnaire showed positive dietary behaviors for breakfast, fruit, vegetable, and olive oil consumption. However, some other aspects can still be improved through specific educational interventions, targeted for example to promoting fish, pulse, and nuts consumption, the intake of which is lower than the national recommendations, consistently with results from other Italian surveys [20,27]. No evidence was found of an association between BMI and MD score, in partial agreement with other studies. Actually, only 10 out of 26 papers published on the topic reported an inverse association of MD adherence with BMI values [28].

A significant association was observed between MD scores and PAL. This result is aligned with the findings of 14 out of 17 studies found in the literature and investigating the association of MD adherence with lifestyle aspects in children and adolescents [28]. Our study population showed a medium-high active lifestyle with only 13% classified as low PAL. This last result is slightly better than the national data [20], reporting 16% of "non-active" children. This may be partially due to the Giocampus experience, during which children received, each school year, a 2-h/week professionally guided program of physical activity that was found to improve their motor abilities [15], and may increase children's sensibility towards active lifestyles. In agreement with national data [20], a significantly more active lifestyle was observed for males.

No evidence was found of any association between BMI and PAL. In contrast, a highly significant negative association was found between BMI and sleep hours, although more than 76% of children declared sleeping the recommended amount of hours per night. Moreover, children with a lower sleep duration were also characterized by a low adherence to the MD, while children with a medium or high adherence to the MD slept for a similar number of hours, considering both mean and weekdays sleep quantity. These finding are aligned with results from the study by Ferranti and colleagues [25], where shorter sleep durations and poor sleep were associated with higher BMI and with unhealthy eating behaviors in adolescents. The results of this study are in agreement with the national survey "Okkio alla salute" [20], where the prevalence of overweight and obesity is significantly higher in children who sleep less hours per night. Moreover, results from the Quebec Longitudinal Study in preadolescents showed that, for each hour less of sleep per night at 10 years of age, a child was 1.5 times more likely of being overweight or 2.1 times of being obese at 13 years of age [30]. Adolescents with a longer wakefulness had a higher intake of high density snacks [31]. Moreover, results from a longitudinal study in the United States highlight bedtime as a potential target for weight management during adolescence and during the transition to adulthood [32]. In general, the importance of sleep patterns in the lifestyle of children is accepted worldwide, despite obvious cultural differences among countries [31].

In our study, we did not find any association between sleep patterns and overweight/obesity in agreement with Ferranti and colleagues [25]. However, He and colleagues [32] found that a high habitual variability in sleep patterns, but not the habitual sleep duration, was related to increased energy and food intake in adolescents, suggesting that the maintenance of a regular sleep pattern may decrease the risk of obesity.

Finally, both high adherence to the MD and normal body weight status seem to be correlated to high school achievement, suggesting a link between healthy lifestyle and academic performance. Recently, Tonetti and colleagues [33] found that a higher BMI was associated with a poorer school performance in Italian high school students when controlling for sleep quality, sleep duration, and socioeconomic status.

The main limitations of this study are linked to the biases inherent in the use of self-reported data, such as dietary habits and physical activity level. Besides, non-response bias shall also be considered a limitation due to the fact that the sample of respondents might not be representative of the entire potential population, and the lack of information on the non-response children (33%) could not allow bias corrections. Another limitation is that children lifestyle behaviors are affected by parental habits, which were not investigated in the present study.

5. Conclusions

In conclusion, this study investigated lifestyle behaviors of a sample of primary school Italian children who were enrolled in the fifth and last year of the Giocampus school program, in Parma, Italy. The prevalence of overweight and obesity was lower in this group when compared to both the regional and national situations. In addition, the adherence to the MD and the PAL were higher than the ones reported in nationwide surveys, suggesting that the Giocampus school programme may represent a relevant contribution to the attainment of healthy lifestyles in children. Additionally, the high/very high mean amount of sleep hours highlighted a healthy lifeslyle pattern and, interestingly, was negatively and significantly associated with body weight.

Based on these observations, the prevention of child obesity requires a multidisciplinary approach that considers not only physical activity and a healthy diet but also great care in defining sleeping habits. Promoting virtuous sleep behaviors may represent an important and relatively low-cost strategy for reducing the incidence of childhood obesity.

Further studies are recommended to better understand the role of sleep duration and sleep related behaviors in child energy balance.

Acknowledgments: We gratefully acknowledge all actors of the GIOCAMPUS Project, including children, teachers and families involved in it. Moreover, we gratefully thank Cinzia Franchini, and Rossella Santoro for their support in data acquisition.

Author Contributions: AR helped in designing research, performed the study, analyzed data, and wrote the manuscript. MVC helped in performed the study and contributed to write the manuscript. LP designed research, helped in data interpretation, and contributed to manuscript revision. GM helped in designing research and in data interpretation. LP analyzed data, helped in data interpretation, and contributed to manuscript revision. EV helped in data acquisition and data interpretation. FB helped in designing research and in data interpretation. FS designed research, contributed to data interpretation, contributed to writing the manuscript, and had primary responsibility for the final version of the manuscript.

Conflicts of Interest: The authors declare no conflict of interest.

References

1. Binkin, N.; Fontana, G.; Lamberti, A.; Cattaneo, C.; Baglio, G.; Perra, A.; Spinelli, A. A national survey of the prevalence of childhood overweight and obesity in Italy. *Obes. Rev.* **2010**, *11*, 2–10. [CrossRef] [PubMed]

2. Nardone, P.; Buoncristiano, M.; Lauria, L. OKkio alla SALUTE: Sintesi dei Risultati 2016. Italian Ministry of Health, 2017. Available online: http://www.salute.gov.it/imgs/C_17_notizie_2935_listaFile_itemName_24_file.pdf (accessed on 17 April 2017).

3. Di Renzo, L.; Tyndall, E.; Gualtieri, P.; Carboni, C.; Valente, R.; Ciani, A.S.; Tonini, M.G.; De Lorenzo, A. Association of body composition and eating behavior in the normal weight obese syndrome. *Eat. Weight Disord.* **2016**, *21*, 99–106. [CrossRef] [PubMed]

4. Golley, R.K.; Maher, C.A.; Matricciani, L.; Olds, T.S. Sleep duration or bedtime[quest] Exploring the association between sleep timing behavior, diet and BMI in children and adolescents. *Int. J. Obes.* **2013**, *37*, 546–551. [CrossRef] [PubMed]

5. Granich, J.; Rosenberg, M.; Knuiman, M.; Timperio, A. Understanding children's sedentary behavior: A qualitative study of the family home environment. *Health Educ. Res.* **2010**, *25*, 199–210. [CrossRef] [PubMed]

6. Serra-Majem, L.; Trichopoulou, A.; de la Cruz, J.N.; Cervera, P.; Álvarez, A.G.; La Vecchia, C.; Lemtouni, A.; Trichopoulos, D. Does the definition of the Mediterranean diet need to be updated? *Public Health Nutr.* **2004**, *7*, 927–929. [CrossRef] [PubMed]

7. Sofi, F.; Macchi, C.; Abbate, R.; Gensini, G.F.; Casini, A. Mediterranean diet and health status: An updated meta-analysis and a proposal for a literature-based adherence score. *Public Health Nutr.* **2014**, *17*, 2769–2782. [CrossRef] [PubMed]

8. St-Onge, M.-P.; Shechter, A. Sleep Restriction in Adolescents: Forging the Path Towards Obesity and Diabetes? *Sleep* **2013**, *36*, 813–814. [CrossRef] [PubMed]

9. St-Onge, M.P. The role of sleep duration in the regulation of energy balance: Effects on energy intakes and expenditure. *J. Clin. Sleep Med.* **2013**, *9*, 73–80. [CrossRef] [PubMed]

10. Westerlund, L.; Ray, C.; Roos, E. Associations between sleeping habits and food consumption patterns among 10–11-year-old children in Finland. *Br. J. Nutr.* **2009**, *102*, 1531–1537. [CrossRef] [PubMed]

11. Miller, A.L.; Lumeng, J.C.; LeBourgeois, M.K. Sleep patterns and obesity in childhood. *Curr. Opin. Endocrinol. Diabetes Obes.* **2015**, *22*, 41–47. [CrossRef] [PubMed]

12. WHO Regional Office for Europe. *WHO European Action Plan for Food and Nutrition Policy, 2007–2012*; WHO Regional Office for Europe: Copenhagen, Danmark, 2008.

13. Tremblay, A.; Lachance, É. Tackling obesity at the community level by integrating healthy diet, movement and non-movement behaviors. *Obes. Rev.* **2017**, *18*, 82–87. [CrossRef] [PubMed]

14. Rosi, A.; Brighenti, F.; Finistrella, V.; Ingrosso, L.; Monti, G.; Vanelli, M.; Vitale, M.; Volta, E.; Scazzina, F. Giocampus school: A "learning through playing" approach to deliver nutritional education to children. *Int. J. Food Sci. Nutr.* **2016**, *67*, 207–215. [CrossRef] [PubMed]

15. Chiodera, P.; Volta, E.; Gobbi, G.; Milioli, M.A.; Mirandola, P.; Bonetti, A.; Delsignore, R.; Bernasconi, S.; Anedda, A.; Vitale, M. Specifically designed physical exercise programs improve children's motor abilities. *Scand. J. Med. Sci. Sports* **2008**, *18*, 179–187. [CrossRef] [PubMed]

16. WHO. *Physical Status: The Use and Interpretation of Anthropometry*; WHO, Technical Report Series N 854; WHO: Geneva, Switzerland, 1995.

17. Censi, L.; Spinelli, A.; Roccaldo, R.; Bevilacqua, N.; Lamberti, A.; Angelini, V.; Nardone, P.; Baglio, G. Dressed or undressed? How to measure children's body weight in overweight surveillance? *Public Health Nutr.* **2013**, *17*, 2715–2720. [CrossRef] [PubMed]

18. Cole, T.J.; Lobstein, T. Extended international (IOTF) body mass index cut-offs for thinness, overweight and obesity. *Pediatr. Obes.* **2012**, *7*, 284–294. [CrossRef] [PubMed]

19. Serra-Majem, L.; Ribas, L.; Ngo, J.; Ortega, R.M.; Garcia, A.; Perez-Rodrigo, C.; Aranceta, J. Food, youth and the Mediterranean diet in Spain. Development of KIDMED, Mediterranean Diet Quality Index in children and adolescents. *Public Health Nutr.* **2004**, *7*, 931–935. [CrossRef] [PubMed]

20. Nardone, P.; Spinelli, A.; Buoncristiano, M.; Lauria, L.; Pizzi, E.; Andreozzi, S.; Galeone, D. *Il Sistema di Sorveglianza OKkio alla SALUTE: Risultati 2014. [Surveillance System OKkio alla SALUTE: 2014 Results.]*; Istituto Superiore di Sanità: Firenze, Italy, 2016; p. 63.

21. Kowalski, K.C.; Crocker, P.R.E.; Donen, R.M. The Physical Activity Questionnaire for Older Children (PAQ-C) and Adolescents (PAQ-A) Manual. Available online: http://www.dapa-toolkit.mrc.ac.uk/documents/en/PAQ/PAQ_manual.pdf (accessed on 17 April 2017).

22. SINU. *Livelli di Assunzione di Riferimento di Nutrienti ed Energia per la Popolazione Italiana—IV Revisione*; Società Italiana di Nutritione Umana: Firenze, Italy, 2014.

23. Institute of Medicine. *Dietary Reference Intakes for Energy, Carbohydrate, Fiber, Fat, Fatty Acids, Cholesterol, Protein, and Amino Acids (Macronutrients)*; The National Academies Press: Washington, DC, USA, 2005; pp. 1–1331.

24. Hirshkowitz, M.; Whiton, K.; Albert, S.M.; Alessi, C.; Bruni, O.; DonCarlos, L.; Hazen, N.; Herman, J.; Adams Hillard, P.J.; Katz, E.S.; et al. National Sleep Foundation's updated sleep duration recommendations: Final report. *Sleep Health* **2015**, *1*, 233–243. [CrossRef]

25. Ferranti, R.; Marventano, S.; Castellano, S.; Giogianni, G.; Nolfo, F.; Rametta, S.; Matalone, M.; Mistretta, A. Sleep quality and duration is related with diet and obesity in young adolescent living in Sicily, Southern Italy. *Sleep Sci.* **2016**, *9*, 117–122. [CrossRef] [PubMed]

26. Touchette, É.; Mongrain, V.; Petit, D.; Tremblay, R.E.; Montplaisir, J.Y. Development of sleep-wake schedules during childhood and relationship with sleep duration. *Arch. Pediatr. Adolesc. Med.* **2008**, *162*, 343–349. [CrossRef] [PubMed]

27. Roccaldo, R.; Censi, L.; D'Addezio, L.; Toti, E.; Martone, D.; D'Addesa, D.; Cernigliaro, A. Adherence to the Mediterranean diet in Italian school children (The ZOOM8 Study). *Int. J. Food Sci. Nutr.* **2014**, *65*, 621–628. [CrossRef] [PubMed]

28. Iaccarino Idelson, P.; Scalfi, L.; Valerio, G. Adherence to the Mediterranean Diet in children and adolescents: A systematic review. *Nutr. Metab. Cardiovasc. Dis.* **2017**, *27*, 283–299. [CrossRef] [PubMed]

29. Grosso, G.; Marventano, S.; Buscemi, S.; Scuderi, A.; Matalone, M.; Platania, A.; Giorgianni, G.; Rametta, S.; Nolfo, F.; Galvano, F.; et al. Factors associated with adherence to the Mediterranean diet among adolescents living in Sicily, southern Italy. *Nutrients* **2013**, *5*, 4908–4923. [CrossRef] [PubMed]

30. Seegers, V.; Petit, D.; Falissard, B.; Vitaro, F.; Tremblay, R.E.; Montplaisir, J.; Touchette, E. Short Sleep Duration and Body Mass Index: A Prospective Longitudinal Study in Preadolescence. *Am. J. Epidemiol.* **2011**, *173*, 621–629. [CrossRef] [PubMed]

31. Chaput, J.P.; Katzmarzyk, P.T.; LeBlanc, A.G.; Tremblay, M.S.; Barreira, T.V.; Broyles, S.T.; Fogelholm, M.; Hu, G.; Kuriyan, R.; Kurpad, A.; et al. Associations between sleep patterns and lifestyle behaviors in children: An international comparison. *Int. J. Obes. Suppl.* **2015**, *5* (Suppl. 2), S59–S65. [CrossRef] [PubMed]

32. He, F.; Bixler, E.O.; Berg, A.; Imamura Kawasawa, Y.; Vgontzas, A.N.; Fernandez-Mendoza, J.; Yanosky, J.; Liao, D. Habitual sleep variability, not sleep duration, is associated with caloric intake in adolescents. *Sleep Med.* **2015**, *16*, 856–861. [CrossRef] [PubMed]

33. Tonetti, L.; Fabbri, M.; Filardi, M.; Martoni, M.; Natale, V. The association between higher body mass index and poor school performance in high school students. *Pediatr. Obes.* **2016**, *11*, e27–e29. [CrossRef] [PubMed]

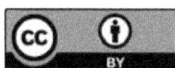

nutrients

MDPI

Article

Food and Nutrients Intake in the School Lunch Program among School Children in Shanghai, China

Zhenru Huang, Runying Gao, Nadila Bawuerjiang, Yali Zhang, Xiaoxu Huang and Meiqin Cai *

School of Public Health, Shanghai Jiao Tong University,227 South Chongqing Rd, Huangpu Qu, Shanghai 200025, China; hzhenru@163.com (Z.H.); dly-slyj@hotmail.com (R.G.); nadirah@126.com (N.B.); abeney@126.com (Y.Z.); xiaoxuhuang0909@126.com (X.H.)
* Correspondence: caimeiqin@sjtu.edu.cn; Tel.: +86-021-63846590

Received: 9 April 2017; Accepted: 2 June 2017; Published: 7 June 2017

Abstract: This study aimed to evaluate the intake of food and nutrients among primary, middle, and high schools students in Shanghai, and provide recommendations for possible amendments in new school lunch standards of Shanghai. Twenty schools were included in the school lunch menu survey. Of those, seven schools enrolled 5389 students and conducted physical measurement of plate waste and a questionnaire survey. The amount of food and nutrients was compared according to the new China National Dietary Guideline for School Children (2016) and Chinese Dietary Reference Intakes (2013). The provision of livestock and poultry meat in menus was almost 5–8 times the recommended amount. The amount of seafood was less than the recommended amount, and mostly came from half-processed food. The average percentage of energy from fat was more than 30% in students of all grades. The greatest amount of food wasted was vegetables with 53%, 42%, and 31%, respectively, among primary, middle and high school students. Intake of Vitamin A, Vitamin B_2, calcium, and iron was about 50% of the recommended proportion. Only 24.0% students were satisfied with the taste of school lunches. Higher proportions of livestock and poultry meat and low intake of vegetables have become integral problems in school lunch programs. Additionally, more attention needs to be paid to the serving size in primary schools with five age groups.

Keywords: students; school lunch; nutrient; intake; plate waste

1. Introduction

Children and adolescents are in a crucial period of body growth and maturation. Adequate nutrition during this period is of great importance. A number of studies has revealed that inappropriate nutrition in childhood is related to both the occurrence of diseases in youth [1] and the risks of developing obesity, cardiovascular diseases, and cancer in adulthood [2–4].

Lunch becomes a very important issue when it comes to school-aged children since a large number of students have lunch at school. The National School Lunch Program (NSLP) in the United States operates in more than 101,000 public and nonprofit private schools, and provides over 28 million low-cost or free lunches to children on a typical school day [5]. In Japan, more than 10 million schoolchildren in 32,400 schools participate in the lunch program [6]. China launched the first School Lunch Program in Hangzhou, Zhejiang Province in 1987 [7], and then expanded it to a number of cities. Shanghai, as a developed city in China, started the program in 1993, and now has more than 95% students having lunch at school [8], which is a total of 1.4 million students according to Shanghai Statistic Yearbook (2016) [9].

Since lunch is correlated to the health of young generations and involves so many students, it has drawn much attention worldwide. In developed countries, such as the US and Japan, they have called a legislative action to ensure well implemented school lunch programs. The U.S. signed the National School Lunch Act (NSLA) in 1946 and the Child Nutrition Act (CAN) in 1966, as well as subsequent amendments to the two acts that guide the program's administration [5]. Japan also introduced the School Lunch Act in 1954 and revised it in 2008 to change its aim to promote Shokuiku, which emphasizes food education. These acts clearly demonstrate the daily food and nutrient reference intake for each age group so that schools and companies that prepare lunches are able to provide adequate nutrition to students. China released the Amount of Nutritional Provision for School Lunch (ANPSL-1998) as the national standard for school lunches in 1998; there have been no amendments to date [10].

However, the health status and dietary structure of Chinese people have undergone tremendous changes within the last 20 years. Excessive intake of meat and insufficient consumption of dairy products and vegetables have emerged as concerns in Chinese dining habits [11]. Hence, it is very urgent and necessary to draw up an updated and feasible standard for the school lunch program, which requires on in-depth evaluation of the available data on the present status of school lunches. The former evaluation studies were all based on the ANPSL-1998, which might be inaccurate since China has published the new China National Dietary Guideline for School Children (2016) (CNDG-Children 2016) [12] and the Chinese Dietary Reference Intakes (2013) (DRIs-2013) [13]. To the best of our knowledge, this is the first study that applied the new guideline and DRIs to assess lunch intake in China. Additionally, unlike in the existing studies, we separated elementary, middle, and high school students into several sub-groups to obtain more information, as recommended by a recently published study by the NSLP in the US [14]. This is also the first time a comprehensive and regional-level investigation of school lunch program that involves multiple districts all over Shanghai has been conducted. As the study team of the new school lunch standardization commission in Shanghai, we aim to provide more evidence and scientific recommendations for updates.

Therefore, the objectives of this study were to evaluate the intake of food and nutrients among primary, middle and high schools students in Shanghai in reference to the CNDG-Children 2016 and the DRIs-2013 and to provide recommendations for possible amendments on new school lunch standards of Shanghai.

2. Methods

2.1. Sample Selection

Eight primary schools, five middle schools, and five high schools, two combined middle-high schools, making up a total of 20 schools, from seven districts of Shanghai, participated in the three-day lunch menu survey in 2015. Simultaneously, the intake survey and questionnaire survey were conducted among 5389 students from three primary schools (2936 students), three middle schools (1841 students), and one high school (612 students). The study population consisted of 2765 boys (51.3%) and 2624 girls (48.7%).

Signed informed consents were obtained from the students as well as their parents. No experiment and biological sample collection were conducted in this study. At no time were individual students associated with any particular lunch, and the questionnaire was anonymous without any personal identifying information, except for the students' grade and sex.

2.2. Data Collection

2.2.1. Menu Survey

Menu survey was a very common and easy way to assess the provision of school lunch [15,16]. Three-day lunch menus were obtained from 20 schools. Menus were analyzed with nutrient analysis software Fei Hua (2.a), Beijing Bowenshixun Technology Ltd., Beijing, China, which provided daily averages for staple food (including rice, noodles, and other cereal food), livestock and poultry meat, egg, seafood, bean products, and vegetables, as well as energy, protein, fat, carbohydrates, vitamins, and minerals. The oil, salt, and sugar used were also considered.

2.2.2. Intake Survey

In seven schools, menu survey was also applied. And plate waste measures were conducted over three days, using a previously validated physical measurement of aggregate selective plate waste [17,18]. Two randomly selected sample of school lunch trays were taken from each age group serving line before lunch. Meanwhile, the weights of food before and after cooking were recorded to calculate the raw/cooked ratio (Ration of r/c). Separate trash bins with plastic bags were prepared for each food category before lunch. The research team members waited at the designated spots and separated the leftovers into the corresponding trash bin when the students finished eating and brought their trays. The number of students who had lunch at school of every day was recorded.

Food Intake per Student (cooked) in grams for each food category was calculated as follows (1):

$$\text{Food Intake per student(cooked)} = \text{Sample Weight} - \frac{\text{Total Plate Waste}}{\text{Number of students}} \qquad (1)$$

Since the nutrient analysis software and the reference standard both require raw food data, the Food Intake per Student (cooked) was transformed with the raw/cooked ratio (Ration of r/c) as shown in Formula (2) below.

$$\text{Food Intake per student(raw)} = \text{Food Intake per student(cooked)} \times \text{Ration of r/c} \qquad (2)$$

Plate waste is defined as the quantity percentage of edible food served as part of the lunch but not consumed, as shown in Formula (3) below.

$$\%\text{Plate Waste} = \frac{\text{Total Plate waste/Number of students}}{\text{Sample weight}} \times 100 \qquad (3)$$

Both menu and intake evaluation were based on the CNDG-Children 2016 for food category and the DRIs-2013 for nutrient assessment. To evaluate the lunch and nutrition intake, 40% of daily recommended intake in the CNDG-Children 2016 and the DRIs-2013 was used, as the CNDG 2016 distributes daily energy and nutrients into breakfast, lunch and dinner at the ratio 3:4:3 [19].

2.2.3. Questionnaire Survey

The aim of the questionnaire survey was to find out the reason for plate waste and the existing problems in the School Lunch Program.

Validity: Three nutrition and survey research experts were invited to evaluate the appropriateness of the survey questions and response options; then, face-to-face interviews were conducted with 36 students (three students from each grade level ranging from Grades 1–12) as a pilot. The students were asked to talk about the clarity of each question to ensure the targeted respondents understand what each question is asking as well as what each response means.

The questionnaire included the following information: (1) demographic background (i.e., age, sex); (2) knowledge and attitudes: basic knowledge of food and nutrients (including six questions, one point for each correct answer, six points in total), attitude towards healthy behaviors (including four behaviors, two points for very positive attitude, one point for positive attitude and zero point for neutral or negative attitude, eight points in total); and (3) opinions on food served at the school canteen (i.e., appearance, flavor, temperature, and portion size of the food served).

Reliability: Internal consistency reliability was calculated using Cronbach's alpha coefficient formula. Reliability of the questions related to knowledge, attitude and views on the school lunches were thus calculated to be 0.866, 0.807, and 0.792, respectively. This suggests that the reliability of this survey was adequate, since $\alpha \geq 0.7$ is generally considered to be the minimum for adequate internal consistency [20].

2.3. Data Analysis

Excel 2010 (Microsoft Corporation, Redmond, WA, USA) was used to record and calculate the food provided and intake. The nutrient analysis software Fei Hua (2.a) (Beijing Bowenshixun Technology Ltd., Beijing, China) was used to analyze nutrient contents. EpiData 3.1 (A comprehensive tool for validated entry and documentation of data. EpiData Association, Odense, Denmark) was used for double recording of questionnaire data. Data that presented abnormal distribution were analyzed using two independent samples via Wilcoxon rank sum test, while categorical variables were analyzed via chi-Square test using SPSS 21.0 (IBM SPSS Inc., Chicago, IL, USA). Differences found were determined to be statistically significant at $p \leq 0.05$.

3. Results

3.1. Evaluation of Food Provision

Amounts of staple food, livestock, and poultry meat in menus exceeded the recommended amount in all school grades; livestock and poultry meat were particularly high, almost 5–8 times the recommended amounts. On the contrary, the provision of seafood was insufficient. Additionally, we found the seafood supplied for lunch was mostly fish ball or other half-processed foods, instead of fresh products. Egg provision in the diet was higher than recommended for primary and middle school students. The amount of bean products and vegetables was generally adequate for all grades (see Table 1).

Table 1. Provision of food in the menus of twenty schools as compared to CNDG-Children 2016/g.

Category	Primary School		Middle School		High School	
	Recommended	Menu	Recommended	Menu	Recommended	Menu
Staple Food	60–80	99.6 ± 31.8	90–100	104.7 ± 42.7	100–120	154.3 ± 60.4
Livestock & Poultry Meat	16	123.4 ± 38.4	20	101.3 ± 44.9	20–30	135.4 ± 51.6
Egg	10–16	26.0 ± 27.8	16–20	22.8 ± 25.8	20	15.1 ± 20.6
Seafood	16	11.4 ± 23.7	20	28.3 ± 49.4	20–30	13.2 ± 24.5
Bean Product	6	9.0 ± 17.0	6	15.8 ± 25.5	6–10	32.2 ± 35.6
Vegetable	120	130.6 ± 60.8	160–180	189.2 ± 63.7	180–200	178.4 ± 84.5

Recommended amount is 40% of daily recommended intake in China National Dietary Guideline for School Children (2016) (CNDG-Children 2016).

Energy indicated in the menus was aligned with the recommendations. However, the proportion of fat in total energy exceeded the recommended percentage (20–30%). Protein was served excessively, at nearly twice the recommended amount, especially among primary school students. The percentage of energy from carbohydrate, which is supposed to be 50–65%, was found to be below the lower limit. As for the vitamins and minerals, Vitamin B_2 and calcium were insufficient. Vitamin A, Vitamin B_1, Vitamin C, iron, and zinc contents were consistent with the goals specified in the DRIs-2013 for students in all grades (see Table 2).

Table 2. Provision of energy and nutrients in 20 schools as compared to DRIs-2013/n (%).

Item	Primary School		Middle School		High School	
	DRIs	Menu	DRIs	Menu	DRIs	Menu
Energy (kcal)	621	696 ± 139 (112.0)	783	752 ± 229 (96.0)	844	1005 ± 179 (119.1)
Protein (g)	17.4	35.9 ± 7.5 (206.3)	23.4	32.0 ± 7.9 (136.8)	25.3	41.8 ± 10.0 (165.2)
Protein/%E	-	21 ± 4	-	18 ± 5	-	17 ± 4
Fat/%E	20–30	32 ± 10	20–30	39 ± 10	20–30	37 ± 12
Carbonhydrate/%E	50–65	47 ± 10	50–65	43 ± 7	50–65	46 ± 12
Vitamin A (µgRE)	199	204 ± 184 (102.5)	258	258 ± 173 (100)	272	221 ± 144 (81.3)
Vitamin B$_1$ (mg)	0.39	0.48 ± 0.21 (123.1)	0.5	0.49 ± 0.20 (98.0)	0.54	0.60 ± 0.21 (111.1)
Vitamin B$_2$ (mg)	0.39	0.33 ± 0.09 (84.6)	0.48	0.32 ± 0.08 (66.7)	0.51	0.37 ± 0.09 (72.5)
Vitamin C (mg)	26	39 ± 29 (150.0)	36	60 ± 34 (166.7)	38	54 ± 32 (142.1)
Calcium (mg)	390	140 ± 85 (35.9)	413	217 ± 196 (52.5)	375	226 ± 183 (60.3)
Iron (mg)	5.14	5.65 ± 1.77 (109.9)	6.28	6.91 ± 4.71 (110.0)	6.38	8.50 ± 4.71 (133.2)
Zinc (mg)	2.81	4.42 ± 1.65 (157.3)	3.66	4.28 ± 1.25 (116.9)	3.75	5.52 ± 1.52 (147.2)

DRIs are 40% of average of daily recommended intake in different age and sex group according to Chinese Dietary Reference Intakes (2013) (DRIs-2013). The value in brackets was the proportion that provision amount took up in the correspondent recommendation.

3.2. Evaluation of Food Intake and Plate Waste

The intake of staple food for grades 1–2 and middle school students was insufficient (with plate waste ranging from 15–24%), but was adequate for grades 3–5 and high school students (with 16–21% of plate waste). All students consumed livestock and poultry meat in amounts exceeding the recommended amount. Egg intake was in accordance with the recommended amounts, except among high school students. Seafood intake was in a severe shortage for primary school and high school students since their provision was also insufficient. Bean product consumption was deficient among primary school students, but reasonable among middle and high school students. Vegetable consumption was the lowest and the accompanying plate waste levels ranked the highest, with 53%, 42%, and 31%, of waste among primary, middle, and high school students, respectively. Livestock and poultry meat, and egg followed as the second ranking plate waste among all food categories (see Table 3). Additionally, students of lower grades in primary school seemed to waste more food than students of higher grades ($p < 0.05$). Girls tended to waste more food and nutrients than boys ($p < 0.05$).

Table 3. Actual food intake and plate waste percentage in seven schools among different age groups and sexes/g (%).

Stage		Staple Food	Livestock & Poultry Meat	Egg	Seafood	Bean Product	Vegetable
Primary School	Recommended	60–80	16	10–16	16	6	120
	Menu	79.5	141.6	24.9	0.4	5.0	101.6
	Grades 1–2	52.9 (34%)	73.7 (46%)	10.5 (50%)	0.2 (50%)	2.4 (50%)	38.9 (57%)
	Grades 3–5	63.1 (21%)	75.0 (45%)	14.8 (30%)	0.2 (50%)	3.2 (33%)	45.1 (50%)
	Average Intake	58.8 (27%)	74.5 (46%)	13.0 (38%)	0.2 (50%)	2.9 (40%)	42.5 (53%)
Middle School	Recommended	90–100	20	16–20	20	6	160–180
	Menu	93.4	119.4	34.9	27.9	14.9	176.7
	Grades 6–7 (Male)	74.5 (11%)	106.3 (14%)	16.2 (29%)	25.8 (12%)	10.5 (20%)	118.2 (35%)
	Grades 6–7 (Female)	64.4 (23%)	96.7 (22%)	14.1 (38%)	21.7 (26%)	7.9 (40%)	104.1 (43%)
	Grades 8–9 (Male)	81.0 (3%)	95.1 (23%)	16.3 (28%)	25.6 (13%)	9.0 (32%)	105.3 (42%)
	Grades 8–9 (Female)	61.5 (26%)	82.1 (34%)	15.2 (33%)	24.9 (15%)	8.8 (33%)	87.8 (52%)
	Average Intake	70.9 (15%)	96.7 (22%)	15.5 (32%)	24.6 (16%)	9.2 (30%)	105.9 (42%)
High School	Recommended	100–120	20–30	20	20–30	6–10	180–200
	Menu	140.4	164.3	18.4	2.0	23.0	198.1
	Grades 10–12 (Male)	149.0 (1%)	161.0 (0%)	17.6 (24%)	2.0 (0%)	18.6 (18%)	154.2 (27%)
	Grades 10–12 (Female)	103.0 (31%)	141.1 (12%)	13.4 (42%)	1.3 (35%)	14.4 (37%)	139.4 (34%)
	Average Intake	126.7 (16%)	151.3 (6%)	15.5 (33%)	1.6 (20%)	16.6 (27%)	147.0 (31%)

Energy intake for students in Grades 1–9 was under the recommended amount. The intakes of protein and fat for all students were excessive, while the carbohydrate intake was deficient. Primary school students were facing a lack of vitamins in their diet, including Vitamin B_1, Vitamin B_2, and Vitamin C. Calcium intake was very low for all students. Iron intake was low except for boys in high school. Zinc intake was matched with the recommended amount. In summary, Vitamin A, Vitamin B_2, calcium, and iron were the most deficient micronutrients in school lunches, which corresponded to about 50% of the recommendation (see Table 4).

Table 4. Actual intake and proportion to the recommended amounts of energy and nutrients in seven schools among different age groups and sexes/n (%).

Stage		Energy kcal	Protein g	Fat %E	Carbonhydrate %E	Vitamin A µgRE	Vitamin B₁ mg	Vitamin B₂ mg	Vitamin C mg	Calcium mg	Iron mg	Zinc mg
	Recommended	662	19	20–30	50–65	212	0.42	0.42	28	416	5.5	3.0
	Menu	638 (96.4)	35 (188.2)	35	42	156 (73.6)	0.38 (91.3)	0.32 (76.9)	28 (100.0)	95 (22.8)	4.7 (85.4)	4.3 (143.3)
Primary School	Grades 1–2	409 (61.8)	20 (107.5)	37	43	58 (27.4)	0.19 (45.7)	0.19 (45.7)	10 (35.7)	48 (11.5)	2.9 (52.2)	2.5 (83.3)
	Grades 3–5	480 (72.5)	22 (118.3)	38	43	79 (37.3)	0.25 (60.1)	0.21 (50.5)	12 (42.9)	60 (14.4)	3.1 (56.6)	2.8 (93.3)
	Average Intake	451 (68.1)	21 (112.9)	37	43	70 (33.0)	0.23 (55.3)	0.20 (48.1)	11 (39.3)	55 (13.2)	3.0 (54.7)	2.7 (90.0)
	Recommended	835	25	20–30	50–65	275	0.53	0.51	38	440	6.7	3.9
	Menu	665 (79.6)	32 (128.0)	38	43	232 (84.4)	0.59 (111.3)	0.30 (58.8)	55 (144.7)	168 (38.2)	5.1 (76.1)	3.8 (97.4)
	Grades 6–7 (Male)	612 (73.3)	29 (116.0)	42	39	148 (53.8)	0.63 (118.9)	0.25 (49.0)	35 (92.1)	117 (26.6)	4.0 (59.6)	3.2 (82.1)
Middle School	Grades 6–7 (Female)	542 (64.9)	26 (104.0)	43	38	127 (46.2)	0.60 (113.2)	0.23 (45.1)	30 (78.9)	104 (23.6)	3.5 (52.8)	2.9 (74.4)
	Grades 8–9 (Male)	599 (71.7)	28 (112.0)	40	41	131 (47.6)	0.58 (109.4)	0.24 (47.1)	32 (84.2)	105 (23.9)	3.8 (56.7)	3.2 (82.1)
	Grades 8–9 (Female)	499 (59.8)	24 (96.0)	42	39	112 (40.7)	0.48 (90.6)	0.20 (39.2)	26 (68.4)	89 (20.2)	3.2 (48.1)	2.6 (66.7)
	Average Intake	570 (68.3)	27 (108.0)	42	39	132 (48.0)	0.58 (109.4)	0.23 (45.1)	31 (81.6)	106 (24.1)	3.7 (55.2)	3.0 (76.9)
	Recommended	900	27	20–30	50–65	290	0.58	0.54	40	400	6.8	4.0
	Menu	924 (102.7)	46 (170.4)	35	46	242 (83.4)	0.71 (121.9)	0.40 (74.1)	61 (152.5)	180 (45.0)	7.5 (110.3)	5.4 (135.0)
High School	Grades 10–12 (Male)	910 (101.1)	45 (166.7)	30	51	190 (65.5)	0.70 (120.7)	0.39 (72.2)	45 (112.5)	146 (36.5)	6.9 (101.5)	5.3 (132.5)
	Grades 10–12 (Female)	697 (77.4)	36 (133.3)	33	46	158 (54.5)	0.55 (94.8)	0.31 (57.4)	40 (100.0)	112 (28.0)	5.0 (73.5)	4.1 (102.5)
	Average Intake	807 (89.7)	40 (148.1)	32	49	175 (60.3)	0.62 (106.9)	0.35 (64.8)	43 (107.5)	129 (32.3)	6.0 (88.2)	4.7 (117.5)

The value in brackets was the proportion that actual intake took up in the correspondent recommendation.

3.3. Analysis for Possible Reasons for Plate Waste

A total of 5937 students from seven schools were administered questionnaires, of which 5389 (90.8%) valid responses were included in this study.

Results from the questionnaire showed that the percentage of students who often or always had leftovers was 56.3%. The main reason for plate waste among primary school students was food being too much (43.3%) and unpalatable food (43.4%). However, the main reason for plate waste in 54.5% of the middle school and 61.9% of the high school students was unpalatable food.

As for knowledge about nutrition, students from primary, middle, and high schools scored 4.44 ± 1.50, 4.69 ± 1.21 and 4.92 ± 0.98, respectively, with accuracy over 70%. However, their scores towards healthy behaviors were relatively low, at 5.80 ± 2.10, 4.25 ± 2.46, and 3.15 ± 2.18, for primary, middle, and high school students, respectively.

Students rated the food temperature and portion size as satisfactory; however, they were not satisfied with food appearance and flavor. Only 24% of the students marked the overall food taste as good (see Table 5).

Table 5. Students' opinion on school lunches/n (%).

Rank	Good	Neutral	Bad
Appearance	1067 (19.8%)	2689 (49.9%)	1633 (30.3%)
Flavor	1515 (28.1%)	2705 (50.2%)	1169 (21.7%)
Temperature	2716 (50.4%)	2177 (40.4%)	496 (9.2%)
Adequate in Portion Size	2792 (51.8%)	1918 (35.6%)	679 (12.6%)
Overall Food Taste	1293 (24.0%)	2905 (53.9%)	1191 (22.1%)

4. Discussion

The latest report on nutrition status and chronic diseases of Chinese people issued in 2015 revealed that the wasting percentage of Chinese adolescents aged 6–17 years was 9%, while the overweight and obesity percentages were 9.6% and 6.4%, respectively [21]. Diet-related problems including anorexia and obesity have been increasing among school children [6]. School lunch, as one of the important meals in a day, also provides direct access to nutrition for students.

Nevertheless, problems continue to exist in the School Lunch Program. In the present study, we evaluated the provision and actual intake, as well as the students' opinion on school lunches to uncover the existing problems and come up with feasible recommendations when amending the new school lunch standards of Shanghai. In particular, the provision of livestock and poultry meat was too excessive while seafood was in a severe shortage. This study highlighted the fact that excessive provision of animal protein in school lunch diets may be associated with a greater intake of fat. This high-level of fat content in school lunches is a common issue worldwide. To decrease children's access to lunches with a high fat content, the US Department of Agriculture implemented School Meals Initiative for Healthy Children in 1995 [22]. However, this program did not show favorable results, since the three School Nutrition Dietary Assessment Studies showed that the average percentages of energy from total fat were 38% (school year 1991–1992), 33–34% (school year 1998–1999) and 33.8% (school year 2004–2005), respectively [23–25]. The higher-fat provision in school lunch should be given more attention as obesity has become a global public health threat [26].

The actual food intake was also unsatisfying. The plate waste of livestock and poultry meat, eggs and vegetables was higher than other food category. The provision of livestock and poultry meat, as well as eggs, far exceeded the recommended amounts, and this may be the reason for high plate waste. However, the situation for vegetables was different. The vegetable provision was within the recommended range, but accounted for the highest plate waste. Having further investigated, we found that vegetables were prepared in a large cauldron, in a manner that resulted in overcooking. Additionally, the time between cooking and consumption was about 1.5–2 h, and individual lunch sets were covered with a plastic covering to prevent contamination. This may have resulted in the vegetables gaining an unpleasant color and unpalatable flavor, leading to increased plate waste.

In fact, vegetables were reported to be the food items that are wasted the most, and this is very common all over the world [18,27]. A study involving students from grades 3–8 in four schools in the U.S. showed the waste percentage of vegetables was up to 58.9% [28]. Another study conducted in Beijing, China also indicated that vegetables were the dominant wasted food with 42% of plate waste [29], comparable with the present study ranging from 31–53%.

Due to high plate waste of vegetables and other foods, intake for energy and a majority of nutrients did not meet the recommended targets in this study. The reason for higher intake of fat and protein was the unreasonable high fat content of lunches. Intake of micronutrients, such as Vitamin A, Vitamin B_2 and iron, was also less than the recommended level, which might be a consequence of high plate waste, especially for vegetables. However, we should notice that, for most Chinese people, they are used to eat more at dinner rather than lunch. Hence, the distribution of breakfast, lunch and dinner at the ratio 3:4:3 might not be the occasion and whether the nutrient intake over a full day is adequate remains unknown. Calcium insufficiency was also found in this study. As people usually drink milk in the morning or at night, it is difficult to judge the intake of calcium at lunch. However, the insufficiency of calcium intake has always been a problem among Chinese students because of low-milk dietary habits of Chinese people [21].

A number of factors could influence food intake, causing the unreasonable nutrient intake among students. Previous studies have concluded that students' knowledge, attitude, and eating behaviors [29,30], as well as characteristics of the food itself (including the appearance, flavor, and temperature) [31], were the main influencing factors leading to plate waste. It was inspiring that the students achieved about 70% accuracy when answering nutrition-related questions. However, their attitudes toward healthy behaviors were not very positive. Therefore, future nutrition education should focus more on how to encourage students to turn their good nutrition knowledge into actions. In terms of the characteristics of food, the results revealed a low satisfaction in the appearance of food (19.8%) and flavor (28.1%), which might be a result of comprehensive factors, such as cooking skills of the kitchen staff, food quality, food preparation equipment and storage and so on. Furthermore, 50.4% students were satisfied with the food temperature, showing that the supply chain worked quite successfully.

Plate waste may also be due to serving size. We found that younger students wasted more food than the older ones in primary school. This must be addressed since the lunch patterns and serving sizes for food were similar within school level (primary, middle, and high school). For example, a primary school may contain five grades of different age students, but their serving sizes are the same. In addition, the recommendations for different age groups do not correspond with the actual real-life situation. DRIs-2013 for school children and CNDG-Children 2016 determined the recommendations at three age levels, i.e., 7–10 years, 11–13 years, and 14–17 years. However, the primary, middle, and high schools in Shanghai include students aged from 7–11 years, 12–15 years, and 16–18 years old, respectively. Apparently, the age group in DRIs-2013 and CNDG-Children is different from the actual situation. It should be mentioned that ANPSL-1998 successfully matched the age groups with actual school stage and separated recommendations for two age groups for primary school (i.e., students aged 6–8 years and 9–11 years). However, the recommendation for students older than 15 years is absent in ANPSL-1998. Hence, some gaps between the present recommendations and the actual situation were found. Whether the younger students in primary school need less energy, nutrients, or smaller portion sizes remains unknown. This is in accordance with the opinion of Niaki et al. from the U.S. [14]. Another study from Portugal and Denmark also suggested that portion sizes need to be reconsidered in School Lunch Program [32,33].

The physical measurement of plate waste was recommended and commonly used in dietary surveys in China [17]. Its advantages of providing detailed and accurate plate waste information were also demonstrated in a report to the U.S. Congress [18]. It overcomes the need to rely on students' memory or lack of ability to accurately estimate portion sizes, which are common limitations of 24 h recall investigations [34]. However, the measurement of plate waste in this study was an average estimation based on total plate waste across food items rather than the individual plate waste. We did not take into account any differences in individual behaviors. Measurement of individual plate waste is quite costly and time-consuming, especially for samples over 50–100 persons [35]. Hence, visual estimation and digital photography methods have been applied in some plate waste studies [36–38]. Digital photography was proven to be a more accurate method to estimate plate waste since it can be standardized and offers a way to enhance the reliability and validity of recording dietary intake [36,38]. The digital photography method is worth further development, although it is not used widely in China yet.

This study was conducted in Shanghai so it has limitations to generalize to other cities or at the national level. However, some findings, such as excessive provision of livestock and poultry meat, low intake of vegetables and low satisfaction about school lunches from students, were very common across China.

5. Conclusions

Based the above, the recommendations for the new school lunch standards of Shanghai are as follows: (1) emphasize the provision of less livestock and poultry meat, and more fresh seafood instead of half-processed products; (2) recommend mixed-vegetable dishes. Leafy vegetables could be cooked with other food categories, such as bean products and mushrooms to improve the flavor of vegetables. More importantly, multi-component interventions should be encouraged, which was proven to be an effective way to increase the consumption of vegetables in many countries [6,39,40]; (3) recommend yogurt at lunch or milk at breakfast but this is not compulsory according to Chinese dietary habits; and (4) supplement the recommendations for students aged 15–18 years to cover the missing points in the old standard (ANPSL-1998), while separating the recommendations for primary school students as in the old standard.

Acknowledgments: The authors would like to thank the Shanghai Association Student Nutrition and Health Promotion for funding (Grant #SXYJ-2015) and confirm that the financial supporters had no role in the design and implementation of the study, including data collection, analysis, and interpretation. Additionally, we would like to thank all of the participants who participated in the study. We are also grateful to the teachers and other staff from the schools and companies that prepared lunch in support of our field investigation.

Author Contributions: Z.H., R.G., N.B., Y.Z. and X.H. conceived, designed the study and collected the data in the field; Z.H. and R.G. analyzed the data; Z.H. wrote the first draft of the paper. All the authors participated in the revising of this article. M.C. was the corresponding author and provided professional guidance during the entire study. All authors provided assistance in the completion of the manuscript.

Conflicts of Interest: The authors declare no conflict of interest.

References

1. Papandreou, D.; Makedou, K.; Zormpa, A.; Karampola, M.; Ioannou, A.; Hitoglou-Makedou, A. Are Dietary Intakes Related to Obesity in Children? *Maced. J. Med. Sci.* **2016**, *4*, 194–199. [CrossRef] [PubMed]
2. Liang, Y.; Hou, D.; Zhao, X.; Wang, L.; Hu, Y.; Liu, J.; Cheng, H.; Yang, P.; Shan, X.; Yan, Y.; et al. Childhood obesity affects adult metabolic syndrome and diabetes. *Endocrine* **2015**, *50*, 87–92. [CrossRef] [PubMed]
3. Petkeviciene, J.; Klumbiene, J.; Kriaucioniene, V.; Raskiliene, A.; Sakute, E.; Ceponiene, I. Anthropometric measurements in childhood and prediction of cardiovascular risk factors in adulthood: Kaunas cardiovascular risk cohort study. *BMC Public Health* **2015**, *15*, 218. [CrossRef] [PubMed]
4. Wiseman, M. The second World Cancer Research Fund/American Institute for Cancer Research expert report. Food, nutrition, physical activity, and the prevention of cancer: A global perspective. *Proc. Nutr. Soc.* **2008**, *67*, 253–256. [CrossRef] [PubMed]
5. Ralston, K.; Newman, C.; Clauson, A.; Guthrie, J.; Buzby, J.C. *The National School Lunch Program: Background, Trends, and Issues*; Economic Research Report Number 61; U.S. Department of Agriculture: Washington, DC, USA, 2008; p. 2.

6. Tanaka, N.; Miyoshi, M. School lunch program for health promotion among children in Japan. *Asia Pac. J. Clin. Nutr.* **2012**, *21*, 155–158. [PubMed]

7. Hu, C.K. The current situation and future development perspective of School Lunch Program in China. *Food Nutr. China* **2008**, *2*, 4–6. (In Chinese).

8. Guo, P.; Yang, M.Y.; Chen, D.M. The analysis of school lunch industries in Shanghai. *Chin. J. Sch. Health* **2004**, *25*, 376–377. (In Chinese).

9. Shanghai Bureau of Statistics. Shanghai Statistic Yearbook. 2016. Available online: http://www.stats-sh.gov.cn/tjnj/nj16.htm?d1=2016tjnj/C2003.htm (accessed on 17 February 2017).

10. Ministry of Health People's Republic of China. *Amount of Nutritional Provision for School Lunch*; WS/T 100-1998; Ministry of Health People's Republic of China: Beijing, China, 1998; pp. 78–82.

11. Zhang, B.; Zhai, F.Y.; Du, S.F.; Popkin, B.M. The China Health and Nutrition Survey, 1989–2011. *Obes. Rev.* **2014**, *15* (Suppl. 1), 2–7. [CrossRef] [PubMed]

12. Chinese Nutrition Society. *China National Dietary Guideline for School Children (2016)*, 1st ed.; People's Medical Publishing House: Beijing, China, 2016; p. 49. (In Chinese)

13. Chinese Nutrition Society. *Chinese Dietary Reference Intakes (2013)*, 1st ed.; Science Press: Beijing, China, 2014; pp. 649–660. (In Chinese)

14. Niaki, S.F.; Moore, C.E.; Chen, T.A.; Weber Cullen, K. Younger Elementary School Students Waste More School Lunch Foods than Older Elementary School Students. *J. Acad. Nutr. Diet.* **2017**, *117*, 95–101. [CrossRef] [PubMed]

15. Smith, S.L.; Cunningham-Sabo, L. Food choice, plate waste and nutrient intake of elementary-and middle-school students participating in the US National School Lunch Program. *Public Health Nutr.* **2014**, *17*, 1255–1263. [CrossRef] [PubMed]

16. Condon, E.M.; Crepinsek, M.K.; Fox, M.K. School Meals: Types of Foods Offered to and Consumed by Children at Lunch and Breakfast. *J. Am. Diet. Assoc.* **2009**, *109*, S67–S78. [CrossRef] [PubMed]

17. Sun, C.H.; Ling, W.H.; Huang, G.W. *Nutrition and Food Hygiene*, 7th ed.; People's Medical Publishing House: Beijing, China, 2012; p. 201. (In Chinese)

18. Buzby, J.C.; Guthrie, J.F. *Plate Waste in School Nutrition Programs: Report to Congress*; E-FAN-02-009; Economic Research Service, U.S. Department of Agriculture: Washington, DC, USA, 2002.

19. Chinese Nutrition Society. *China National Dietary Guideline (2016)*, 1st ed.; People's Medical Publishing House: Beijing, China, 2016; p. 309. (In Chinese)

20. Bland, J.M.; Altman, D.G. Statistics notes: Cronbach's alpha. *BMJ* **1997**, *314*, 572. [CrossRef] [PubMed]

21. National Health and Family Planning Commission of the People's Republic of China. Report on Nutrition Status and Chronic Diseases of Chinese People. 2015. Available online: http://www.nhfpc.gov.cn/xcs/s3574/201506/6b4c0f873c174ace9f57f11fd4f6f8d9.shtml (accessed on 17 February 2017).

22. Office of the Federal Register, National Archives and Records Administration. *National School Lunch Program and School Breakfast Program: School Meals Initiative for Healthy Children*; Office of the Federal Register: Washington, DC, USA, 1995; pp. 31188–31222.

23. Crepinsek, M.K.; Gordon, A.R.; McKinney, P.M.; Condon, E.M.; Wilson, A. Meals offered and served in US public schools: Do they meet nutrient standards? *J. Am. Diet. Assoc.* **2009**, *109* (Suppl. 2), S31–S43. [CrossRef] [PubMed]

24. Clark, M.A.; Fox, M.K. Nutritional quality of the diets of US public school children and the role of the school meal programs. *J. Am. Diet. Assoc.* **2009**, *109* (Suppl. 2), S44–S56. [CrossRef] [PubMed]

25. Fox, M.K. School nutrition dietary assessment study-II. *Math. Policy Res. Rep.* **2001**, *67* (Suppl. 1), 67–69.

26. NCD Risk Factor Collaboration (NCD-RisC). Trends in adult body-mass index in 200 countries from 1975 to 2014: A pooled analysis of 1698 population-based measurement studies with 19.2 million participants. *Lancet* **2016**, *387*, 1377–1396.

27. Byker, C.J.; Farris, A.R.; Marcenelle, M.; Davis, G.C.; Serrano, E.L. Food Waste in a School Nutrition Program After Implementation of New Lunch Program Guidelines. *J. Nutr. Educ. Behav.* **2014**, *46*, 406–411. [CrossRef] [PubMed]

28. Cohen, J.F.; Richardson, S.; Parker, E.; Catalano, P.J.; Rimm, E.B. Impact of the New U.S. Department of Agriculture School Meal Standards on Food Selection, Consumption, and Waste. *Am. J. Prev. Med.* **2014**, *46*, 388–394. [CrossRef] [PubMed]

29. Liu, Y.; Cheng, S.; Liu, X.; Cao, X.; Xue, L.; Liu, G. Plate Waste in School Lunch Programs in Beijing, China. *Sustainability* **2016**, *8*, 1288. [CrossRef]

30. Baik, J.Y.; Lee, H. Habitual plate-waste of 6-to 9-year-olds may not be associated with lower nutritional needs or taste acuity, but undesirable dietary factors. *Nutr. Res.* **2009**, *29*, 831–838. [CrossRef] [PubMed]

31. Marlette, M.A.; Templeton, S.B.; Panemangalore, M. Food Type, Food Preparation, and Competitive Food Purchases Impact School Lunch Plate Waste by Sixth-Grade Students. *J. Am. Diet. Assoc.* **2005**, *105*, 1779–1782. [CrossRef] [PubMed]

32. Thorsen, A.V.; Lassen, A.D.; Andersen, E.W.; Christensen, L.M.; Biltoft-Jensen, A.; Andersen, R.; Damsgaard, C.T.; Michaelsen, K.F.; Tetens, I. Plate waste and intake of school lunch based on the new Nordic diet and on packed lunches: A randomised controlled trial in 8-to 11-year-old. *J. Nutr. Sci.* **2015**, *4*, e20. [CrossRef] [PubMed]

33. Dinis, D.; Martins, M.L.; Rocha, A. Plate Waste as an Indicator of Portions Inadequacy at School Lunch. *Int. Sch. Sci. Res. Innov.* **2013**, *7*, 477–480.

34. Warren, J.M.; Henry, C.J.; Livingstone, M.B.; Lightowler, H.J.; Bradshaw, S.M.; Perwaiz, S. How well do children aged 5–7 years recall food eaten at school lunch? *Public Health Nutr.* **2003**, *6*, 41–47. [CrossRef] [PubMed]

35. Comstock, E.M.; St Pierre, R.G.; Mackiernan, Y.D. Measuring individual plate waste in school lunches. Visual estimation and children's ratings vs. actual weighing of plate waste. *J. Am. Diet. Assoc.* **1981**, *79*, 290–296. [PubMed]

36. Swanson, M. Digital photography as a tool to measure school cafeteria consumption. *J. Sch. Health* **2008**, *78*, 432–437. [CrossRef] [PubMed]

37. Nicklas, T.A.; O'Neil, C.E.; Stuff, J.; Goodell, L.S.; Liu, Y.; Martin, C.K. Validity and Feasibility of a Digital Diet Estimation Method for Use with Preschool Children: A Pilot Study. *J. Nutr. Educ. Behav.* **2012**, *44*, 618–623. [CrossRef] [PubMed]

38. Martins, M.L.; Cunha, L.M.; Rodrigues, S.S.P.; Rocha, A. Determination of plate waste in primary school lunches by weighing and visual estimation methods: A validation study. *Waste Manag.* **2014**, *34*, 1362–1368. [CrossRef] [PubMed]

39. Thomson, C.A.; Ravia, J. A systematic review of behavioral interventions to promote intake of fruit and vegetables. *J. Am. Diet. Assoc.* **2011**, *111*, 1523–1535. [CrossRef] [PubMed]

40. Blanchette, L.; Brug, J. Determinants of fruit and vegetable consumption among 6–12-year-old children and effective interventions to increase consumption. *J. Hum. Nutr. Diet.* **2005**, *18*, 431–443. [CrossRef] [PubMed]

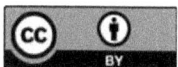

nutrients

MDPI

Article

A Socio-Ecological Examination of Weight-Related Characteristics of the Home Environment and Lifestyles of Households with Young Children

Virginia Quick [1,*], Jennifer Martin-Biggers [1], Gayle Alleman Povis [2], Nobuko Hongu [2], John Worobey [1] and Carol Byrd-Bredbenner [1]

[1] Department of Nutritional Sciences, Rutgers University, 26 Nichol Avenue, New Brunswick, NJ 08901, USA; jmartin@aesop.rutgers.edu (J.M.-B.); worobey@rci.rutgers.edu (J.W.); bredbenner@aesop.rutgers.edu (C.B.-B.)
[2] Department of Nutritional Sciences, University of Arizona, 406 Shantz Building, 1177 E. 4th Street, Tucson, AZ 85721, USA; gpovis@email.arizona.edu (G.A.P.); hongu@email.arizona.edu (N.H.)
* Correspondence: vquick@njaes.rutgers.edu; Tel.: +1-848-932-0965

Received: 23 April 2017; Accepted: 9 June 2017; Published: 14 June 2017

Abstract: Home environment and family lifestyle practices have an influence on child obesity risk, thereby making it critical to systematically examine these factors. Thus, parents ($n = 489$) of preschool children completed a cross-sectional online survey which was the baseline data collection conducted, before randomization, in the HomeStyles program. The survey comprehensively assessed these factors using a socio-ecological approach, incorporating intrapersonal, interpersonal and environmental measures. Healthy intrapersonal dietary behaviors identified were parent and child intakes of recommended amounts of 100% juice and low intakes of sugar-sweetened beverages. Unhealthy behaviors included low milk intake and high parent fat intake. The home environment's food supply was found to support healthy intakes of 100% juice and sugar-sweetened beverages, but provided too little milk and ample quantities of salty/fatty snacks. Physical activity levels, sedentary activity and the home's physical activity and media environment were found to be less than ideal. Environmental supports for active play inside homes were moderate and somewhat better in the area immediately outside homes and in the neighborhood. Family interpersonal interaction measures revealed several positive behaviors, including frequent family meals. Parents had considerable self-efficacy in their ability to perform food- and physical activity-related childhood obesity protective practices. This study identified lifestyle practices and home environment characteristics that health educators could target to help parents promote optimal child development and lower their children's risk for obesity.

Keywords: socio-ecological model; home environment; parents; child; nutrition; diet; physical activity; sleep; obesity

1. Introduction

The high prevalence of obesity, especially among young children, continues to be of great public health concern given obesity's long-term negative health effects on child growth, development and lifelong health [1–3]. Research suggests the pervasiveness of obesity is at least partly due to myriad socio-ecological factors that, unlike genetic factors, may be modifiable via public health interventions [4]. The socio-ecological model considers the complex interplay between intrapersonal factors (e.g., values, self-efficacy, outcome expectations), interpersonal factors (e.g., social norms, social support), and environmental factors (e.g., physical environment related to food and physical activity availability and accessibility). Understudied socioecological factors critical to childhood obesity prevention are the weight-related aspects of the home environment and family interpersonal factors and lifestyle patterns [5,6].

The socio-ecological model is a graphic depiction of the ecological theory of a specific health behavior or outcome [4,5]. It illustrates how the health and well-being of an individual is determined by multiple influences that interact at both the macro-level and micro-level environments [7]. At the macro-level, factors such as social norms, economic policies and advertising have a more indirect influence on behaviors. Micro-level factors, such as an individual's physical and social environment (i.e., interpersonal level) and personal factors (i.e., intrapersonal level), more directly influence behaviors. In obesity research, socio-ecological theory is conceptualized as being influenced by factors across multiple levels: individual and family characteristics, and characteristics of the home, community, and region [8]. Environments that do not support healthy weight-management behaviors (e.g., access to safe parks and sidewalks for physical activity) make it difficult for individuals to engage in behaviors that prevent, limit, or reverse weight gain. To date, obesity interventions focused on prevention of weight gain in children under 5 years of age have shown limited effectiveness in reducing or limiting weight gain [9]. A systematic review of obesity prevention interventions among preschool children suggest the failure to show an intervention effect may be partly due to the lack of focus on social and environmental factors within which diet and physical activity behaviors are enacted [10].

The currently available research on the prevention and treatment of obesity among preschool-aged children and adults highlight the importance of considering the environment [11]. The micro-level of the home is the prominent shared environment of parents and their children. Parents act as 'gate keepers' of the home and role models for their children; they strongly influence food and physical activity behaviors and practices that may increase or decrease their child's obesity risk [12–21]. Additionally, physical attributes of the home environment (e.g., availability of healthy foods) and parental behaviors (e.g., parent feeding practices) have been found to be associated with preschool children's weight-related behaviors (e.g., physical activity, dietary patterns) [22]. Prior research has suggested that a number of intra- and inter-personal factors in the home environment are also associated with children's overweight status, such as parent overweight status [23], limited daily physical activity [24], frequent family meals [25], low household availability of fruits and vegetables [26], greater daily television viewing time [25], and less parental modeling of healthy behaviors [27].

Given the home environment (intra- and inter-personal factors) may greatly influence child obesity risk, it is critical to systematically examine these factors. Few studies have comprehensively assessed the home environment and lifestyles of parents of preschool-aged children using a socio-ecological approach with reliable and validated intrapersonal, interpersonal, and environmental measures [28], which are necessary for understanding the potential influencers of obesity risk on families with young children [29]. To expand our understanding, the objective of this study was to utilize a baseline dataset collected prior to randomization to describe the socio-ecological factors related to the obesogenic home environments of parents with preschool-aged children (2 to 5 years of age) in a program called HomeStyles [30–33].

2. Materials and Methods

Details of the protocol for the HomeStyles program are reported elsewhere [34] and are described in brief in this section. The Institutional Review Board at the authors' universities approved this study (ethical approval code is #11-294Mc). All participants gave informed consent.

2.1. Sample & Recruitment

Parents of preschool children (ages 2 to <6 years) who resided in the catchment areas of New Jersey and Arizona in the U.S. were recruited to participate in a program that would help them build closer family bonds and raise healthier families. Recruitment notices were distributed as flyers, posters, and/or email announcements to community centers, workplaces, schools, daycare programs, doctor's offices, and places of worship. In-person recruiting was conducted at these sites and community events. To be eligible to participate, parents had to have at least one preschool child, be able to read and write English or Spanish at about the 4th to 5th grade level, be the key decision maker with regard to family food purchases and preparation, and have consistent access to the Internet. Recruited participants began by completing a brief online eligibility screener survey. Those who were eligible were then directed to complete the online baseline survey. The online baseline survey dataset utilized in this study was collected before parents began the intervention.

2.2. Instruments

2.2.1. Survey Development & Implementation

Development of the online survey and implementation is described in detail elsewhere [34]. In brief, the survey included an array of valid, reliable measures assessing parent and household psychographic characteristics (e.g., personal organization, family conflict) as well as parent and child weight-related behaviors (i.e., diet, physical activity, sleep) and parent weight-related cognitions (e.g., values, self-efficacy) that are described further below. Measures were selected to yield an understanding of intrapersonal and interpersonal/social behaviors and cognitions and environmental conditions in and near participants' homes pertaining to diet and physical activity. All measures were self-report and underwent rigorous selection or development procedures to ensure they were valid and reliable, matched the goals of HomeStyles, and acceptable and accurately interpreted by the target audience [5,6,35,36]. Prior to data collection, the survey was pre-tested ($n = 48$) to identify refinements needed to improve clarity and verify accuracy of scale scoring algorithms. The survey was also pilot tested ($n = 550$) to confirm scale unidimensionality and internal consistency, and further reviewed by a panel of experts to confirm measures were of integrity and suitability to the study purpose [6]. After undergoing rigorous testing, recruitment and implementation of the survey was conducted online over a 15-month period [34]. Parents with more than one preschool child were instructed to report data for one "target" child, defined as the child born closest to a randomly selected date specified in the survey (i.e., noon on 1 June). The measures in the survey, including scale type, number of items, possible score range, and Cronbach's alpha (as applicable), are organized by level of the socio-ecological model as presented in Table 1.

2.2.2. Sociodemographic Characteristics

Sociodemographic characteristics of the sample (e.g., parent race/ethnicity, education level, age, sex) were collected. Family socio-economic status was assessed with both the 4-item Family Affluence Scale [37,38] and annual median household income based on U.S. Census Bureau zip code data. Parents rated their own and their child's health status (poor, fair, good, very good, or excellent) using the Centers for Disease Control and Prevention's Health-Related Quality of Life questionnaire [39,40].

2.2.3. Intrapersonal Factors

Intrapersonal measures included three scales assessing the extent of parents' personal organization [41], their need for cognition (e.g., enjoyment of thinking) [42,43], and control of stress [44]. Intrapersonal weight-related assessments included food frequency questionnaires evaluating dietary intake (e.g., fruits and vegetables, milk, sugar-sweetened beverages, fat) [45–50], physical activity level [51–53], screentime [54–56], and sleep duration [57,58] of parents and children.

2.2.4. Interpersonal/Social Factors

Interpersonal/social characteristics assessed included household chaos [41,59], family conflict [60], family support for healthy eating and physical activity, frequency of family meals [61], frequency of eating family meals in various locations (e.g., in the car) [54,62,63], and frequency with which television or other media devices were used during family meals [6,22,54]. Other interpersonal/social characteristics included appraisals of the emotional environment at family mealtime [22,62–64], meal planning behaviors [65], self-efficacy for preparing family meals [66], and parental modeling of healthy eating behaviors and self-efficacy for childhood obesity-protective practices [6,55,67–70]. Interpersonal/social characteristics associated with physical activity included frequency of parent and child actively playing together [6], parental modeling of physical activity [22,50–52,71], and parental encouragement of and self-efficacy for promoting children's physical activity [6,22,52,67,68,72,73]. The importance and value parents placed on dietary and physical activity practices and cognitions linked to obesity prevention [66,72,74] also were evaluated.

2.2.5. Environmental Factors

Food-frequency questionnaires evaluated the typical availability of fruit/vegetable juice, salty/fatty snacks, sugar-sweetened beverages, and milk in the home [46,47,50,75,76]. The availability of space and supports for physical activity inside the home, immediately outside the home (yard), and neighborhood, along with perceived neighborhood safety and frequency of outdoor active play, were appraised with the HOP-Up (Home Opportunities for Physical activity check-Up) Checklist [77]. The home media environment (i.e., media devices in the home and child bedroom [22,54–56], amount of daily screentime children were allowed [22,54–56], and total time TV was on daily [78]) served as a proxy for sedentary behavior supports.

2.3. *Data Analysis*

Descriptive statistics (means, standard deviations, percentages, actual score ranges) were computed to describe the sociodemographic characteristics of study participants and intrapersonal, interpersonal/social, and environmental factors. Internal consistency for continuous scales were also measured (when applicable) using Cronbach's alpha. SPSS software version 24.0 (IBM Corporation, Chicago, IL, USA) was used for all analyses.

3. Results

Of the 1221 individuals who responded to recruitment advertisements, were eligible for the study, and gave informed consent, 489 (40%) completed the baseline survey. [34]. The mean parent age was 32.34 ± 5.71 SD years and the vast majority were female (93%). More than half were white (58%), resided in New Jersey (53%), had earned a baccalaureate degree or higher (51%), and spoke English at home (87%). Slightly more than one-third of participants did not have paid employment (36%) or worked full time (38%), with the remainder working part-time.

Most households had 1 (30%) or 2 children (42%) children less than 18 years old and at least one of these children between the ages of 2 and <6 years. The target children were approximately evenly divided by sex (48% female) and had an average age of 3.85 ± 1.05 SD years. A plurality was white (49%) and most were the biological offspring of the participating parent (91%).

Most participants lived in dual parent households (82%) and had spouses/partners who had at least some post-secondary education (78%) and worked full-time (84%). A total of 17%, 58%, and 25% were low, middle, and high family affluence level [33,34], respectively. Annual median household income was based on U.S. Census Bureau zip code data for each participant's home (mean $63,654.84 ± 24,787.07 SD).

As displayed in Table 1, intrapersonal parent measure scores indicate that participants were somewhat disorganized personally, were fairly neutral about whether they had a need for cognition, and were able to handle most stresses. On average, parents reported good to very good health status. Intake of 100% fruit/vegetable juice and milk servings were low at slightly more than half a serving daily, which was lower than the nearly three-quarters of a serving of sugar-sweetened beverages daily intake. Fat intake exceeded one-third of total daily calories. Overall, physical activity level was low while sedentary screentime was high (~6 h/day).

Table 1. HomeStyles Study Measures and Baseline Scores (n = 489).

Measures	# of Items	Scale Type	Possible Score Range	Cronbach's Alpha	Mean ± SD	Actual Score Range
Intrapersonal Factors						
Parents						
Personal Organization [41]	4	5-point agreement rating A	1-5	0.64	2.60 ± 0.94	1-5
Need for Cognition [42,43]	1	5-point agreement rating A	1-5	*	3.39 ± 0.97	1-5
Control of Stress [44]	2	4-point frequency rating B	1-4	0.76	3.39 ± 0.76	1-4
Health Status [37,38]	1	5-point excellence rating C	1-5	*	3.45 ± 0.94	1-5
100% Fruit/Vegetable Juice (servings/day) [45,47–50]	2	9-point servings drank scale D	0-2.3	*	0.57 ± 0.57	0-2.29
Milk (servings/day) [45,47–50]	1	9-point servings drank scale D	0-8	*	0.57 ± 0.45	0-1.14
Sugar-sweetened Beverages [46,50] (servings/day)	4	9-point servings eaten scale D	0-4.6	*	0.71 ± 0.81	0-4.57
% Total Calories from Fat [45,47–49]	17	5-point servings eaten scale E	0-100	*	36.66 ± 6.00	22.10–56.90
Physical Activity Level [51–53]	3	8-point exercise scale F	0-42	*	13.8 ± 9.87	0-42
Screentime [6,56] (minutes/day)	1	minutes/day	0-1440	*	354.69 ± 279.54	0-1425
Sleep Duration (minutes/day) [57,58] ¥	1	hours/day	0-24	*	7.08 ± 1.21	4-12
Children						
Health Status [37,38]	1	5-point excellence rating C	1-5	*	4.36 ± 0.77	2-5
Fruit/Vegetable Juice (servings/day) [45–50,76]	2	9-point servings drank scale D	0-2.3	*	0.75 ± 0.56	0-2.29
Milk (servings/day) [45–50,76]	1	9-point servings drank scale D	0-8	*	0.85 ± 0.35	0-1.14
Sugar-sweetened Beverage (servings/day) [45–50,76]	2	9-point servings drank scale D	0-2.3	*	0.28 ± 0.42	0-2.29
Physical Activity Level [51–53]	3	8-point Exercise scale F	0-42	*	25.83 ± 11.53	0-42
Screentime minutes/day [6,56]	1	minutes	0-1440	*	294.57 ± 261.98	
Sleep Duration (hours/day) [57,58] †	1	hours	0-24	*	10.68 ± 1.41	8-15
Interpersonal/Social Factors						
Household Chaos [41,57]	2	5-point agreement rating A	1-5	0.86	2.51 ± 1.07	1-5
Family Conflict [60]	5	5-point agreement rating A	1-5	0.86	1.99 ± 0.76	1-5
Family Support for Healthy Eating and Physical Activity [61]	4	5-point frequency rating G	1-5	0.79	3.55 ± 1.35	1-5
Food-Related						
Family Meal frequency/week [61]	3	0-7 days for breakfast, lunch, dinner; score is sum of 3 meals	0-21	*	12.40 ± 5.02	0-21

Table 1. Cont.

Measures	# of Items	Scale Type	Possible Score Range	Cronbach's Alpha	Mean ± SD	Actual Score Range
Family Meal Location [54,62,63]						
In Car (days/week)	1	0–7 days	0–7	*	0.55 ± 1.4	0–7
At Fast Food Restaurant (days/week)	1	0–7 days	0–7	*	0.88 ± 1.27	0–7
At Dining Table (days/week)	1	0–7 days	0–7	*	4.64 ± 2.5	0–7
In Front of TV (days/week)	1	0–7 days	0–7	*	2.36 ± 2.52	0–7
Media Device Use at Family Meals [6,22,52] (days/week)	1	0–7 days	0–7	*	1.69 ± 2.4	0–7
TV Use at Family Meals & Snacking Occasions [6,22,52] (days/week)	1	0–7 days	0–7	*	3.50 ± 2.67	0–7
Family Mealtime Emotional Environment [22,63]	2	5-point agreement rating [A]	1–5	0.62	4.06 ± 0.85	1–5
Family Meals are Planned [65,66]	2	5-point agreement rating [A]	1–5	0.77	3.38 ± 1.02	1–5
Parent Family Meal Preparation Self-Efficacy [66]	2	5-point agreement rating [A]	1–5	0.56	3.95 ± 0.9	1–5
Parent Modeling of Healthy Eating [55,69,70]	4	5-point agreement rating [A]	1–5	0.74	3.61 ± 0.81	1–5
Parent Self-efficacy for Food-Related Childhood Obesity-Protective Practices [6,67,68]	6	5-point confidence rating [H]	1–5	0.81	3.78 ± 0.71	1–5
Physical Activity-Related						
Parent: Child Co-Physical Activity (days/week) [6]	2	8-point modeling scale [I]	0–7	0.68	3.64 ± 1.85	0–7
Parent Modeling of Physical Activity (days/week) [22,54,55,70]	2	8-point modeling scale [I]	0–7	0.59	3.20 ± 1.31	0–6.67
Parent Modeling of Sedentary Activity (days/week) [22,54,55,70]	2	8-point modeling scale [I]	0–7	0.72	3.51 ± 2.33	0–7
Parent Encouragement of Child Physical Activity [6,22,55,72,73]	5	5-point agreement rating [A]	1–5	0.85	4.02 ± 0.67	1–5
Parent Self-Efficacy for Physical-Activity Related Childhood Obesity-Protective Practices [6,67,68]	3	5-point confidence rating [H]	1–5	0.84	3.49 ± 1.01	1–5
Parent Values Related to Obesity-Protective Practices						
Healthy Eating Outcome Expectations [66,74]	6	5-point agreement rating [A]	1–5	0.92	4.55 ± 0.54	2–5
Physical Activity Outcome Expectations [66,74]	6	5-point agreement rating [A]	1–5	0.94	4.44 ± 0.61	2–5
Value Placed on Modeling Physical Activity [6,22,71–73]	2	5-point agreement rating [A]	1–5	0.73	3.86 ± 0.86	1–5
Valued Placed on Not Modeling Sedentary Behavior [6]	1	5-point agreement rating [A]	1–5	*	3.81 ± 0.97	1–5
Value Placed on Physical Activity for Children [72,73]	2	5-point agreement rating [A]	1–5	0.71	3.70 ± 0.88	1–5
Environmental Factors						
Household Food Availability [46,47,50,75,76]						

Table 1. *Cont.*

Measures	# of Items	Scale Type	Possible Score Range	Cronbach's Alpha	Mean ± SD	Actual Score Range
100% Fruit/Vegetable Juice (servings/household member/week)	2	9-point servings scale^J	0–8	*	3.19 ± 2.06	0–8
Salty/fatty snacks (servings/household member/week)	4	9-point servings scale^J	0–32	*	7.9 ± 7.19	0–32
Sugar-sweetened Beverages (servings/household member/week)	4	9-point servings scale^J	0–8	*	1.62 ± 1.8	0–8
Milk (servings/household member/week)	1	9-point servings scale^J	0–8	*	6.60 ± 2.04	0–8
Physical Activity Environment [77]						
Indoor Home Space & Supports For Physical Activity	6	Varies by item; 2 items are counts; 1 item is a 5-point agreement rating;^A 3 items are 5-point occurrence ratings^K	1–5	0.74	3.31 ± 0.87	1–5
Outdoor/Yard Space & Supports For Physical Activity ‡	4	5-point agreement rating^A	1–5	0.75	4.31 ± 0.7	1–5
Neighborhood Space & Supports For Physical Activity §	4	5-point agreement rating^A	1–5	0.88	4.01 ± 0.99	0.50–5
Neighborhood Environment Safety	2	5-point agreement rating^A	1–5	0.42	3.41 ± 0.87	1–5
Frequency of Active Play Outdoors	2	5-point occurrence ratings^K	1–5	0.54	2.55 ± 0.97	1–5
Media Environment						
Total Number of Inactive Media Devices (including TV) in the Home [22,54,55]	6	Total devices^L	0–66	*	10.51 ± 4.53	1–27
Total Number of Inactive Media Devices (including TV) in Children's Bedrooms	7	Total # of media device types^M	0–7	*	1.32 ± 1.57	0–7
Time Children are Allowed to Watch TV/Movies & Use Inactive Media Devices (e.g., computers, tablets, smart phones) [6] (minutes/day)	1	minutes	0–1440	*	475.98 ± 701.11	0–1440
Total Time TV is on When No One is Watching [6,22,78] (minutes/day)	1	minutes	0–1440	*	130.18 ± 214.95	0–1410

* Not applicable. ¥ n = 477. † n = 448. ‡ n = 437. § n = 482. ^A 5-point Agreement Rating: strongly disagree, disagree, neither agree nor disagree, agree, strongly agree; scored 1 to 5 respectively with scoring reversed for negatively worded statements; scale score equals average of item scores; higher scale score indicates greater expression of the trait. ^B 4-point Frequency Rating: not at all, several days, more than half the days, nearly every day; scored 1 to 4; higher score indicates greater frequency. ^C 5-point Excellence Rating: poor, fair, good, very good, excellent; scored 1 to 5 respectively; higher score indicates better health. ^D 9-point Beverage Servings Rating: <1 time/week, 1 day/week, 2 days/week, 3 days/week, 4 days/week, 5 days/week, 6 days/week, 7 days/week, >1 time/day; scored 0 to 8 respectively; higher score indicates greater frequency. ^E 5-point Fatty Food Servings Rating: 1 time/month or less, 2 to 3 times/month, 1 to 2 times/week, 3 to 4 times/week, 5 or more times/week; scored 0 to 4 respectively; scale scoring algorithm is protected by copyright and described in detail elsewhere [79]; higher score indicates greater intake. ^F 8-point Exercise Days/week: 0, 1, 2, 3, 4, 5, 6, and 7; days/week weighted by exercise intensity (weights of 1, 2, 3 for walking, moderate, and vigorous activity, respectively) and summed to create scale score; higher scale score indicates greater activity level. ^G 5-point Frequency Rating: never, rarely, sometimes, most of the time, always; scored 1 to 5; higher score indicates greater frequency. ^H 5-point Confidence Rating: not at all confident, not confident, confident, quite confident, very confident; scored 1 to 5 respectively; higher scale score indicates greater confidence. ^I 8-point Modeling Days/week: 0 (almost never), 1, 2, 3, 4, 5, 6, and 7; days averaged to create scale score; higher score indicates more frequent modeling. ^J 9-point Household Servings Rating: <1 time/week, 1 day/week, 2 days/week, 3 days/week, 4 days/week, 5 days/week, 6 days/week, 7 days/week, >1 time/day; scored 0 to 8 respectively; higher score indicates greater frequency. ^K 5-point Occurrence Rating: almost never, 1-2 times/week, 3 to 4 times/week, 5 to 6 times/week, every day; scored 1 to 5 respectively; scale score equals average of items; higher scale score indicates greater occurrence of behavior. ^L 11-point Media Device Count: 1 = 1 to 10 = 10, 11 = more than 10; scale score equals sum of items; higher score indicates greater number of media devices. ^M Response for each media device in child's bedroom was 0 = no and 1 = yes; scale score equals sum of items; higher score indicates greater number of different media device types.

Child intake of fruit/vegetable juice, milk, and sugar-sweetened beverages all equaled less than one serving per day. Physical activity was moderate while sedentary screentime was high (~5 h/day). Sleep averaged 7 h nightly for parents (~62% meeting sleep recommendations of 7 or more hours per night) and total sleep duration for children (daytime naps and nighttime sleep) was nearly 11 h (62% meeting sleep recommendations (11–14 h/day for 2 year olds; 10–13 h/day for 3–5 year olds).

Psychographic household measures indicated that participants' had somewhat chaotic households and tended to feel their families got along fairly well, disagreeing that they had family conflict. Family meals were eaten nearly twice per day and were eaten at a dining table more often than other locations. On average, TV was watched during family meals or while snacking on half the days in a week. Parents agreed that family meals had a positive emotional environment. They somewhat agreed that they planned family meals, had self-efficacy for preparing family meals, modeled healthy eating behaviors to children, and had self-efficacy for food-related childhood obesity-protective practices. With regard to physical activity, parents agreed that they encouraged children to be physically active, but actively played with children or modeled physical activity to children less than half of the days in a week. Parents strongly agreed that healthy eating and physical activity behaviors lead to positive outcomes, however the value placed on modeling healthy physical activity behaviors tended to be somewhat neutral.

The household food environment provided about 3 servings of 100% fruit/vegetable juice and 1.5 servings of sugar-sweetened beverages per household member per week. Approximately 7 servings of both milk and salty/fatty snacks were available weekly per person. Physical activity space and supports for children inside the home were moderate, with outdoor/yard and neighborhood space and supports for physical activity ratings being higher. Neighborhood safety ratings tended to be neutral, and participants reported the frequency of child active play outdoors occurred 2 to 3 times per week. Households were replete with 'inactive' media devices, and the time spent with these devices equaled about 8 h daily.

4. Discussion

Healthy intrapersonal behaviors identified in this study population include parent and child intakes of 100% fruit/vegetable juice that mirror recommendations of 4 to 6 ounces per day [80,81], with these intake levels corroborated by the household environment's availability of 100% fruit/vegetable juice servings/household member/week. Another positive feature is the intake and household availability of sugar-sweetened beverages (e.g., soft drinks, fruit drinks) were fairly low, contributing only about 90 and 29 calories (and 18 and 6 grams of sugar) to parent and child daily intake, respectively; values which are lower than the per capita intakes found in nationally representative studies [82]. An area in great need of improvement is milk intake and availability in the household, which were far below recommendations for both parents and children [80], thereby potentially placing parents at risk of osteoporosis [83] and children at risk for decreased bone mineralization and associated sequelae [83]. These low milk intakes during childhood are especially worrisome given that milk intake tends to drop off as children, especially females, enter adolescence [82]. Also of concern are the household availability of more than 1 serving/person daily of salty/fatty snacks and the percentage of total calories contributed by fat to parents' diets. Indeed, parents' fat intake exceeded the upper limit of the Acceptable Macronutrient Distribution Ranges (AMDRs) [84] and was somewhat higher than the mean intake of U.S. adults [85].

Physical activity levels, time spent in sedentary activity, and the physical activity and media environment were found to be less than ideal. Much like in national reports [85], adults in this study had limited physical activity, scoring less than one-third of the maximum score possible. One-third of parents reported walking at least 10 minutes continuously and/or engaging in moderate exercise at least 5 times per week, but only 10% engaged in vigorous activity 5 or more times per week. Children had more physical activity, but achieved only about 60% of the highest score possible. Unlike parents, half of the children walked at least 10 minutes continuously, two-thirds engaged in moderate exercise, and 40% received vigorous exercise at least 5 times per week. Environmental supports for active play inside homes were moderate. That is, children had restricted space inside homes to vigorously play (e.g., the amount of active play space for half of the children was insufficient for doing more than 3 continuous somersaults or cartwheels before hitting furniture), few toys that helped them be active inside (37% had less than 5 toys supporting active play inside the home), and engaged in active play inside the home few days per week (one-third actively played indoors less than 3 times weekly). Supports and space for physical activity outdoors and in the neighborhood were higher than indoors. Almost all parents agreed or strongly agreed that the yard or area immediately outside their homes had plenty of room for kids to play games, and more than 8 out of 10 agreed or strongly agreed that there were outdoor areas like parks, pools, and playgrounds nearby where their children could play. However, the frequency of playing outdoors averaged less than 3 to 4 times weekly. (Data were collected year round from both New Jersey and Arizona, hence seasonality should not be an influence on this frequency). The relatively infrequent outdoor play may reflect the young age of the children studied and their need for adult supervision as well as the fairly neutral ratings parents gave their neighborhood for being safe from crime and biting insects and animals.

Parents and children reported 5 to 6 h of daily screentime; children exceeded the 2016 recommendations from the American Academy of Pediatrics by 5 times [86]. The home media environment was clearly conducive to sedentary behavior—children were allowed to watch television or use 'inactive' media devices nearly 8 h daily and television was on for 2 h, even when no one was watching. Despite recommendations to make children's bedrooms media free [86], 56% of children had at least one media device in their bedrooms.

Adequate sleep appears protective against excess weight gain [87–92]. The nightly sleep duration recommendation for adult is 7 to 9 h per night [93]. Nearly two-thirds of parents surveyed met these recommendations, while the remainder got less than the recommendations. The mean sleep time for parents in this study, however, is higher than the 6 h and 31 min average nightly duration for U.S. adults [94]. A comparison of children's sleep with age-specific recommendations [93] indicated that 28% got less daily sleep than recommended for their age group.

Measures of interpersonal or family social interactions indicated several positive behaviors. For example, frequent family meals eaten in a positive emotional environment without distractions, such as television and angry discussions, are associated with healthier dietary intakes [87,95–101]. Parents in this study reported that their families ate together almost twice daily and mealtimes were fairly calm (e.g., low stress, infrequent arguments). Most meals were eaten at a dining or kitchen table, a location associated with fewer problems with child behaviors at mealtime [102], which likely contributed to the positive emotional atmosphere reported. However, television and media devices were used fairly often while eating, and meals were eaten in front of the television more than two days per week.

Although observational learning is an important way that children learn [103,104], parents were neutral about whether they modeled healthy eating to their children. Scores on scales assessing parent modeling of healthy physical activity behaviors, sedentary activity behaviors, and active play with their children indicated that they exhibited these behaviors fewer than three days per week. Parents tended to agree that they valued modeling physical activity and not modeling sedentary behavior to children. Opportunities for parents to learn how to put these values into action are warranted.

Outcome expectations and self-efficacy are key predictors of behavior [104–106]. Parents were firm in their beliefs that healthy eating and physical activity improved health. Their self-efficacy scores for engaging in food-related and physical activity-related childhood obesity protective practices showed that they were confident to very confident in their ability to perform these practices. Providing opportunities for parents to increase their self-efficacy to be "very confident" could help them increase implementation of these childhood obesity protective behaviors.

Although this is one of few studies that has comprehensively assessed obesity-related factors associated with home environment and lifestyle practices among parents of preschool aged children using a socio-ecological approach, findings should be interpreted in the light of study limitations. The cross-sectional study design does not allow for inference of causality in the observed associations. Additionally, the study sample only included parents of preschool-aged children in two geographical areas of the U.S., so findings may not be generalizable to families with children of different ages or living in other areas of the country including geography (rural vs. urban). There also is a potential for self-selection bias as participants were recruited for a behavioral intervention. Lastly, all information from participants was self-reported and may be subject to both reporting error and bias. Future research should examine the relationship of socioecological factors related to the home obesogenic environment with child weight status to determine factors predictive of childhood obesity.

5. Conclusions

In conclusion, this study identified socioecological factors related to the obesogenic home environment of parents with preschool-aged children that could be improved to promote optimal child development while lowering the risk of childhood obesity. However, parents had a constellation of characteristics that likely would make it a challenge for them to orchestrate changes to weight-related characteristics of their home environments and lifestyles. That is, parents indicated they tended to be disorganized (e.g., late for appointments, put off chores, not dependable) and did not enjoy dealing with situations requiring a lot of thinking. Additionally, they reported high stress levels—on at least half the days in a week they felt unable to control important things in their life and felt difficulties were piling up so high they could not overcome them. They also reported households were somewhat chaotic (i.e., a real "zoo", noisy). On a positive note, these families had low family conflict (e.g., fighting, criticizing). These findings suggest that obesity prevention interventions for parents of preschool children need to address not only obesity-protective behaviors (e.g., diet, physical activity, sleep, parent behavior modeling) and cognitions associated with behavior change (e.g., self-efficacy, values), but also should take into consideration behavioral characteristics (e.g., parent organizational skills, need for cognition, stress, household organization) that may affect their ability to realize the benefits of the intervention.

Acknowledgments: This study was funded by USDA NIFA #2011-68001-30170.

Author Contributions: C.B.-B., J.W. and N.H. conceived and designed the study. J.M.-B., C.B.-B. and G.A.P. collected data. V.Q., J.M.-B. and C.B.-B. analyzed the data. All authors were involved in manuscript preparation and revision and approved the final manuscript.

Conflicts of Interest: The authors declare no conflict of interest. The founding sponsors had no role in the design of the study; in the collection, analyses, or interpretation of data; in the writing of the manuscript, and in the decision to publish the results.

References

1. Finkelstein, E.; Trogdon, J.; Cohen, J.; Dietz, W. Annual medical spending attributalbe to obesity: Payer-and service-specific estimates. *Health Aff.* **2009**, *28*, w822–w831. [CrossRef] [PubMed]
2. Pi-Sunyer, F. The obesity epidemic: Pathophysiology and consequences of obesity. *Obes. Res.* **2002**, *10*, 97S–104S. [CrossRef] [PubMed]
3. Ogden, L.; Carroll, M.; Jit, B.; Flegal, K. Prevalence of childhood and adult obesity in the United States. *JAMA* **2014**, *311*, 806–814. [CrossRef] [PubMed]
4. Fairburn, C.; Brownell, K. *Eating Disorders and Obesity*; Guilford Press Inc.: New York, NY, USA, 2002.
5. Martin-Biggers, J.M.; Worobey, J.; Byrd-Bredbenner, C. Interpersonal Characteristics in the Home Environment Associated with Childhood Obesity. In *Recent Advances in Obesity in Children*; Avid Science Publications: Berlin, Germany, 2016; Available online: www.avidscience.com/wp-content/uploads/2016/05/OIC-15-03_May-06-2016.pdf (accessed on 10 April 2017).
6. Martin-Biggers, J. Home Environment Characteristics Associated with Obesity Risk in Preschool-Aged Children and Their Mothers. Ph.D. Thesis, Rutgers, The State University of New Jersey, New Brunswick, NJ, USA, 2016.

7. Story, M.; Kaphingst, K.; Robinson-O'Brien, R.; Glanz, K. Creating healthy food and eating environments: Policy and environmental approaches. *Annu. Rev. Public Health* **2008**, *29*, 253–272. [CrossRef] [PubMed]

8. Hawkins, S.; Cole, T.; Law, C. An ecological systems approach to examine risk factors for early childhood overweight: Findings from the UK millenium cohort. *J. Epidemiol. Community Health* **2009**, *63*, 147–155. [CrossRef] [PubMed]

9. Wang, Y.; Wu, Y.; Wilson, R.; Bleich, S.; Cheskin, L.; Weston, C.; Showell, N.; Fawole, O.; Lau, B.; Segal, J. *Childhood Obesity Prevention Programs: Comparitive Effectiveness Review and Meta-Analysis*; Prepared by the John Hopkins University Evidence-based Practice Center under Contract No. 290-2007-10061-I; Agency for Healthcare Research and Quality: Rockville, MD, USA, 2013.

10. Monasta, L.; Batty, G.; Macaluso, A.; Ronfani, L.; Lutje, V.; Bavcar, A.; van Lenthe, F.; Brug, J.; Cattaneo, A. Interventions for the prevention of overweight and obesity in preschool children: A systematic review of randomized controlled trials. *Obes. Rev.* **2011**, *12*, e107–e118. [CrossRef] [PubMed]

11. Monasta, L.; Batty, G.; Cattaneo, A.; Lutje, V.; Ronfani, L.; Van Lenthe, F.; Brug, J. Early-life determinants of overweigth and obesity: A review of systematic reviews. *Obes. Rev.* **2010**, *11*, 695–708. [CrossRef] [PubMed]

12. Ogata, B.; Hayes, D. Position of the Academy of Nutrition and Dietetics: Nutrition guidance for healthy children ages 2 to 11 years. *J. Acad. Nutr. Diet.* **2014**, *114*, 1257–1276. [CrossRef] [PubMed]

13. Birch, L.; Davison, K. Family environmental factors influencing the developing behavioral controls of food intake and childhood overweight. *Pediatr. Clin. N. Am.* **2001**, *48*, 893–907. [CrossRef]

14. Brustad, R. Attraction to physical activity in urban schoolchildren: Parental socialization and gender influences. *Res. Q. Exerc. Sport* **1996**, *67*, 316–323. [CrossRef] [PubMed]

15. Demsey, J.; Kimiecik, J.; Horn, T. Parental influence on children's moderate to vigorous physical activity participation: An expectancy-value approach. *Pediatr. Exerc.* **1993**, *5*, 151–167. [CrossRef]

16. Gruber, K.; Haldeman, L. Using the family to combat childhood and adult obesity. *Prev. Chronic Dis.* **2009**, *6*, A106. [PubMed]

17. Lau, R.; Quadrell, J.; Hartman, K. Development and change of young adults' preventive health beliefs and behavior: Influence from parents and peers. *J. Health Soc. Behav.* **1990**, *31*, 240–259. [CrossRef] [PubMed]

18. Patterson, T.; Sallis, J.; Nader, P.; Kaplan, R.; Rupp, J. Familial similarities of changes in cognitive, behavioral and physiological variables in a cardiovascular health promotion program. *J. Pediatr. Psychol.* **1989**, *14*, 277–292. [CrossRef] [PubMed]

19. Sahay, T.; Ashbury, F.; Roberts, M.; Rootman, I. Effective components for nutrition interventions: A review and application of the literature. *Health Promot. Pract.* **2006**, *7*, 418–427. [CrossRef] [PubMed]

20. Skouteris, H.; McCabe, M.; Winburn, B.; Newbreen, V.; Sacher, P.; Chadwick, P. Parental influence and obesity prefention in pre-schoolers: A systematic review of interventions. *Obes. Rev.* **2011**, *12*, 315–328. [CrossRef] [PubMed]

21. Wyse, R.; Campbell, E.; Nathan, N.; Wolfenden, L. Associations between characteristics of the home food environment and fruit and vegetable intake in preschool children: A cross-sectional study. *BMC Public Health* **2011**, *11*, 938. [CrossRef] [PubMed]

22. Spurrier, N.; Magarey, A.; Golley, R.; Curnow, F.; Sawyer, M. Relationships between the home environment and physical activity and dietary patterns of preschool children: A cross-sectional study. *Int. J. Behav. Nutr. Phys. Act.* **2008**, *5*, 31. [CrossRef] [PubMed]

23. Whitaker, R.; Wright, J.; Pepe, M.; Seidel, K.; Dietz, W. Predicting obesity in young adulthood from childhood and parental obesity. *N. Engl. J. Med.* **1997**, *337*, 869–873. [CrossRef] [PubMed]

24. Trost, S.; Sirard, J.; Dowda, M.; Pfeiffer, K.; Pate, R. Physical activity in overwegith and nonoverweight preschool children. *Int. J. Obes. Relat. Metab. Disord.* **2003**, *27*, 834–839. [CrossRef] [PubMed]

25. Anderson, S.; Whitaker, R. Household routines and obesity in US preschool-aged children. *Pediatrics* **2010**, *125*, 420–428. [CrossRef] [PubMed]

26. Rolls, B.; Ello-Martin, J.; Tohill, B. What can intervention studies tell us about the relationship between fruit and vegetable consumption and weight management. *Nutr. Rev.* **2004**, *62*, 1–17. [CrossRef] [PubMed]

27. He, M.; Piche, L.; Harris, S. Screen-related sedentary behaviors: children's and parents' attitudes, motivations, and practices. *J. Nutr. Educ. Behav.* **2010**, *42*, 17–25. [CrossRef] [PubMed]

28. Glanz, K. Measuring food environments: A historical perspective. *Am. J. Prev. Med.* **2009**, *36*, S93–S98. [CrossRef] [PubMed]

29. Pinard, C.; Yaroch, A.; Hart, M.; Serrano, E.; McFerre, M.; Estabrooks, P. Measures of the home environment related to childhood obesity: A systematic review. *Public Health Nutr.* **2012**, *15*, 97–109. [CrossRef] [PubMed]

30. Martin-Biggers, J.; Beluska, K.; Quick, V.M.; Byrd-Bredbenner, C. Cover Lines Using Positive, Urgent, Unique language Entice Moms to Read Health Communications. *J. Health Commun.* **2015**, *20*, 766–772. [CrossRef] [PubMed]

31. Martin-Biggers, J.; Spaccarotella, K.; Delaney, C.; Koenings, M.; Alleman, G.; Hongu, N.; Worobey, J.; Byrd-Bredbenner, C. Development of the intervention materials for the homestyles childhood obesity prevention program for parents of preschoolers. *Nutrients* **2015**, *7*, 6628–6669. [CrossRef] [PubMed]

32. Martin-Biggers, J.; Spaccarotella, K.; Hongu, N.; Worobey, J.; Byrd-Bredbenner, C. Translating it into real life: Cognitions, barriers and supports for key weight-related behaviors of parents of preschoolers. *BMC Public Health* **2015**, *15*, 189. [CrossRef] [PubMed]

33. Delaney, C.; Barrios, P.; Lozada, C.; Soto-Balbuena, K.; Martin-Biggers, J.; Byrd-Bredbenner, C. Applying common Latino magazine cover line themes to health communication. *Hisp. J. Behav. Sci.* **2016**, *38*, 546–558. [CrossRef]

34. Byrd-Bredbenner, C.; Martin-Biggers, J.; Koenings, M.; Quick, V.; Hongu, K.; Worobey, J. Homestyles, A web-based childhood obesity prevention program for families with preschool children: Protocol for a randomized controlled trial. *JMIR Res. Protoc.* **2017**, *6*, e73. [CrossRef] [PubMed]

35. Martin-Biggers, J.; Cheng, C.; Spaccarotella, K.; Byrd-Bredbenner, C. The Physical Activity Environment in Homes and Neighborhoods. In *Recent Advances in Obesity in Children*; Avid Science Publications: Berlin, Germany, 2016. Available online: www.avidscience.com/wp-content/uploads/2016/05/OIC-15-04_May-06-2016.pdf (accessed on 10 April 2017).

36. Byrd-Bredbenner, C.; Maurer Abbot, J. Food choice influencers of mothers of young children: Implications for nutrition educators. *Top. Clin. Nutr.* **2008**, *25*, 198–215. [CrossRef]

37. Hartley, J.; Levin, K.; Currie, C. A new version of the HBSC Family Affluence Scale—FAS III: Scottish qualitative findings from the international FAS developments study. *Child Indicat. Res.* **2016**, *9*, 233–245. [CrossRef] [PubMed]

38. Currie, C.; Mollcho, M.; Boyce, W.; Holstein, B.; Torsheim, T.; Richter, M. Researching health inequalities in adolescents: The development of the health behavior in school-aged children (HBSC) family affluence scale. *Soc. Sci. Med.* **2008**, *66*, 1429–1436. [CrossRef] [PubMed]

39. Centers for Disease Control and Prevention. HRQOL Concepts. Why Is Quality of Life Important? Available online: www.cdc.gov/hrqol/concept.htm (accessed on 9 May 2016).

40. Centers for Disease Control and Prevention. HRQOL-14 Healthy Days Measure. Available online: www.cdc.gov/hrqol/hrqol14_measure.htm (accessed on 9 May 2016).

41. Matheny, A.; Wachs, T.; Ludwig, J.; Phillips, K. Bringing order out of chaos: Psychometric characteristics of the confusion, hubbub, and order scale. *J. Appl. Dev. Psychol.* **1995**, *16*, 429–444. [CrossRef]

42. Cacioppo, J.; Petty, R. The need for cognition. *J. Personal. Soc. Psychol.* **1982**, *42*, 116–131. [CrossRef]

43. Cacioppo, J.; Petty, R.; Kao, C.F. The efficient assessment of need for cognition. *J. Personal. Assess.* **1984**, *48*, 306–307. [CrossRef] [PubMed]

44. Cohen, S.; Kamarck, T.; Mermelstein, R. A global measure of perceived stress. *J. Health Soc. Behav.* **1983**, *24*, 385–396. [CrossRef] [PubMed]

45. Wakimoto, P.; Block, G.; Mandel, S.; Medina, N. Development and reliability of brief dietary assessment tools for Hispanics. *Perv. Chronic Dis.* **2006**, *3*, A95.

46. Nelson, M.; Lytle, L. Development and evaluation of a brief screener to estimate fast-food and beverage consumption among adolescents. *J. Am. Diet. Assoc.* **2009**, *109*, 730–734. [CrossRef] [PubMed]

47. Block, G.; Gillespie, C.; Rosenbaum, E.H.; Jenson, C. A rapid food screener to assess fat and fruit and vegetable intake. *Am. J. Prev. Med.* **2000**, *18*, 284–288. [CrossRef]

48. Block, G.; Hartman, A.; Naughton, D. A reduced dietary questionnaire: Development and validation. *Epidemiology* **1990**, *1*, 58–64. [CrossRef] [PubMed]

49. Block, G.; Thompson, F.; Hartman, A.; Larkin, F.; Guire, K. Comparison of two dietary questionnaires validated against multiple dietary records collected during a 1-year period. *J. Am. Diet Assoc.* **1992**, *92*, 686–693. [PubMed]

50. West, D.; Bursac, Z.; Quimby, D.; Prewit, T.; Spatz, T.; Nash, C.; Mays, G.; Eddings, K. Self-reported sugar-sweetened beverage intake among college students. *Obesity* **2006**, *14*, 1825–1831. [CrossRef] [PubMed]

51. Quick, V.; Byrd-Bredbenner, C.; Shoff, S.; White, A.; Lohse, B.; Horacek, T.; Kattlemann, K.; Phillips, B.; Hoerr, S.; Greene, G. A streamlined, enhanced self-report physical activity measure for young adults. *Int. J. Health Promot. Educ.* **2016**, *54*, 245–254. [CrossRef]

52. Lee, P.; Macfarlane, D.; Lam, T.; Stewart, S. Validity of the international physical activity questionnaire short form (IPAQ-SF): A systematic review. *Int. J. Behav. Nutr. Phys. Act.* **2011**, *8*, 115. [CrossRef] [PubMed]

53. Craig, C.; Marshall, A.; Sjostrom, M.; Bauman, A.E.; Booth, M.L.; Ainsworth, B.E.; Pratt, M.; Ekelund, U.; Yngve, A.; Sallis, J.F.; et al. International Physical Activity Questionnaire: 12-country reliability and validity. *Med. Sci. Sport Exerc.* **2003**, *35*, 1381–1395. [CrossRef] [PubMed]

54. Bryant, M.; Ward, D.; Hales, D.; Vaughn, A.; Tabak, R.; Stevens, J. Reliability and validity of the Healthy Home Survey: A tool to measure factors within homes hypothesized to relate to overweight in children. *Int. J. Behav. Nutr. Phys. Act.* **2008**, *5*, 23. [CrossRef] [PubMed]

55. Gattshall, M.; Shoup, J.; Marshall, J.; Crane, L.; Estabrooks, P. Validation of a survey instrument to assess home environments for physical activity and healthy eating in overweight children. *Int. J. Behav. Nutr. Phys. Act.* **2008**, *5*, 3. [CrossRef] [PubMed]

56. Owen, N.; Sugiyama, T.; Eakin, E.; Gardiner, P.; Tremblay, M.; Sallis, J. Adults' sedentary behavior determinants and interventions. *Am. J. Prev. Med.* **2011**, *41*, 189–196. [CrossRef] [PubMed]

57. Buysse, D.; Reynolds, C.; Monk, T.; Berman, S.; Kupfer, D. The Pittsburgh Sleep Quality Index: A new instrument for psychiatric practice and research. *Psychiatry Res.* **1989**, *28*, 193–213. [CrossRef]

58. Carpenter, J.; Andrykowski, M. Psychometric evaluation of the Pittsburgh Sleep Quality Index. *J. Psychosom. Res.* **1998**, *45*, 5–13. [CrossRef]

59. Coldwell, J.; Pike, A.; Dunn, J. Household chaos—Links with parenting and child behaviour. *J. Child Psychol. Psychiatry* **2006**, *47*, 1116–1122. [CrossRef] [PubMed]

60. Moos, R.; Moos, B. *Family Environment Scale Manual: Development, Applications, Research*, 3rd ed.; Consulting Psychologists Press: Palo Alto, CA, USA, 1994.

61. Koszewski, W.; Behrends, D.; Nichols, M.; Sehi, N.; Jones, G. Patterns of family meals and food and nutrition intake in limited resource families. *Fam. Consum. Sci. Res. J.* **2011**, *39*, 431–441. [CrossRef]

62. Neumark-Sztainer, D.; Story, M.; Hannan, P.; Moe, J. Overweight status and eating patterns among adolescents: Where do youths stand in comparison to the Healthy People 2010 Objectives? *Am. J. Public Health* **2002**, *92*, 844–851. [CrossRef] [PubMed]

63. Neumark-Sztainer, D.; Wall, M.M.; Story, M.; Perry, C.L. Correlates of unhealthy weight-control behaviors among adolescents: Implications for prevention programs. *Health Psychol.* **2003**, *22*, 88–98. [CrossRef] [PubMed]

64. Neumark-Sztainer, D.; Story, M.; Hannan, P.; Perry, C.; Irving, L. Weight-Related Concerns and Behaviors Among Overweight and Nonoverweight Adolescents Implications for Preventing Weight-Related Disorders. *Arch. Pediatr. Adolesc. Med.* **2002**, *156*, 171–178. [CrossRef] [PubMed]

65. Neumark-Sztainer, D.; Larson, N.; Fulkerson, J.; Eisenberg, M.; Story, M. Family meals and adolescents: What have we learned from Project EAT (Eating Among Teens)? *Public Health Nutr.* **2010**, *13*, 1113–1121. [CrossRef] [PubMed]

66. Byrd-Bredbenner, C.; Maurer Abbot, J.; Cussler, E. Relationship of social cognitive theory concepts to mothers' dietary intake and BMI. *Matern. Child Nutr.* **2011**, *7*, 241–252. [CrossRef] [PubMed]

67. Kiernan, M.; Moore, S.; Schoffman, D.; Lee, K.; King, A.; Taylor, C.; Kiernan, N.; Perri, M. Social support for healthy behavior: Scale psychometrics and prediction of weight loss among women in a behavioral program. *Obesity* **2012**, *20*, 756–764. [CrossRef] [PubMed]

68. Ball, K.; Crawford, D. An investigation of psychological, social and environmental correlates of obesity and weight gain in young women. *Int. J. Obes.* **2006**, *30*, 1240–1249. [CrossRef] [PubMed]

69. Wardle, J.; Sanderson, S.; Guthrie, C.A.; Rapoport, L.; Plomin, R. Parental feeding style and the inter-generational transmission of obesity risk. *Obes. Res.* **2002**, *10*, 453–462. [CrossRef] [PubMed]

70. Ogden, J.; Reynolds, R.; Smith, A. Expanding the concept of parental control: A role for overt and covert control in children's snacking behaviour? *Appetite* **2006**, *47*, 100–106. [CrossRef] [PubMed]

71. Earls, F.; Brooks-Gunn, J.; Raudenbush, S.; Sampson, R. *Project on Human Development in Chicago Neighborhoods (PHDCN): Home and Life Interview, Wave 2, 1997–2000*; Instruments for ICPSR 13630; Inter-University Consortium for Political and Social Research: Ann Arbor, MI, USA, 2005.

72. Sallis, J.F.; Prochaska, J.J.; Taylor, W.C.; Hill, J.O.; Geraci, J.C. Correlates of physical activity in a national sample of girls and boys in Grades 4 through 12. *Health Psychol.* **1999**, *18*, 410–415. [CrossRef] [PubMed]

73. Trost, S.G.; Sallis, J.F.; Pate, R.R.; Freedson, P.S.; Taylor, W.C.; Dowda, M. Evaluating a model of parental influence on youth physical activity. *Am. J. Prev. Med.* **2003**, *25*, 277–282. [CrossRef]

74. AbuSabha, R.; Achterberg, C. Review of self-efficacy and locus of control for nutrition- and health-related behavior. *J. Am. Diet. Assoc.* **1997**, *97*, 1122–1132. [CrossRef]

75. Martin-Biggers, J.; Koenings, M.; Quick, V.; Abbot, J.; Byrd-Bredbenner, C. Appraising nutrient availability of household food supplies using Block dietary screeners for individuals. *Eur. Clin. Nutr.* **2015**, *69*, 1028–1034. [CrossRef] [PubMed]

76. Hunsberger, M.; O'Malley, J.; Block, T.; Norris, J. Relative validation of Block Kids Food Screener for dietary assessment in children and adolescents. *Matern. Child Nutr.* **2012**, *11*, 260–270. [CrossRef] [PubMed]

77. Cheng, C.; Martin-Biggers, J.; Quick, V.; Spaccarotella, K.; Byrd-Bredbenner, C. Validity and reliability of HOP-Up: A questionnaire to evaluate physical activity environments in homes with preschool-aged children. *Int. J. Behav. Nutr. Phys. Act.* **2016**, *13*, 91. [CrossRef] [PubMed]

78. Lapierre, M.; Piotrowski, J.; Linebarger, D. Background television in the homes of US children. *Pediatrics* **2012**, *130*, 839–846. [CrossRef] [PubMed]

79. Block, G.; Clifford, C.; Naughton, M.; Henderson, M.; McAdams, M. A brief dietary screen for high fat intake. *J. Nutr. Educ.* **1989**, *21*, 199–207. [CrossRef]

80. United States Department of Agriculture. ChooseMyPlate.gov. Available online: https://www.choosemyplate.gov/ (accessed on 9 February 2017).

81. American Academy of Pediatrics Committee on Nutrition, Policy statement: The use and misuse of fruit juices in pediatrics. *Pediatrics* **2006**, *107*, 1210–1213.

82. Lasater, G.; Piernas, C.; Popkin, B. Beverage patterns and trends among school-aged children in the US, 1989–2008. *Nutr. J.* **2011**, *10*, 103. [CrossRef] [PubMed]

83. Committee to Review Dietary Reference Intakes for Vitamin D and Calcium; Food and Nutrition Board; Institute of Medicine; National Academy of Sciences. *Dietary Reference Intakes for Calcium and Vitamin D*; National Academies Press: Washington, DC, USA, 2011.

84. Food and Nutrition Board; Institute of Medicine; National Academy of Sciences. *Dietary Reference Intakes for Energy, Carbohydrate. Fiber, Fat, Fatty Acids, Cholesterol, Protein, and Amino Acids*; National Academies Press: Washington, DC, USA, 2005.

85. U.S. Department of Health and Human Services; Centers for Disease Control and Prevention; National Center for Health Statistics. *Health, United States, 2015 with Special Feature on Racial and Ethnic Health Disparities*; U.S. Government Printing Office: Hyattsville, MD, USA, 2015.

86. Council on Communications and Media; American Academy of Pediatrics. Media and young minds. *Pediatrics* **2016**, *138*, e20162591.

87. Golem, D.; Martin-Biggers, J.; Koenings, M.; Finn Davis, K.; Byrd-Bredbenner, C. An integrative review of sleep for nutrition professionals. *Adv. Nutr.* **2014**, *5*, 742–759. [CrossRef] [PubMed]

88. Hiscock, H.; Scalzo, K.; Canterford, L.; Wake, M. Sleep duration and body mass index in 0–7-year old. *Arch. Dis. Child.* **2011**, *96*, 735–739. [CrossRef] [PubMed]

89. Bell, J.F.; Zimmerman, F.J. Shortened nighttime sleep duration in early life and subsequent childhood obesity. *Arch. Pediatr. Adolesc. Med.* **2010**, *164*, 840–845. [CrossRef] [PubMed]

90. Taveras, E.; Rifas-Shiman, S.; Oken, E.; Gunderson, E.; Gillman, M. Short Sleep Duration in Infancy and Risk of Childhood Overweight. *Arch. Pediatr. Adolesc. Med.* **2008**, *165*, 305–311. [CrossRef] [PubMed]

91. Cappuccio, F.P.; Taggart, F.M.; Ngianga-Bakwin, K.; Currie, A.; Peile, E.; Stranges, S.; Miller, M.A. Meta-analysis of short sleep duration and obesity in children and adults. *Sleep* **2008**, *31*, 619–626. [CrossRef] [PubMed]

92. Chaput, J.-P.; Brunet, M.; Tremblay, A. Relationship between short sleeping hours and childhood overweight/obesity: Results from the 'Québec en Forme' Project. *Int. J. Obes.* **2006**, *30*, 1080–1085. [CrossRef] [PubMed]

93. Hirshkowitz, M.; Whiton, K.; Albert, S.; Alessi, C.; Bruni, O.; DonCarlos, L.; Hazen, N.; Herman, J.; Hillard, P.; Katz, E.; et al. National Sleep Foundation updated sleep duration recommendations: Final report. *Sleep Health* **2015**, *1*, 233–243. [CrossRef]

94. National Sleep Foundation. *International Bedroom Poll: Summary of Findings*; National Sleep Foundation: Arlington, VA, USA, 2013.
95. Burnier, D.; Dubois, L.; Girard, M. Arguments at mealtime and child energy intake. *J. Nutr. Educ. Behav.* **2011**, *43*, 473–481. [CrossRef] [PubMed]
96. Neumark-Sztainer, D.; Hannan, P.J.; Story, M.; Croll, J.; Perry, C. Family meal patterns: Associations with sociodemographic characteristics and improved dietary intake among adolescents. *J. Am. Diet Assoc.* **2003**, *103*, 317–322. [CrossRef] [PubMed]
97. Ayala, G.; Baquero, B.; Arrendondo, E.; Campbell, N.; Larios, M.; Elder, J. Association between family variables and Mexican American children's dietary behaviors. *J. Nutr. Educ. Behav.* **2007**, *39*, 62–69. [CrossRef] [PubMed]
98. Gillman, M.; Rifas-Shiman, S.; Frazier, L.; Rockett, H.; Camargo, C.; Field, A.; Berkey, C.; Colditz, G. Family dinner and diet quality among older children and adolescents. *Arch. Fam. Med.* **2000**, *9*, 235–240. [CrossRef] [PubMed]
99. Guthrie, J.; Lin, B.; Frazao, E. Role of food prepared away from home in the American diet, 1977–78 versus 1994–96: Changes and consequences. *J. Nutr. Educ. Behav.* **2002**, *34*, 140–150. [CrossRef]
100. Boutelle, K.; Fulkerson, J.; Neumark-Sztainer, D.; Story, M.; French, S. Fast food for family meals: Relationships with parent and adolescent food intake, home food availability, and weight status. *Public Health Nutr.* **2007**, *10*, 16–23. [CrossRef] [PubMed]
101. McIntosh, W.; Kubena, K.; Tolle, G.; Dean, W.; Jan, J.; Anding, J. Mothers and meals. The effects of mothers. meal planning and shopping motivations on children's participation in family meals. *Appetite* **2010**, *55*, 623–628. [CrossRef] [PubMed]
102. Anderson, S.; Must, A.; Curtin, C.; Bandini, L. Meals in our household: Reliability and initial validation of a questionnaire to assess child mealtime behaviors and family mealtime environments. *J. Acad. Nutr. Diet* **2012**, *112*, 276–284. [CrossRef] [PubMed]
103. Bandura, A. *Social Learning Theory*; Prentice-Hall: Englewood Cliffs, NJ, USA, 1977.
104. Kelder, S.; Hoelscher, D.; Perry, C. How individuals, environments, and health behavior interact; Social Cognitive Theory. In *Health Behavior and Health Education. Theory, Research, and Practice*, 4th ed.; Glanz, K., Rimer, B., Viswanath, K., Eds.; Jossey-Bass: San Francisco, CA, USA, 2015.
105. Montano, D.; Kasprzyk, D. Theory of reasoned action, theory of planned behavior, and the integrated behavioral model. In *Health Behavior and Health Education. Theory, Research, and Practice*, 4th ed.; Glanz, K., Rimer, B., Viswanath, K., Eds.; Jossey-Bass: San Francisco, CA, USA, 2015.
106. Bandura, A. *Self-Efficacy: The Exercise of Control*; W.H. Freeman: New York, NY, USA, 1997.

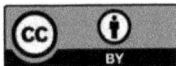

nutrients

MDPI

Review

Preschool and School Meal Policies: An Overview of What We Know about Regulation, Implementation, and Impact on Diet in the UK, Sweden, and Australia

Patricia Jane Lucas [1,*], Emma Patterson [2,3], Gary Sacks [4], Natassja Billich [4] and Charlotte Elizabeth Louise Evans [5]

[1] School for Policy Studies, University of Bristol, Bristol BS8 1TZ, UK
[2] Department of Public Health Sciences, Karolinska Institutet, SE-171 77 Stockholm, Sweden;
     Emma.Patterson@ki.se
[3] Centre for Epidemiology and Community Medicine, Stockholm County Council,
     SE-113 65 Stockholm, Sweden
[4] Global Obesity Centre, School of Health and Social Development, Deakin University,
     Geelong VIC 3220, Australia; gary.sacks@deakin.edu.au (G.S.); natassja.billich@deakin.edu.au (N.B.)
[5] Nutritional Epidemiology Group, School of Food Science and Nutrition, University of Leeds,
     Leeds LS2 9JT, UK; C.E.L.Evans@leeds.ac.uk
* Correspondence: patricia.lucas@bristol.ac.uk; Tel.: +44-117-331-0866

Received: 22 April 2017; Accepted: 3 July 2017; Published: 11 July 2017

Abstract: School meals make significant contributions to healthy dietary behaviour, at a time when eating habits and food preferences are being formed. We provide an overview of the approaches to the provision, regulation, and improvement of preschool and primary school meals in the UK, Sweden, and Australia, three countries which vary in their degree of centralisation and regulation of school meals. Sweden has a centralised approach; all children receive free meals, and a pedagogical approach to meals is encouraged. Legislation demands that meals are nutritious. The UK system is varied and decentralised. Meals in most primary schools are regulated by food-based standards, but preschool-specific meal standards only exist in Scotland. The UK uses food groups (starchy foods, fruit and vegetables, proteins and dairy) in a healthy plate approach. Australian States and Territories all employ guidelines for school canteen food, predominantly using a "traffic light" approach outlining recommended and discouraged foods; however, most children bring food from home and are not covered by this guidance. The preschool standards state that food provided should be nutritious. We find that action is often lacking in the preschool years, and suggest that consistent policies, strong incentives for compliance, systematic monitoring, and an acknowledgement of the broader school eating environment (including home provided food) would be beneficial.

Keywords: school; preshool; children; school meals; nutrition intake; policy

---

1. Introduction

1.1. Background and Aims

There is increasing interest in policies aimed at establishing schools and Early Education and Care (EEC) as health promoting environments [1], including health education within the school curriculum, and schools as a site for healthy eating [2]. Food eaten in education and care settings makes a significant contribution to children's total diet. Some have even suggested that a failure to provide healthy foods in schools is a breach of children's human rights [3]. Policy, guidance, and regulation in this field has considerable potential to impact on the dietary intake of young children [4].

This paper aims to compare the school meal policies in preschool and primary educational settings in three high-income country contexts: UK, Australia, and Sweden. These were selected to illustrate the variation in OECD countries in approaches to regulation and standard setting at the regional and national level, from entirely centralised (Sweden) to entirely federal (Australia), and from highly standardised (Sweden) to highly varied (UK). We provide an overview [5] of policy and research in the field. Policy documents and regulatory tools do not lend themselves to systematic approaches, and require expert knowledge to locate the associated (grey) literature. We used our local policy knowledge to locate much of the literature included here. In addition, we searched Medline for studies published within the last 10 years in each of our target countries, with search terms for school food/meals and evaluations (the search terms are available from the corresponding author on request). The UK government is unusual in providing a searchable database of policy and government publications, and we reviewed the latest relevant policy documents using the search terms "school meals" and "school food".

We asked: what is the current policy in each country, how many children does it reach, what do we know about how it is implemented, and what evidence exists for the impact of this approach on children's health? We focus here on policy interventions at the national or regional level, not on research or pilot programmes.

1.2. School Food as a Public Health Nutrition Intervention

The diet of preschool and primary children in all three countries leaves room for improvement, with higher than recommended intakes of sugar and saturated fats [6,7], and lower intakes of fruits and vegetables [8]. Moreover, there are stark inequalities with respect to dietary quality, with lower income families reporting poorer diets [6,9–12].

The provision of meals during school hours has a long history as a public health measure [2,13]. Patterns of school food consumption mirror total diet, suggesting both that dietary choices are consistent and that school is an important eating occasion in terms of total intake [14,15]. The contribution of weekday meals for school children is approximately 30% of daily intake in both the UK [16] and Sweden [17]. There is very limited data to comment on the total contribution to diet from meals consumed in preschool [13,18].

Good quality school meals have the potential to improve children's diets and health. The availability of healthy nutritious choices influences diet positively in school children [19]. The provision of fruit and vegetables to children in schools increases their fruit and vegetable consumption [20], and has been shown to level family differences in fruit and vegetable intakes among 11-year-old children [21]. Changes to school cafeteria environments can improve food choices at school [22]. In the earliest years, the behaviour of childcare workers themselves has a positive impact on preschool children's intake of fruit and vegetables [23].

Health promoting schools successfully provide health education and a healthier environment for school aged children across the world [1,24,25]. Health education is an important part of the curriculum in both the primary and preschool years, and in both the UK and Sweden EEC settings are tasked to help children understand their own health choices [26,27].

1.3. Country Contexts

The UK has a total population of 64 million, of whom 18% are aged less than 15; 19% of Australia's population of 24 million are children, and 17% of the 10 million people in Sweden are children [28].

Sweden is a Nordic European nation with a well-developed welfare system and relatively high taxes. Legislation is made centrally, but the 290 local authorities are responsible for the delivery of many services, including education. Preschool care/education for 1–5 year-olds is heavily subsidized (free for many or capped at ~€150 per child per month, even when privately run), and over 90% of children attend, often from 18 months of age. Primary school education covers the ages six to fifteen, is free (even when privately run), and parents incur no charges for education-related expenses, including meals.

The UK is a Western European nation. It has three devolved regions: Scotland, Wales, and Northern Ireland. National policy always applies to England, but applies to different degrees in each devolved region. Children aged 3–4 years in all regions are entitled to 15 h/week in EEC (due to rise to 30 h/week in England in September 2017); parents decide where to spend this provision from within public, private, or voluntary sector settings [29]. In England, Northern Ireland, and Scotland 2 years old in the greatest need (including those living in poverty and those with disabilities) receive the same allocation [29–31]. The government pays a flat rate of £55/week, which is not intended to cover food or other additional costs. Primary education is compulsory for 5–11 years old, but most children begin school aged 4 years. Primary schools may be state funded and maintained, state funded but independently run (academies, free, and church schools), or privately funded and run.

Australia is a Federation of States and Territories (New South Wales, Victoria, South Australia, Western Australia, Queensland, Tasmania, Australian Capital Territory, and Northern Territory). Education in Australia is primarily the responsibility of the states and territories. Early childhood education in Australia is not compulsory and is delivered to children through a range of settings, including childcare centres, kindergartens, and preschools in the year before full-time schooling (age 5 or 6). The Australian Government pays part of the cost of some childcare through the social security system. Compulsory education in Australia starts at around the age of five or six years. Government schools educate approximately 60% of Australian primary school students, with approximately 40% in either private or independent (including Catholic) schools.

Since policy follows organisational structures, not chronological age, we adopt the educational stage cut offs of preschool and primary school in this paper. Thus, for example, 5-year-olds attend school in England but preschool in Sweden. It is important to remember these age differences when comparing between countries. Countries apply adequacy requirements (Table 1) and limits (Table 2), which vary in their regulation, reach, cost to families, and systems of monitoring (Table 3).

Table 1. School food adequacy standards in the UK, Australia, and Sweden.

Food	Standard or Guidance	Level, Country (Jurisdiction)
Fruit and vegetables	Minimum number portions per day/meal	School and Preschool, UK (England, Scotland)
Meat, fish, eggs, and non-dairy protein		
Starchy foods	Recommended number of portions per day	School and Preschool, UK (England, Scotland)
Milk and dairy		
Drinks	Fresh water to be freely available	School and Preschool, UK (England, Scotland)
	Diluted fruit juice or fresh cows' milks	Preschool, UK (England, Scotland)
Traffic Light: "Green" foods	Minimum of 60% of food and snacks sold should be "Green"	School, Australia (WA *)
	Should be available every day the canteen is open	School, Australia (NT, SA, Q, V *)
Every-day (Core) foods	Recommended to make up 75% of food and drinks sold	School, Australia (NSW *)
"Nutritious" meals	Meals must be "nutritious". Preschool meals must also be "varied", and "evenly distributed over the day"	School and Preschool, Sweden
"Good meals in preschool"	Suggestions provided for meal components and nutritional content (e.g., serve fatty fish twice within 4 weeks, serve only milk and water to drink, provide a wide selection of salads, include wholegrain versions of products etc.)	School and Preschool, Sweden
"Good school meals"		

* Northern Territory (NT); South Australia (SA); Queensland (Q); Victoria (V); New South Wales (NSW); Western Australia (WA).

Table 2. School food limiting standards in the UK, Australia, and Sweden.

Food	Standard or Guidance	Level, Country (Jurisdiction)
Meat, fish, eggs, and non-dairy protein	Maximum number portions	School, UK (England), Preschool UK (Scotland)
Starchy foods	Maximum number of occasions higher fat versions offered (fried starchy foods and cheese as protein)	School, UK (England)
Milk and dairy food		
Traffic Light: "Amber" foods	Maximum of 40% of foods and drinks sold should be "Amber"	School, Australia (WA *)
	"Amber" foods should be limited and sold in smaller serve sizes	School, Australia (NT, SA, Q, V *)
Desserts & Puddings	To be served only once per day with main meal	School and Preschool UK (England, Scotland)
Occasional (non-core) foods	Maximum of 25% of food and drinks sold should be "occasional" and least healthy not sold	School, Australia (NSW *)

Table 2. *Cont.*

Food	Standard or Guidance	Level, Country (Jurisdiction)
Foods high in fat, salt, and sugar	Avoided or limited	School and Preschool, UK (England, Scotland)
Traffic Light: "Red" foods	"Red" foods prohibited or limited to special occasions (no more than twice per term)	School, Australia (NT, SA, Q, V*)
	"Red" foods prohibited	School, Australia (NT, SA, Q, V*)
Salt and condiments	Reduced or not salt in cooking. No salt available to add. Condiments avoided or size limited.	School and Preschool, UK (England, Scotland)
	Should not be available to students	School and Preschool, Sweden
Drinks	All those not specified to be excluded	School and Preschool, UK (England, Scotland)
	"Amber" drinks should be avoided and sold in smaller serve sizes	School, Australia (NT, SA, Q, V*)
	"Red" drinks (sugary) not to be sold and not permitted	School, Australia (all states and territories)
	No sweet drinks containing sugar or sweetener	School and Preschool, Sweden
Confectionary	Not permitted	School and Preschool, UK (England, Scotland)
	Not permitted	School, Australia (all states and territories)
	Should not be provided	School and Preschool, Sweden

* Northern Territory (NT); South Australia (SA); Queensland (Q); Victoria (V); New South Wales (NSW); Western Australia (WA).

Nutrients **2017**, *9*, 736

Table 3. School food policy regulation and monitoring in the UK, Sweden, and Australia. Abbreviation: EEC, early education and care.

Policy	Country (Jurisdiction)	Level	Reach	Cost to Families	System of Monitoring
Food Based Standards for Schools in England	UK (England)	School	Mandatory for local government controlled schools and schools that became academies before 2010 and after June 2014. Recommended for remaining academies and private schools.	Free for 4–7 years Paid for other years	Included in the Office of Standards in Education (OFSTED) inspection report on healthy eating.
Voluntary Guidance	UK (England)	Preschool	Voluntary	Paid	Not monitored in OFSTED inspections, although the Early Years Foundation Stage (EYFS) requires that provided food must be "healthy balanced and nutritious" (EYFS 2017).
Preschool standards	UK (Scotland)	Preschool	Mandatory for all settings registered with the Care Inspectorate.	Paid	Inspected by the Care Inspectorate. EEC must show they provide opportunities for children to learn about diet and health. EEC must show children have access to a well-balanced and healthy diet. For example, through use of a food policy.

Table 3. *Cont.*

Policy	Country (Jurisdiction)	Level	Reach	Cost to Families	System of Monitoring
Traffic light food groups	Australia (Australia Capital Territory)	School	Policy applies to all food services activities within a school setting. Mandatory for government schools. In independent and Catholic schools, it is not mandatory but highly recommended.	Paid	Independent compliance monitoring. Free assessment, resources and training available for canteens. Facilitate government license agreements with school canteens.
	Australia (Northern Territory)	School	Policy applies to all food services activities within a school setting. Mandatory for government schools	Paid	Independent compliance monitoring, schools responsible for oversight.
	Australia (South Australia)	School	Policy applies to all food services activities within a school setting. Mandatory for government schools. Catholic and independent school sectors support implementation of the policy.	Paid	Independent compliance monitoring, schools responsible for oversight. Resources provided to canteens.
	Australia (Queensland)	School	Policy applies to all food services activities within a school setting. Mandatory for government schools.	Paid	Independent compliance monitoring, schools responsible for oversight. Training and resources provided to canteens.
	Australia (Tasmania)	School	Schools are recommended (not mandatory) to apply to have their canteen accredited.	Paid	Training, resources and monitoring available to canteens.
	Australia (Victoria)	School	Policy applies to all food services activities within a school setting. Mandatory for government schools.	Paid	Independent compliance monitoring, schools responsible for oversight. Optional monitoring and assessment of canteens available. Training and resources provided to canteens.
Every-day vs. occasional foods	Australia (New South Wales)	School	Policy applies to all food services activities within a school setting. Mandatory for government schools. Catholic and independent schools are also encouraged to participate.	Paid	Independent compliance monitoring, schools responsible for oversight. Resources provided to canteens.
Traffic light and core vs. non-core foods	Australia (Western Australia)	School	Policy applies to all food services activities within a school setting. Mandatory for government schools. Catholic schools have a similar mandatory policy.	Paid	Principals are required to develop and implement a whole school-based policy on the provision of healthy food and drinks and ensure that the school canteen/food service menu complies with the requirements of the policy.
Nutritious preschool meals	Sweden	Preschool	Legislation. Mandatory for all (whether local authority or privately run).	Free or subsidized *	Monitoring of provision and cost is not required. Monitoring of nutritional quality falls to the management (i.e., the local authority or owner).
Nutritious school meals	Sweden	School	Legislation. Mandatory for all (whether local authority or privately run).	Free	Monitoring of provision and cost is not required. Monitoring of nutritional quality falls under the School Inspectorate, but is delegated to the school management (i.e., the local authority or owner).
"Good meals in preschool", "Good school meals"	Sweden	Preschool, School	Guidelines. Voluntary for all.	Free or subsidized *	Not applicable, but for schools, compliance with several of the guidelines can be demonstrated using "School Food Sweden" tool.

* Some parents pay a capped low fee for preschool; meals are provided for all.

2. UK National Preschool and Primary Food Policy

In the UK, the provision of a nutritious meal at lunch time in schools dates back over 150 years [32]. Three national school food policies apply UK-wide, while the remainder have some regional variation. Firstly, under the Nursery Milk Scheme, all children under 5 years attending EEC in all UK regions are entitled to 189 mL/day (1/3 pint) of fresh cows' milk for free. Secondly, the Free School Fruit and Vegetable Scheme provides fruit and vegetables (3 times per week) to all state funded schools for 4–6 years old. Thirdly, Free School Meals (FSM) are provided to all children living in low income households, and since 2014, to all 4–7 year-olds in England and all 4–8 year-olds in Scotland.

2.1. UK Regional Preschool Food Policies

In Northern Ireland and Wales, state registered EEC settings must follow the nutritional standards set out for under 12 s (see schools below). England and Scotland have preschool-specific guidance, but while these link to compulsory standards in Scotland, in England they are voluntary.

In England, national voluntary guidelines based on four food groups (starchy foods, fruit and vegetables, non-dairy sources of protein, and dairy) apply [33] (see Tables 1–3, and Table S1). The guidance focuses on balancing intake across the day, suggesting, for instance, that lunch should contribute 30% of energy needs. Nutrient based standards are also provided [34]. For children aged 1–4 years attending full daycare, the food served should provide approximately 116 kcals, 45 g fat, and 155 g carbohydrates; no more than 34.2 Non Milk Extrinsic Sugar (NMES), 810 mg Sodium, and 2.1 g Salt; at least 14 g protein, 7.2 mg Iron, 5.7 mg Zinc, 330 mg Calcium, 390 µg Vit A, and 27 mg Vit C. The guidance makes some provision for foods brought from home (packed meals), including for meal composition, food safety guidance, and the consideration of common allergens.

The Scottish Standards follow the same nutritional guidance as the English model, and include the same food groups (see Tables 1 and 2, and Table S1) [35]. The standards require that the provided food is "well-balanced and healthy" (p. 7) [35], and set out required portions, where a portion is "what a young child can hold in their hand" (p. 50). The standards do not cover home provided food, although additional guidance suggests food items for healthy packed lunches [35].

2.2. UK Regional School Food Policies

The School Food Plan introduced updated food-based standards in England in January 2014. These standards stipulate that a school meal should include an adequate provision of fruit and vegetables, dairy food, low fat proteins, and low fat starchy food (see Table 1, and Table S1). Fried foods, foods high in fats and sugars, and sweetened beverages are restricted (see Table 2). The School Food Plan applies to all state-run schools, and to those state funded but independently run Academies and Free schools created since 2015. Independent schools, along with Academies and Free schools created prior to 2015, are not covered by this policy.

There are no national policies for packed lunches, although some local government and individual schools do recommend foods to include or restrict in packed lunches, such as drinks, fruit and vegetables, and sweet and savoury snacks [36].

2.3. UK Reach and Implementation of Preschool and Primary Food Policy

Policy reach, cost, and monitoring is summarized in Table 3. The majority of English children now attend an EEC setting (93% 3–4 years old in 2012) [37], but we know little about how many are covered by this policy. Given part-time attendance, we do not know how many meals are eaten in EEC. Furthermore, many of these meals may be home-provided. The use of packed meals is under-recognised in preschool children, but estimates in studies have found that between 39% and 49% of Early Years Settings use only packed lunches [38,39]. We do not know whether the guidelines are adhered to in either case.

The school population is very nearly the entire child population [40], so nearly all children eat meals at school. The most recent data on the take up of school meals in England predates the introduction of universal FSM for the youngest children. At that time, 42.6% of children in primary schools ate provided meals, although it was much higher for those eligible for FSM on the basis of household income (75.1%). The average lunch cost was £2.04, and price was predictive of take up, reducing by 1.9% for every 10p more charged for the school meal [41]. The extension of FSM has high take up in Scotland (76% of children) [42].

Both primary and preschools are monitored by the Office for Standards in Education (OFSTED). Inspections should ensure standards are met where they are statutory, but not where voluntary.

2.4. UK Impact of Policy on Diet Quality

There is limited evidence on the quality of food provision in UK EEC, and almost none on consumption [38]. Most nurseries in England are providing meals that contain too much salt and insufficient energy [43]. There is no independent evaluation of the use of the guidelines in England nor the standards in Scotland. A before and after study conducted in England suggests that the guidelines improve staff knowledge and confidence of healthy eating guidelines, and EECs self-report a greater diversity of food and a reduced use of high sugar and salt foods [44]. However, we cannot say whether children's diets have improved as a result of the policy in either region.

The evidence of the use of packed lunches in preschools is worrying, and probably undermines gains in provided meal quality. In one study of preschool packed lunches in the UK, 42% included crisps, 24% confectionary, and most provided a sugar-sweetened drink [38]. In the USA, preschool packed lunches are high in salt, and low in minerals, vegetables, fruit, and dietary fibre [45,46].

A number of evaluations of the primary school meal standards in the UK have demonstrated that lunchtime and whole day intake have improved with the introduction of a high quality school meal. The research mainly includes cross-sectional studies of food intake carried out after the introduction of standards and compared with intakes before the introduction of the standards [47–50]. These suggest that there may have been improvements in food provision, including increases in fruit and vegetables and reductions in non-permitted foods [51–53], but mixed evidence on portion size [54]. Children in schools included in Jamie Oliver's "feed me better campaign" achieved better in standard testing relative to neighbouring schools, and authorised absences (usually for illness or planned appointments) fell [55]. A pilot trial was carried out in two areas of England looking at free meals for infants, which reported better behaviour in pupils in the classroom and healthier food at lunchtime [56].

Packed lunches in primary schools are known to be of poor quality [57], and cross-sectional studies of children across England reported that diet quality over the whole day is higher for children having a school meal compared to a packed lunch [58,59]. To the extent that meal standards and FSM extension increase school meal uptake relative to packed lunches, they therefore probably improve diet.

3. Swedish Preschool and Primary Meals Provision

To our knowledge, Sweden and Finland are the only countries that currently provide free school meals to all children in all years of primary school, regardless of parental income or school form. School meals are regulated by the Education Act, which states that all children attending primary school (age 6–16 years) are entitled to free and nutritious school meals [60], and by extension preschools [61]. All children are offered a prepared warm dish, salad buffet, bread, and a drink at no cost, which should be nutritionally adequate (Table 1); soft drinks are not provided (Table 2), and desserts and fried foods are rare; there are few if any vending machines, and where tuck shops exist these are often closed during lunch. Variation exists in implementation; food can be prepared on site or in an external kitchen, from scratch or from semi-processed components, and local authority or privately run.

Although not an official policy, the concept of "the pedagogic lunch" is well-established in Sweden and Finland. Teachers eat together with the children, and ideally use this opportunity to teach about food and health [62]. Preschools serve food "family style" in communal dishes to tables of approximately 10 children.

3.1. Swedish Preschool and Primary School Meals Guidelines

The provision of free school meals has been required by law since 1997 (Table 3), although most have done so since the 1970s, and charging for meals has not been permitted since 1946. The requirement that meals be "nutritious" (Table 1) was added in 2011, but school meals are not inspected (Table 3). The National Food Agency issues non-binding national guidelines and advice [63,64]. The guidelines focus on the whole meal experience, including quality, timing, composition, and environment. Meals are considered as more than a source of nutrition; and should be tasty, nutritious, safe, pleasant, sustainable, and integrated within the preschool/school day.

In 2010, an audit-and-feedback tool was developed by researchers and stakeholders (SkolmatSverige: School Food Sweden) to assess all of the elements of the meal experience (Figure 1) [65]. The tool aims to aid the evaluation of the impact of the 2011 law, create a nationally representative database of school meal quality, and support schools to undertake their own monitoring and evaluation and thereby improve their own school meal quality. It is web-based, free to use, and requires no training. Feedback is tailored and fully automatic.

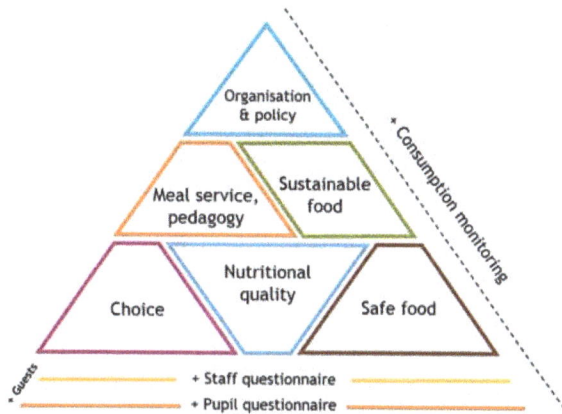

Figure 1. Components of SkolmatSverige instrument.

3.2. Sweden: Reach, Implementation and Impact of Preschool and Primary School Meals Policy

Since policy and provision in Sweden is universal, all children in preschool/school are reached. However, there is some evidence that older children may eat lunch outside of school premises or choose to skip lunch [17]. The very fact of free provision means there are no data available to record uptake (i.e., no till or reimbursement receipts), much less to track the composition of the school meals that students choose. The nature of the traditional Swedish school lunch means that many unhealthy foods (e.g., fried foods) will simply not appear, although the implementation of the newest requirements for nutritious meals is not complete. Sociable, educational interactions modelling good eating habits have been observed in the pedagogic meal, but not among all teachers [62].

The SkolmatSverige instrument is the only current source of national data. To date, 40% of primary schools use it, but the figure is increasing [66]. In a small, but nationally representative, study of schools using the tool before and after the introduction of the law requiring "nutritious" school meals, nutritional quality increased significantly, but remained low [67]. Over a 4-week period in 2014/2015, most schools provided meals that fulfilled iron and fibre requirements (86% and 96%, respectively), but less often met requirements for vitamin D and fat (51% and 41%, respectively). Most schools (71%) offered a choice of warm meals daily, and a salad buffet with at least five components (93%) [68]. Improvements in other aspects of meal quality have not been as marked [68]. These are encouraging signs, although from a self-selecting sample.

The universal nature of Sweden's school meal policy makes evaluation challenging because comparisons can only be historical. While the law may have had some effect, the new national guidelines, national concern about the issue, and related educational activities probably have a role too. Knowledge of the national guidelines for school meals is high [69], and three-quarters of local authorities have developed meal policies. The preliminary results from the first few years of data gathered by SkolmatSverige suggest that the repeated use of the tool results in improvements. As new data becomes available, it will be possible to validate this finding. The tool has also recently been expanded (November 2016) to include a module that helps schools measure uptake and the average amount of food that students actually consume, taking into account plate waste.

No national data on current preschool meal quality are available, and the instrument School Food Sweden was only developed for primary schools [66].

4. Australian Preschool and Primary School Meals

4.1. Australian Preschool Meal Policies

In Australia, EEC services are offered by government, community, and private providers, and are the responsibility of the states and territories (the Federal Government contributes funding to Indigenous preschool services). A National Quality Framework was agreed on by the Council of Australian Governments (COAG), and includes a National Law and Regulations that apply in all States and Territories [70]. National Quality Standards are a key element of the regulations, and apply to most forms of day care and EEC. The standards are overseen by the Australian Children's Education and Care Quality Authority (ACEQUA), and each State and Territory is a regulatory authority with monitoring, compliance, and quality assessment roles.

Food and drink provided in EEC must comply with the legislation, regulations, and standards within the National Quality Framework. Specifically, standard 2.2 states that "healthy eating is embedded in the program for children", and "food and drinks provided by the service are nutritious and appropriate for each child". The meaning of "nutritious and appropriate" is not further stipulated. Each State/Territory provides guidance (see Table 1) and training to support these services to adopt nutrition and healthy eating policies. For example, the Victorian government provides a Healthy Eating Advisory Service [71], the NSW government runs the Munch & Move program [72], and the ACT has a Nutrition Support Service [73]. None of the State/Territory guidelines are mandated (Table 3).

4.2. Australian Primary and Secondary School Meal Policies

In Australia, most school-aged children bring their lunch from home [74,75], but the canteen or "tuckshop" plays an integral role in educating and modelling a healthy food environment [76]. The canteen in Australian schools serves as a small shop where students can purchase lunch, snacks, and drinks, and operate anywhere from one to five days per week [77]. They are operated either by canteen managers, volunteer parents, or are outsourced to external food manufacturing and supply companies.

National voluntary guidelines (based on the Australian Dietary Guidelines [78]) have been published to guide States and Territories in developing healthy school food provision policies. From these, each State/Territory has developed a set of independent healthy canteen guidelines [79–86]. Seven States and Territories have implemented mandatory standards based on their guidelines (Tables 1 and 2).

In the majority of States/Territories, the traffic light system is used in the canteen guidelines to categorise foods into "Green", healthy foods which are encouraged (see Table 1), "Amber" (less healthy), and "Red" (least healthy) items which are discouraged (see Table 2) based on their nutritional quality. The traffic light system is relatively consistent across all States/Territories, and follows the principles outlined in the National Healthy School Canteens Traffic Light criteria (Figure 2). This system enables schools to assess their canteen menu and any other school food provision, and align food and drinks provision to these guidelines. New South Wales (NSW) has recently updated their policy in a move away from the traffic light system, to classify foods as "everyday" or "occasional". The NSW policy mandates that even "occasional" foods are required to maintain a certain degree of healthiness (based on the government-endorsed Health Star Rating system for food labelling).

All of the other States and Territories identify "red category" foods, which are either completely banned in schools or heavily restricted (see Table 2). Guidelines are generally mandatory for government schools in each State/Territory, and are highly encouraged for Independent/Catholic schools (see Table 3).

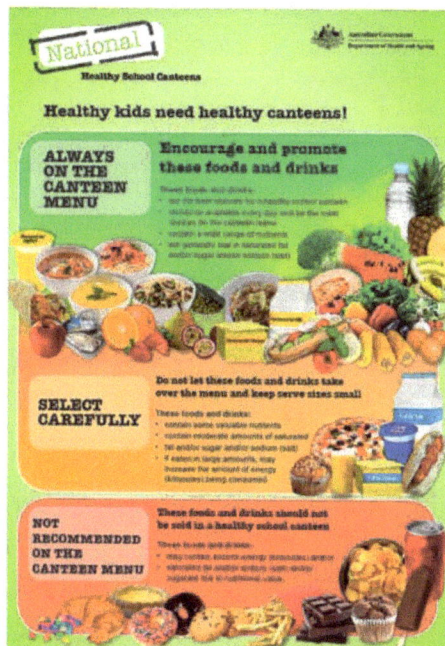

Figure 2. National healthy school canteens traffic light labelling guidelines. © Commonwealth of Australia 2017.

4.3. Australian Reach, Implementation, and Impact of Preschool and School Meals Policies

The monitoring and compliance of policy guidelines in schools varies by State/Territory. In general, the policies are not actively enforced or routinely monitored by government. There is variable implementation across the different jurisdictions, and poor rates of adherence.

A cross-sectional study conducted by Woods et al. collected data in 2012 to assess whether schools were adhering to healthy canteen guidelines. The study explored the compliance of a convenience sample of government schools to healthy canteen guidelines, the proportion of "Green", "Amber", and "Red" on each menu, and the presence of discretionary items [87]. Woods et al. found low to moderate levels of adherence to state canteen guidelines, with the highest rate of compliance in Western Australia (62% of primary and secondary schools) [87]. Four studies report low to moderate rates of compliance with government healthy canteen policies [88–91]. The self-reported implementation of guidelines was demonstrated to be high in one Queensland study [92]. However, Principal and canteen manager self-reporting has been demonstrated to be in poor agreement with the gold standard of compliance assessment [93]. A recently published randomised controlled trial further found that a menu audit and feedback system made only moderate impacts on compliance, although some improvements were seen [94].

Since most school children bring lunch from home, evidence about the content of these and any spillover effect for the canteen guidelines is needed.

Similarly, there is very limited evidence about food provided or eaten in preschool settings. Since the standard is simply that food is "nutritious", monitoring compliance is not particularly meaningful. One qualitative study suggests that the guidelines are not used [95]. Furthermore, due to the highly disparate nature and uptake of EEC services in Australia, it is difficult to know how many children are using preschool provision and how many meals are eaten there.

5. Discussion

Quite different approaches to ensuring school meal quality are taken in the three countries reviewed here. Sweden has almost universal provision and uptake of school meals from preschool through primary years, and a requirement for nutritious meals, but this requirement is not strictly monitored and the guidelines issued for the meals are non-binding. In contrast, Australia largely relies on home-provided meals in the primary years supplemented by in-school canteens. National "traffic light" guidance for canteen food in primary schools exists, but implementation is at a state level and adherence is poor. Preschools in Australia have state-specific support for the provision of healthy food, but national standards simply stipulate food and drinks provided must be "nutritious and appropriate", which makes this standard too vague to be enforceable. The UK uses food-based standards in both the primary and preschool years, but these are only statutory in some contexts. Free school meal uptake is high, but where meals are paid for (including in preschools), the use of home provided meals is common, undermining the positive contribution of food standards to diet. In none of the three countries are the mechanisms for the monitoring of these food standards clearly enforced, limiting our knowledge and potentially limiting impact on diet and health. In both the UK and Australia, there is little regulation and provision for the youngest children.

In the UK, researchers have been active in using opportunistic research designs to estimate the impact of policy changes in the primary years. The introduction of food-based standards for primary school meals combined with an increased uptake following the introduction of universal free meals in the infant years appears to have had positive impacts on children's diet.

The range and breadth of additional guidance and supporting materials available are a strength of the current policy approaches [26,33,71–73]. The wealth of information supplied particularly to preschools is valued by some providers and parents [44], and has the potential to influence diet outside of school too. The ambition to integrate food into the pedagogic environment in Sweden, and to a lesser extent in the UK's preschools, is also a strength. Evidence suggests that embedding discussions about healthy eating and exposing children to healthy food choices is likely to be useful in shaping their long term eating preferences [13,96].

Two core weakness emerge, however. The first is that provided school meals are only part of the picture of food consumed during school hours. Packed lunches commonly provide alternate meals in both Australia and the UK, but additional food sources in all countries include vending machines, tuck shops, bake sales, other foods brought from home, and food provided in care before and after school. As children age, they may also be leaving school premises to purchase food from local food retailers. The nutritional advantages of high quality meal provision are undermined where few children take up this offer and/or where food from other sources is not included in healthy eating plans.

Secondly, all three countries appear to have weak mechanisms for monitoring compliance with healthy eating policies, and lack provisions for monitoring children's actual intake. This means that they are unable to comment with certainty on the extent to which schools provide food as envisaged in the policy, and are unable to assess whether policy changes have resulted in improved nutritional intake. Importantly, we also cannot comment on whether these initiatives counteract health inequalities. The voluntary self-monitoring system in Sweden could enable a comparison of school meal quality between catchment areas of differing socio-economic position in the future, but its use is not widespread enough for this to be the case yet. Where free meals are provided for the most disadvantaged (as is the case among older primary aged children in the UK), nutritionally sound meals have the potential to decrease inequalities, but policy complexity makes this difficult to assess. In England, a particular oddity of the policy evolution is that the youngest children are not included in free meal provision, so although the most disadvantaged children are preferentially provided with free preschool places, their meals are neither free nor covered by school food standards. Anecdotally, we note that some nurseries are providing free meals to the most deprived 2 years old from within their own budget, but this micro-level solution is neither testable nor scalable.

5.1. Implications for Policy

The improvement of school food through national or state nutritional guidelines or standards is ongoing in many countries [2,13,97]. We believe that these policies are likely to be important for the long-term health of our populations through their influence on dietary intake and food habits. Two systematic reviews of methods to increase fruit and vegetable intake in children [20,98] suggest the best evidence for success is for provision through schools.

The implications for school meal policies are that: (a) enforcement of policy is necessary to see improvements; (b) uptake of provided food is crucial to deliver benefits; and (c) monitoring of uptake, nutritional intake, and differential intake by social groups is needed to demonstrate whether provided school food is, in fact, a public health success. Others have reached similar conclusions [4], particularly considering the value of monitoring and evaluation for policy success [99]. Overly burdensome data collection can interfere with policy implementation [51], but light touch regulation, using existing education inspection mechanisms, that requires schools to report on their compliance with guidelines and their uptake of provided food could achieve much with little additional effort. In addition, mechanisms to provide clear accountability for compliance with standards, and strong incentives for compliance (e.g., tied to budget mechanisms, or individual Principal performance assessments) need to be explored. The Swedish self-monitoring tool is working well to encourage quality improvements, and it provides a model for efficient audit.

We also need whole-school approaches to healthy eating which are broader than school meals. This should include the consideration of meals and snacks brought from home, but also wider actions to address attitudes towards healthy foods. Banning adults (staff and visitors) from smoking or using tobacco products on the premises or at any school-related activities is a key feature of tobacco free schools [100]. Adopting similar "whole school" approaches to junk-food free schools may be appropriate.

Population-level improvements in health need population-level responses, and political and policy actions addressing the food environment are needed [101]. Reductions in the extensive marketing of unhealthy food in children's immediate environment (fast food outlets and convenience stores) [102], and increases in the relative price of unhealthy compared to healthy food are needed [103], and would support schools in their efforts.

5.2. Implications for Practice

Canteen-style provision now dominates in primary schools in all three countries, but the pedagogic model used in Sweden deserves greater attention [62]. The use of school meal times as an opportunity to talk about food and food choices may be valuable [104], but only if used by teachers [62]. Although further research is needed, we would consider this to be areas of promising practice.

Similarly, involving parents and carers in changes in school food may promote the generalisability of change [20,105]. Food policies that focus only on safety aspects and the avoidance of allergens are unlikely to engage parents as partners in improving diet. Top down policy has little effect if it is not coupled with, and sensitive to, local implementation [106].

5.3. Implications for Research

We know of few published high quality longitudinal studies or randomised controlled trials evaluating the impact of school meal policies on nutrition behaviour, diet quality, and health [107–111], although some are currently underway [112–114]. A more rigorous evaluation of the benefits of school meals on diet quality and health outcomes (such as obesity), including longitudinal studies or randomised controlled trials, are needed to assess the impact of policies, particularly on reducing inequalities in diet and health.

Much of the practice outlined in this paper has not been monitored or evaluated. While guidelines themselves are often based on extensive and expert review of nutritional needs in children, the evidence to support the implementation of such guidelines is regrettably lacking. The research needs are many in this field, but we propose the most urgent ones here: (a) the exploitation of routinely collected data to comment on the impact of policy roll-out when innovation occurs; (b) research on the implementation of nutritional and food-based guidelines; (c) research into the contribution of foods consumed during school hours to total diet across the preschool and primary years; and (d) research into the long term effects of healthy school meal provision on diet and educational achievement. Core to this would be (e) the introduction of standard measures and indicators to assess food intake [97].

6. Conclusions

There is good evidence to suggest that meals eaten in the preschool and primary years should be a target for improving children's dietary habits and preferences. In the three countries reviewed, action in the preschool years generally lags behind schools, and policies tend to lack enforceability. Policies are needed which have clear standards, systems for monitoring compliance and reach, and which acknowledge the whole school eating environment including home provided meals. While important, school food policies will have limited impact in the absence of broader public health and political action to improve our food environment.

Supplementary Materials: The following are available online at www.mdpi.com/2072-6643/9/7/736/s1. Table S1: School Food Standards in England, and Preschool Standards for England and Scotland.

Acknowledgments: G.S. is the recipient of an Australian Research Council Discovery Early Career Researcher Award (project number DE160100307). No other funds supported the preparation of this manuscript.

Author Contributions: P.J.L. and C.E.L.E. conceived of the paper. P.J.L. and C.E.L.E. wrote the UK sections, E.P. the Swedish and G.S. and N.B. the Australian. All authors contributed to the introduction and discussion sections. All authors reviewed and agreed on the final version.

Conflicts of Interest: The authors declare no conflict of interest.

References

1. WHO. What Is a Health Promoting School? Available online: http://www.who.int/school_youth_health/ gshi/hps/en/ (accessed on 12 April 2017).
2. McKenna, M.L. Policy options to support healthy eating in schools. *Can. J. Public Health* **2010**, *101*, S14–S17. [PubMed]
3. Mikkelsen, B.E.; Engesveen, K.; Afflerbach, T.; Barnekow, V. The human rights framework, the school and healthier eating among young people: A European perspective. *Public Health Nutr.* **2016**, *19*, 15–25. [CrossRef] [PubMed]
4. Nelson, M.; Breda, J. School food research: Building the evidence base for policy. *Public Health Nutr.* **2013**, *16*, 958–967. [CrossRef] [PubMed]
5. Grant, M.J.; Booth, A. A typology of reviews: An analysis of 14 review types and associated methodologies. *Health Inf. Libr. J.* **2009**, *26*, 91–108. [CrossRef] [PubMed]
6. Public Health England. *National Diet And Nutrition Survey Results from Years 5 and 6 Combined of the Rolling Programme for 2012 and 2013 to 2013 and 2014: Report*; Public Health England: London, UK, 2016.
7. Barbieri, H.E.; Pearson, M.; Becker, W. *Riksmaten—Barn 2003. Livsmedels-och Näringsintag Bland Barn i Sverige [Food and Nutrient Intake of Children in Sweden]*; Livsmedelsverket: Uppsala, Sweden, 2006. (In Swedish)

8. Australian Bureau of Statistics. *Australian Health Survey: Nutrition First Results—Food and Nutrients, 2011–2012*; Australian Bureau of Statistics: Canberra, Australia, 2014.

9. Public Health England. *National Diet And Nutrition Survey: Results from Years 1 to 4 (Combined) of the Rolling Programme (2008/2009–2011/12): Executive Summary*; Public Health England and Food Standards Agency: London, UK, 2015.

10. Nelson, M.; Erens, B.; Bates, B.; Church, S.; Boshier, T. *Low Income Diet and Nutrition Survey*; The Stationary Office: London, UK, 2007; Volume 3.

11. Rasmussen, M.; Krolner, R.; Klepp, K.; Lytle, L.A.; Brug, J.; Bere, E.; Due, P. Determinants of fruit and vegetable consumption among children and adolescents: A review of the literature. Part I: Quantitative studies. *Int. J. Behav. Nutr. Phys. Act.* **2006**, *3*, 22. [CrossRef] [PubMed]

12. Mattisson, I. *Socioekonomiska Skillnader i Matvanor i Sverige [Socioeconomic Differences in Food Habits in Sweden]*; Livsmedelsverket: Uppsala, Sweden, 2016. (In Swedish)

13. Brambila-Macias, J.; Shankar, B.; Capacci, S.; Mazzocchi, M.; Perez-Cueto, F.J.; Verbeke, W.; Traill, W.B. Policy interventions to promote healthy eating: A review of what works, what does not, and what is promising. *Food Nutr. Bull.* **2011**, *32*, 365–375. [CrossRef] [PubMed]

14. Tilles-Tirkkonen, T.; Pentikainen, S.; Lappi, J.; Karhunen, L.; Poutanen, K.; Mykkanen, H. The quality of school lunch consumed reflects overall eating patterns in 11–16-year-old schoolchildren in Finland. *Public Health Nutr.* **2011**, *14*, 2092–2098. [CrossRef] [PubMed]

15. Raulio, S.; Roos, E.; Prattala, R. School and workplace meals promote healthy food habits. *Public Health Nutr.* **2010**, *13*, 987–992. [CrossRef] [PubMed]

16. Rogers, I.S.; Ness, A.R.; Hebditch, K.; Jones, L.R.; Emmett, P.M. Quality of food eaten in English primary schools: School dinners vs. packed lunches. *Eur. J. Clin. Nutr.* **2007**, *61*, 856–864. [CrossRef] [PubMed]

17. Persson Osowski, C.; Lindroos, A.K.; Enghardt Barbieri, H.; Becker, W. The contribution of school meals to energy and nutrient intake of swedish children in relation to dietary guidelines. *Food Nutr. Res.* **2015**, *59*, 27563. [CrossRef] [PubMed]

18. Syrad, H.; Llewellyn, C.H.; van Jaarsveld, C.H.; Johnson, L.; Jebb, S.A.; Wardle, J. Energy and nutrient intakes of young children in the UK: Findings from the gemini twin cohort. *Br. J. Nutr.* **2016**, *115*, 1843–1850. [CrossRef] [PubMed]

19. Bevans, K.B.; Sanchez, B.; Teneralli, R.; Forrest, C.B. Children's eating behavior: The importance of nutrition standards for foods in schools. *J. Sch. Health* **2011**, *81*, 424–429. [CrossRef] [PubMed]

20. De Costa, P.; Moller, P.; Frost, M.B.; Olsen, A. Changing children's eating behaviour—A review of experimental research. *Appetite* **2017**, *113*, 327–357. [CrossRef] [PubMed]

21. Ray, C.; Roos, E.; Brug, J.; Behrendt, I.; Ehrenblad, B.; Yngve, A.; te Velde, S.J. Role of free school lunch in the associations between family-environmental factors and children's fruit and vegetable intake in four European countries. *Public Health Nutr.* **2013**, *16*, 1109–1117. [CrossRef] [PubMed]

22. Williamson, D.A.; Han, H.; Johnson, W.D.; Martin, C.K.; Newton, R.L., Jr. Modification of the school cafeteria environment can impact childhood nutrition. Results from the wise mind and la health studies. *Appetite* **2013**, *61*, 77–84. [CrossRef] [PubMed]

23. Gubbels, J.S.; Gerards, S.M.; Kremers, S.P. Use of food practices by childcare staff and the association with dietary intake of children at childcare. *Nutrients* **2015**, *7*, 2161–2175. [CrossRef] [PubMed]

24. Mukoma, W.; Flisher, A.J. Evaluations of health promoting schools: A review of nine studies. *Health Promot. Int.* **2004**, *19*, 357–368. [CrossRef] [PubMed]

25. Lister-Sharp, D.; Chapman, S.; Stewart-Brown, S.; Sowden, A. Health promoting schools and health promotion in schools: Two systematic reviews. *Health Technol. Assess.* **1999**, *3*, 1–207. [PubMed]

26. Skolverket [Swedish National Agency for Education]. *Curriculum for the Preschool Lpfö 98 Revised 2010*; Skolverket: Stockholm, Sweden, 2010.

27. Department for Education. *Statutory Framework for the Early Years Foundation Stage. Setting the Standards for Learning, Development and Care for Children from Birth to Five*; Department for Education: London, UK, 2012.

28. The Organisation for Economic Co-operation and Development (OCED). *Country Statistical Profiles: Key Tables from OECD*; The Organisation for Economic Co-operation and Development (OECD): Paris, France, 2017.

29. Gov.Uk. Help Paying for Childcare. Available online: https://www.gov.uk/help-with-childcare-costs/free-childcare-and-education-for-2-to-4-year-olds (accessed on 22 April 2017).

30. Department for Education. Will I Qualify for 30 h Free Childcare? Available online: https://www.gov.uk/government/uploads/system/uploads/attachment_data/file/600592/30_h_free_childcare_eligibility.pdf (accessed on 22 April 2017).

31. Family and Childcare Trust. Help with My Childcare Costs. Available online: https://www.familyandchildcaretrust.org/help-my-childcare-costs (accessed on 10 July 2017).

32. Evans, C.E.; Harper, C.E. A history and review of school meal standards in the UK. *J. Hum. Nutr. Diet.* **2009**, *22*, 89–99. [CrossRef] [PubMed]

33. The Children's Food Trust. *Eat Better Start Better, Voluntary Food and Drink Guidelines for Early Years Settings in England—A Practical Guide*; Children's Food Trust: Sheffield, UK, 2012; p. 80.

34. Advisory Panel on Food and Nutrition in Early Years. *Laying the Table. Recommendations for National Food and Nutrition Guidance for Early Years Settings in England*; Main Report; Schools Food Trust: Sheffield, UK, 2010; Volume 1.

35. NHS Scotland. *Setting the Table. Nutritional Guidance and Food Standards for Early Years Childcare Providers in Scotland*; NHS Scotland: Edinburgh, UK, 2015.

36. Children's Food Trust. Available online: http://www.childrensfoodtrust.org.uk/childrens-food-trust/parents/your-childs-food-at-school/packed-lunches/packed-lunch-information/ (accessed on 10 July 2017).

37. Department for Education. *Provision for Children under Five Years of Age in England*; Statistical First Release; Department for Education: London, UK, 2013.

38. Nicholas, J.; Stevens, L.; Briggs, L.; Wood, L. *Pre-School Food Survey*; Children's Food Trust: Sheffield, UK, 2013.

39. Lucas, P.; Richards, H.; Johnson, L. How common are packed or sack lunches in English early education and care? (Bristol, England). Personal communication, 2017.

40. FOI Directory. Reference from Freedom of Information Directory. Available online: http://www.foi.directory/updates/foi-reveals-rising-numbers-of-pupils-home-educated/ (accessed on 10 July 2017).

41. Wollny, I.; Lord, C.; Tanner, E.; Fry, A.; Tipping, S.; Kitchen, S. *School Lunch Take-Up Survey 2013 to 2014 Research Report*; Department for Education: London, UK, 2015.

42. Chambers, S.; Ford, A.; Boydell, N.; Moore, L.; Stead, M.; Eadie, D. Universal free school meals in Scotland: A process evaluation of implementation and uptake. *Eur. J. Public Health* **2016**, *26*, ckw169. [CrossRef]

43. Parker, M.; Lloyd-Williams, F.; Weston, G.; Macklin, J.; McFadden, K. Nursery nutrition in liverpool: An exploration of practice and nutritional analysis of food provided. *Public Health Nutr.* **2011**, *14*, 1867–1875. [CrossRef] [PubMed]

44. Mucavele, P.; Sharp, L.; Wall, C.; Nicholas, J. Children's food trust 'eat better, start better' programme: Outcomes and recommendations. *Perspect. Public Health* **2014**, *134*, 67–69. [PubMed]

45. Sweitzer, S.J.; Briley, M.E.; Robert-Gray, C. Do sack lunches provided by parents meet the nutritional needs of young children who attend child care? *J. Am. Diet. Assoc.* **2009**, *109*, 141–144. [CrossRef] [PubMed]

46. Romo-Palafox, M.J.; Ranjit, N.; Sweitzer, S.J.; Roberts-Gray, C.; Hoelscher, D.M.; Byrd-Williams, C.E.; Briley, M.E. Dietary quality of preschoolers' sack lunches as measured by the healthy eating index. *J. Acad. Nutr. Diet.* **2015**, *115*, 1779–1788. [CrossRef] [PubMed]

47. Spence, S.; Delve, J.; Stamp, E.; Matthews, J.N.; White, M.; Adamson, A.J. Did school food and nutrient-based standards in England impact on 11–12Y olds nutrient intake at lunchtime and in total diet? Repeat cross-sectional study. *PLoS ONE* **2014**, *9*, e112648. [CrossRef] [PubMed]

48. Spence, S.; Delve, J.; Stamp, E.; Matthews, J.N.; White, M.; Adamson, A.J. The impact of food and nutrient-based standards on primary school children's lunch and total dietary intake: A natural experimental evaluation of government policy in England. *PLoS ONE* **2013**, *8*, e78298. [CrossRef] [PubMed]

49. Golley, R.; Pearce, J.; Nelson, M. Children's lunchtime food choices following the introduction of food-based standards for school meals: Observations from six primary schools in sheffield. *Public Health Nutr.* **2011**, *14*, 271–278. [CrossRef] [PubMed]

50. Adamson, A.; Spence, S.; Reed, L.; Conway, R.; Palmer, A.; Stewart, E.; McBratney, J.; Carter, L.; Beattie, S.; Nelson, M. School food standards in the UK: Implementation and evaluation. *Public Health Nutr.* **2013**, *16*, 968–981. [CrossRef] [PubMed]

51. Moore, L.; Tapper, K. The impact of school fruit tuck shops and school food policies on children's fruit consumption: A cluster randomised trial of schools in deprived areas. *J. Epidemiol. Commun. Health* **2008**, *62*, 926–931. [CrossRef] [PubMed]

52. Haroun, D.; Harper, C.; Wood, L.; Nelson, M. The impact of the food-based and nutrient-based standards on lunchtime food and drink provision and consumption in primary schools in England. *Public Health Nutr.* **2011**, *14*, 209–218. [CrossRef] [PubMed]

53. Nicholas, J.; Wood, L.; Harper, C.; Nelson, M. The impact of the food-based and nutrient-based standards on lunchtime food and drink provision and consumption in secondary schools in England. *Public Health Nutr.* **2013**, *16*, 1052–1065. [CrossRef] [PubMed]

54. Pearce, J.; Wood, L.; Stevens, L. Portion weights of food served in english schools: Have they changed following the introduction of nutrient-based standards? *J. Hum. Nutr. Diet.* **2013**, *26*, 553–562. [CrossRef] [PubMed]

55. Belot, M.; James, J. Healthy school meals and educational outcomes. *J. Health Econom.* **2011**, *30*, 489–504. [CrossRef] [PubMed]

56. Department for Education. Available online: www.gov.uk/government/publications/evaluation-of-the-free-school-meals-pilot-impact-report (accessed on 10 July 2017).

57. Evans, C.E.; Greenwood, D.C.; Thomas, J.D.; Cade, J.E. A cross-sectional survey of children's packed lunches in the UK: Food- and nutrient-based results. *J. Epidemiol. Commun. Health* **2010**, *64*, 977–983. [CrossRef] [PubMed]

58. Evans, C.E.; Mandl, V.; Christian, M.S.; Cade, J.E. Impact of school lunch type on nutritional quality of english children's diets. *Public Health Nutr.* **2016**, *19*, 36–45. [CrossRef] [PubMed]

59. Harrison, F.; Jennings, A.; Jones, A.; Welch, A.; van Sluijs, E.; Griffin, S.; Cassidy, A. Food and drink consumption at school lunchtime: The impact of lunch type and contribution to overall intake in british 9–10-year-old children. *Public Health Nutr.* **2013**, *16*, 1132–1139. [CrossRef] [PubMed]

60. Sveriges Riksdag [The Swedish Parliament]. *Den nya Skollagen—för Kunskap, Valfrihet och Trygghet [The New School Law—For Knowledge, Choice and Security]*; Sveriges Riksdag, Ed.; Sveriges Riksdag: Stockholm, Sweden, 2010. (In Swedish)

61. Skolverket [Swedish National Agency for Education]. *Måluppfyllelse i förskolan [Goal Achievement in Preschool]*; Skolverket: Stockholm, Sweden, 2017. (In Swedish)

62. Persson Osowski, C.; Goranzon, H.; Fjellstrom, C. Teachers' interaction with children in the school meal situation: The example of pedagogic meals in Sweden. *J. Nutr. Educ. Behav.* **2013**, *45*, 420–427. [CrossRef] [PubMed]

63. Swedish National Food Agency. *Good School Meals*; Livsmedelsverket: Uppsala, Sweden, 2014.

64. Livsmedelsverket [Swedish National Food Agency]. *Bra måltider i Förskolan [Good Meals in Preschool]*; Livsmedelsverket: Uppsala, Sweden, 2016. (In Swedish)

65. Patterson, E.; Quetel, A.-K.; Lilja, K.; Simma, M.; Olsson, L.; Schäfer Elinder, L. Design, testing and validation of an innovative web-based instrument to evaluate school meal quality. *Public Health Nutr.* **2013**, *16*, 1028–1036. [CrossRef] [PubMed]

66. SkolmatSverige. What Is Skolmatsverige? Available online: www.skolmatsverige.se/in-english (accessed on 22 June 2017).

67. Patterson, E.; Elinder, L.S. Improvements in school meal quality in Sweden after the introduction of new legislation-a 2-year follow-up. *Eur. J. Public Health* **2015**, *25*, 655–660. [CrossRef] [PubMed]

68. Patterson, E.; Regnander, M.; Elinder, L.S. *SkolmatSveriges Kartläggning av Skolmåltidens Kvalitet—Läsåret 2014/15 [School Food Sweden's Survey of School Meal Quality—For the School Year 2014/15]*; Centrum för Epidemiologi och Samhällsmedicin, Stockholms Läns Landsting: Stockholm, Sweden, 2015. (In Swedish)

69. Skolmatens Vänner; Livsmedelsverket. Kartläggning av Sveriges Kommuner Gällande Skolmaten i Grundskolan [Survey of Sweden's Municpalities Concerning School Food in Primary School]. Available online: https://www.livsmedelsverket.se/globalassets/rapporter/2016/rapport-2016---maltidsverksamheten-i-kommunala-grundskolor.pdf (accessed on 10 July 2017).

70. Australian Children's Education and Care Quality Authority (ACEQUA). The National Quality Framework. Available online: http://www.acecqa.gov.au/national-quality-framework (accessed on 10 July 2017).

71. Nutrition Australia Victoria Division. Healthy Eating Advisory Service. Available online: http://heas.health.vic.gov.au/ (accessed on 10 July 2017).

72. New South Wales Office of Preventative Health. The Munch & Move Program. Available online: http://www.preventivehealth.net.au/munch--move.html (accessed on 10 July 2017).

73. Nutrition Australia ACT Division. Act Nutrition Support Service. Available online: http://www.actnss.org/ (accessed on 10 July 2017).

74. Bell, A.C.; Swinburn, B.A. What are the key food groups to target for preventing obesity and improving nutrition in schools? *Eur. J. Clin. Nutr.* **2004**, *58*, 258–263. [CrossRef] [PubMed]

75. Sanigorski, A.M.; Bell, A.C.; Kremer, P.J.; Swinburn, B.A. Lunchbox contents of Australian school children: Room for improvement. *Eur. J. Clin. Nutr.* **2005**, *59*, 1310–1316. [CrossRef] [PubMed]

76. Department of Health. Role of the School Canteen in Contributing to a Health Promoting School. Available online: http://health.gov.au/internet/publications/publishing.nsf/Content/canteen-mgr-tr1~role-school-canteen (accessed on 10 July 2017).

77. Lawlis, T.; Knox, M.; Jamieson, M. School canteens: A systematic review of the policy, perceptions and use from an Australian perspective. *Nutr. Diet.* **2016**, *73*, 389–398. [CrossRef]

78. NHMRC. *Australian Dietary Guidelines*; NHMRC: Canberra, Australia, 2013.

79. NSW School Canteen Advisory Committee. *Fresh Tastes @ School: NSW Healthy School Canteen Strategy*; NSW School Canteen Advisory Committee: Sydney, Australia, 2006.

80. Department of Education. *Healthy Food And Drink Policy*; Department of Education: Perth, Australia, 2014.

81. Department of Education. *Smart Choices: Healthy Food and Drink Supply Strategy for Queensland Schools*; Department of Education: Brisbane, Australia, 2016.

82. Victorian Government. *Healthy Canteen Kit: School Canteens and Other School Food Services Policy*; Victorian Government: Melbourne, Australia, 2012.

83. Department of Education. *Canteen, Nutrition and Healthy Eating*; Department of Education: Darwin, Australia, 2013.

84. Tasmanian School Canteen Association Inc. *School Canteen Handbook: A Whole School Approach to Healthy Eating*; Tasmanian School Canteen Association Inc.: Hobart, Australia, 2014.

85. Department of Health. *National Healthy School Canteens: Guidelines for Healthy Foods and Drinks Supplied in School Canteens*; Department of Health: Canberra, Australia, 2014.

86. Department for Education and Child Development. *Right Bite, Easy Guide to Healthy Food and Drink Supply for South Australian Schools and Preschools*; Department for Education and Child Development: Adelaide, Australia, 2008.

87. Woods, J.; Bressan, A.; Langelaan, C.; Mallon, A.; Palermo, C. Australian school canteens: Menu guideline adherence or avoidance? *Health Promot. J. Aust.* **2014**, *25*, 110–115. [CrossRef] [PubMed]

88. Ardzejewska, K.; Tadros, R.; Baxter, D. A descriptive study on the barriers and facilitators to implementation of the NSW (Australia) healthy school canteen strategy. *Health Educ. J.* **2012**, *72*, 136–145. [CrossRef]

89. De Silva-Sanigorski, A.; Breheny, T.; Jones, L.; Lacy, K.; Kremer, P.; Carpenter, L.; Bolton, K.; Prosser, L.; Gibbs, L.; Waters, E.; et al. Government food service policies and guidelines do not create healthy school canteens. *Aust. N. Z. J. Public Health* **2011**, *35*, 117–121. [CrossRef] [PubMed]

90. Pettigrew, S.; Donovan, R.J.; Jalleh, G.; Pescud, M. Predictors of positive outcomes of a school food provision policy in Australia. *Health Promot. Int.* **2014**, *29*, 317–327. [CrossRef] [PubMed]

91. Hills, A.; Nathan, N.; Robinson, K.; Fox, D.; Wollfenden, L. Improvement in primary school adherence to the NSW healthy school canteen strategy in 2007 and 2010. *Health Promot. J. Aust.* **2015**, *26*, 89–92. [CrossRef] [PubMed]

92. Dick, M.; Lee, A.; Bright, M.; Turner, K.; Edwards, R.; Dawson, J.; Miller, J. Evaluation of implementation of a healthy food and drink supply strategy throughout the whole school environment in queensland state schools, Australia. *Eur. J. Clin. Nutr.* **2012**, *66*, 1124–1129. [CrossRef] [PubMed]

93. Reilly, K.; Nathan, N.; Wolfenden, L.; Wiggers, J.; Sutherland, R.; Wyse, R.; Yoong, S.L. Validity of four measures in assessing school canteen menu compliance with state-based healthy canteen policy. *Health Promot. J. Aust.* **2016**, *27*, 215–221. [CrossRef] [PubMed]

94. Yoong, S.L.; Nathan, N.; Wolfenden, L.; Wiggers, J.; Reilly, K.; Oldmeadow, C.; Wyse, R.; Sutherland, R.; Delaney, T.; Butler, P.; et al. Cafe: A multicomponent audit and feedback intervention to improve implementation of healthy food policy in primary school canteens: A randomised controlled trial. *Int. J. Behav. Nutr. Phys. Act.* **2016**, *13*, 126. [CrossRef] [PubMed]

95. Cole, A.; Vidgen, H.; Cleland, P. Food provision in early childhood education and care services: Exploring how staff determine nutritional adequacy. *Nutr. Diet.* **2017**, *74*, 105–110. [CrossRef]
96. Council on School Health; Committee on Nutrition. Snacks, sweetened beverages, added sugars, and schools. *Pediatrics* **2015**, *135*, 575–583.
97. Perez-Cueto, F.J.; Aschemann-Witzel, J.; Shankar, B.; Brambila-Macias, J.; Bech-Larsen, T.; Mazzocchi, M.; Capacci, S.; Saba, A.; Turrini, A.; Niedzwiedzka, B.; et al. Assessment of evaluations made to healthy eating policies in Europe: A review within the eatwell project. *Public Health Nutr.* **2012**, *15*, 1489–1496. [CrossRef] [PubMed]
98. Ganann, R.; Fitzpatrick-Lewis, D.; Ciliska, D.; Peirson, L.J.; Warren, R.L.; Fieldhouse, P.; Delgado-Noguera, M.F.; Tort, S.; Hams, S.P.; Martinez-Zapata, M.J.; et al. Enhancing nutritional environments through access to fruit and vegetables in schools and homes among children and youth: A systematic review. *BMC Res. Notes* **2014**, *7*, 422. [CrossRef] [PubMed]
99. Treasury, H. *The Magenta Book. Guidance for Evaluation*; HM Treasury: London, UK, 2011.
100. Campaign for Tobacco Free Kids. How Schools Can Help Students Stay Tobacco-Free. Available online: http://www.tobaccofreekids.org/research/factsheets/pdf/0153.pdf (accessed on 27 June 2017).
101. Oliver, T.R. The politics of public health policy. *Annu. Rev. Public Health* **2006**, *27*, 195–233. [CrossRef] [PubMed]
102. Centre for Disease Control. Zoning to Encourage Healthy Eating. Available online: https://www.cdc.gov/phlp/winnable/zoning_obesity.html (accessed on 27 June 2017).
103. Parliamentary Office for Science and Technology (POST). *Barriers to Healthy Food*; Parliamentary Office for Science and Technology: London, UK, 2016.
104. Dudley, D.A.; Cotton, W.G.; Peralta, L.R. Teaching approaches and strategies that promote healthy eating in primary school children: A systematic review and meta-analysis. *Int. J. Behav. Nutr. Phys. Act.* **2015**, *12*, 28. [CrossRef] [PubMed]
105. Sansolios, S.; Mikkelsen, B.E. Views of parents, teachers and children on health promotion in kindergarten—First results from formative focus groups and observations. *J. Paediatr. Obes.* **2011**, *6*, 28–32. [CrossRef] [PubMed]
106. Moore, S.; Murphy, S.; Tapper, K.; Moore, L. From policy to plate: Barriers to implementing healthy eating policies in primary schools in Wales. *Health Policy* **2010**, *94*, 239–245. [CrossRef] [PubMed]
107. Evans, C.E.; Greenwood, D.C.; Thomas, J.D.; Cleghorn, C.L.; Kitchen, M.S.; Cade, J.E. Smart lunch box intervention to improve the food and nutrient content of children's packed lunches: UK wide cluster randomised controlled trial. *J. Epidemiol. Commun. Health* **2010**, *64*, 970–976. [CrossRef] [PubMed]
108. Sweitzer, S.J.; Briley, M.E.; Roberts-Gray, C.; Hoelscher, D.M.; Staskel, D.M.; Almansour, F.D. How to help parents pack better preschool sack lunches: Advice from parents for educators. *J. Nutr. Educ. Behav.* **2011**, *43*, 194–198. [CrossRef] [PubMed]
109. Sweitzer, S.J.; Ranjit, N.; Calloway, E.E.; Hoelscher, D.M.; Almansor, F.; Briley, M.E.; Roberts-Gray, C.R. Examining how adding a booster to a behavioral nutrition intervention prompts parents to pack more vegetables and whole gains in their preschool children's sack lunches. *Behav. Med.* **2016**, *42*, 9–17. [CrossRef] [PubMed]
110. Williams, P.A.; Cates, S.C.; Blitstein, J.L.; Hersey, J.; Gabor, V.; Ball, M.; Kosa, K.; Wilson, H.; Olson, S.; Singh, A. Nutrition-education program improves preschoolers' at-home diet: A group randomized trial. *J. Acad. Nutr. Diet.* **2014**, *114*, 1001–1008. [CrossRef] [PubMed]
111. Hutchinson, J.; Christian, M.S.; Evans, C.E.; Nykjaer, C.; Hancock, N.; Cade, J.E. Evaluation of the impact of school gardening interventions on children's knowledge of and attitudes towards fruit and vegetables. A cluster randomised controlled trial. *Appetite* **2015**, *91*, 405–414. [CrossRef] [PubMed]
112. De Silva-Sanigorski, A.; Prosser, L.; Carpenter, L.; Honisett, S.; Gibbs, L.; Moodie, M.; Sheppard, L.; Swinburn, B.; Waters, E. Evaluation of the childhood obesity prevention program Kids—'Go for your life'. *BMC Public Health* **2010**, *10*, 288. [CrossRef] [PubMed]

113. Williams, C.M.; Nathan, N.; Delaney, T.; Yoong, S.L.; Wiggers, J.; Preece, S.; Lubans, N.; Sutherland, R.; Pinfold, J.; Smith, K.; et al. Cafe: A multicomponent audit and feedback intervention to improve implementation of healthy food policy in primary school canteens: Protocol of a randomised controlled trial. *BMJ Open* **2015**, *5*, e006969. [CrossRef] [PubMed]

114. Waling, M.; Olafsdottir, A.S.; Lagstrom, H.; Wergedahl, H.; Jonsson, B.; Olsson, C.; Fossgard, E.; Holthe, A.; Talvia, S.; Gunnarsdottir, I.; et al. School meal provision, health, and cognitive function in a nordic setting—The promeal-study: Description of methodology and the nordic context. *Food Nutr. Res.* **2016**, *60*, 30468. [CrossRef] [PubMed]

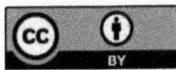

nutrients

MDPI

Article

Changes in Dietary Patterns from Childhood to Adolescence and Associated Body Adiposity Status

Danielle Biazzi Leal [1,2,*] , Maria Alice Altenburg de Assis [1,2], Patrícia de Fragas Hinnig [1], Jeovani Schmitt [3] , Adriana Soares Lobo [1] , France Bellisle [4], Patrícia Faria Di Pietro [1] , Francilene Kunradi Vieira [1] , Pedro Henrique de Moura Araujo [3]and Dalton Francisco de Andrade [5]

[1] Post Graduate Program in Nutrition, Health Sciences Center, Federal University of Santa Catarina, CCS/UFSC, Campus Trindade, Florianopolis 88040-900, Brazil; malicedeassis@gmail.com (M.A.A.d.A.); phinnig@yahoo.com.br (P.d.F.H.); adri_lobo@hotmail.com (A.S.L.); fariadipietro@gmail.com (P.F.D.P.); frankunradi@gmail.com (F.K.V.)
[2] Post Graduate Program in Physical Education, Sports Center, Federal University of Santa Catarina, CDS/UFSC, Campus Trindade, Florianopolis 88040-900, Brazil
[3] Post Graduate Program in Production Engineering, Technological Center, Federal University of Santa Catarina, University Campus Trindade, Florianopolis 88040-900, Brazil; jeovani.schmitt@yahoo.com.br (J.S.); phma05@gmail.com (P.H.d.M.A.)
[4] Equipe de Recherche en Epidémiologie Nutritionnelle, Centre de Recherche en Epidémiologie et Statistiques, Université Paris 13, Inserm (U1153), Inra (U1125), Cnam, COMUE Sorbonne Paris Cité, Bobigny 93017, France; bellisle@uren.smbh.univ-paris13.fr
[5] Informatics and Statistics Department, Technological Center, Federal University of Santa Catarina, University Campus Trindade, Florianopolis 88040-900, Brazil; daltoncasa@hotmail.com
* Correspondence: danibiazzi@yahoo.com.br; Tel.: +55-48-3721-2279

Received: 9 August 2017; Accepted: 8 September 2017; Published: 6 October 2017

Abstract: The aims of this study were to identify cross-sectional dietary patterns (DPs) in a representative sample of 7–10-year-old schoolchildren, to examine how scores for these DPs tracked over a time period of five years (from age 7–10 years to 12–15 years), and to investigate longitudinal associations between changes in DPs scores and changes in BMI (Body Mass Index) z-scores. Children aged 7–10-years were examined in 2007 (n = 1158) and a subset of the sample participated in a follow-up in 2012 (n = 458). Factor analysis (FA) was applied to derive DPs at baseline. The change in DP from childhood to adolescence was analyzed by comparing factor scores using the complete cases, in which factor loadings were the ones evaluated at baseline. Associations of BMI change with DP change were assessed by multivariate linear regression. At baseline, four DP were identified that explained 47.9% of the food intake variance. On average, the factor scores of "DP II" (salty snacks, French fries, fast-food, sugary beverages) decreased in follow-up, while no changes were observed for "DP I" (rice, cooked beans, beef/poultry, leafy vegetables), "DP III" (fruits, cooked and leafy vegetables, fruit juices, pasta, milk, cheese), and "DP IV" (milk, coffee with milk, cheese, breads/biscuits). No significant linear association was shown between changes in BMI z-scores and changes in DP scores from childhood to adolescence. In conclusion, three out of four DP scores identified at baseline tracked slightly in adolescence.

Keywords: dietary patterns; tracking; children; adolescents; factor analysis

1. Introduction

Establishing healthy eating habits is important during childhood and adolescence, given that these behaviors may have cumulative effects on health and tend to be continued into adulthood [1,2]. The transition in diet from childhood to adolescence marks important changes due to individual factors such as physiological development related to growth and maturation, changes in parental influence, as well as the increasing independence and interaction of adolescents with their social environment [3,4]. Investigating eating behaviors in children longitudinally during the transition into adolescence is important in order to provide information on the nature of individual-level change over time and when, how, and why dietary changes occur [4].

The transition in a child's diet may be affected by socioeconomic and demographic changes within the family [4,5]. In addition, in many emerging and developing countries, as incomes rise and populations experience urbanization, there is a shift from traditional fiber and grain-rich diets to fat, sugar-rich, refined grains, animal fat, and protein diets [6], leading to obesity and diet-related chronic diseases [7].

In epidemiology, tracking is defined as the stability or maintenance of a given constant over time [8]. Dietary tracking values can therefore be considered to demonstrate the preservation of dietary habits, and the consumption of food or nutrients over a period of time [1]. Dietary patterns (DPs) are found to track during infancy [9], to older childhood [10], and from children to adults [1], and then remain stable in adulthood [11]. In children and adolescents there are mixed findings, with some studies reporting stability [1,4,12,13], and others showing changes in DPs [14–17]. The limited available prospective epidemiological evidence consistently indicates that DPs that are high in energy-dense, high-fat, and low-fiber foods predispose young people to overweight and obesity later in life [18–20].

DPs have been identified in some cross-sectional studies in Brazilian children and adolescents [21–26]. None of these studies has investigated the stability of DPs specifically from childhood to adolescence, and their relationship with changes in body mass index.

We have previously reported the association between dietary patterns (derived by latent class analysis) and overweight/obesity in a cross-sectional study of 7 to 10-year-old Brazilian schoolchildren [25]. In the present study, we assessed the stability of DPs in the same children five years later, using confirmatory factor analysis (FA). FA was also used at baseline, as this is currently the most popular method for identifying DPs.

The aims of the present study were (a) to identify cross-sectional DPs in a representative sample of schoolchildren aged 7–10 years old; (b) to examine how scores for these DPs tracked over a time period of five years (from age 7–10 years to 12–15 years) and (c) to investigate longitudinal associations between changes in DPs scores and changes in body mass index (BMI) z-scores.

2. Materials and Methods

2.1. Design and Study Population

A cross-sectional survey designed to investigate the prevalence of overweight/obesity and related behaviors of schoolchildren was conducted in Florianopolis (Brazil) from April to October 2007. The final sample consisted of 1232 children from 17 schools (782 children from 11 public schools and 450 children from six private schools). Detailed sampling procedures have been described elsewhere [27].

In 2012, an active search of all adolescents (12–15 years) surveyed in 2007 was performed using the Brazilian School Census (EducaCenso). However, the collection of data for this second study was restricted to students still enrolled in the same schools as the 2007 survey or transferred to other schools in the metropolitan area of the city. As the schoolchildren search did not occur in other regions of the state or the country, the eligible sample decreased. A total of 494 cohort members from 65 schools were identified and interviewed in 2012 (40.1% of the 2007 participants).

After excluding 74 children at baseline (boys *n* = 44, girls *n* = 30) and 36 adolescents at follow-up (boys *n* = 21, girls *n* = 15) with outlier's data for food intake (i.e., reporting fewer than three food items or with a total daily frequency intake of foods/beverages exceeding three standard deviation scores), 1158 children (581 boys and 577 girls) at baseline and 458 adolescents (213 boys and 245 girls) at follow-up were included in the dietary pattern analyses. Detailed sampling and reasons for follow-up losses are shown in the flowchart (Figure 1).

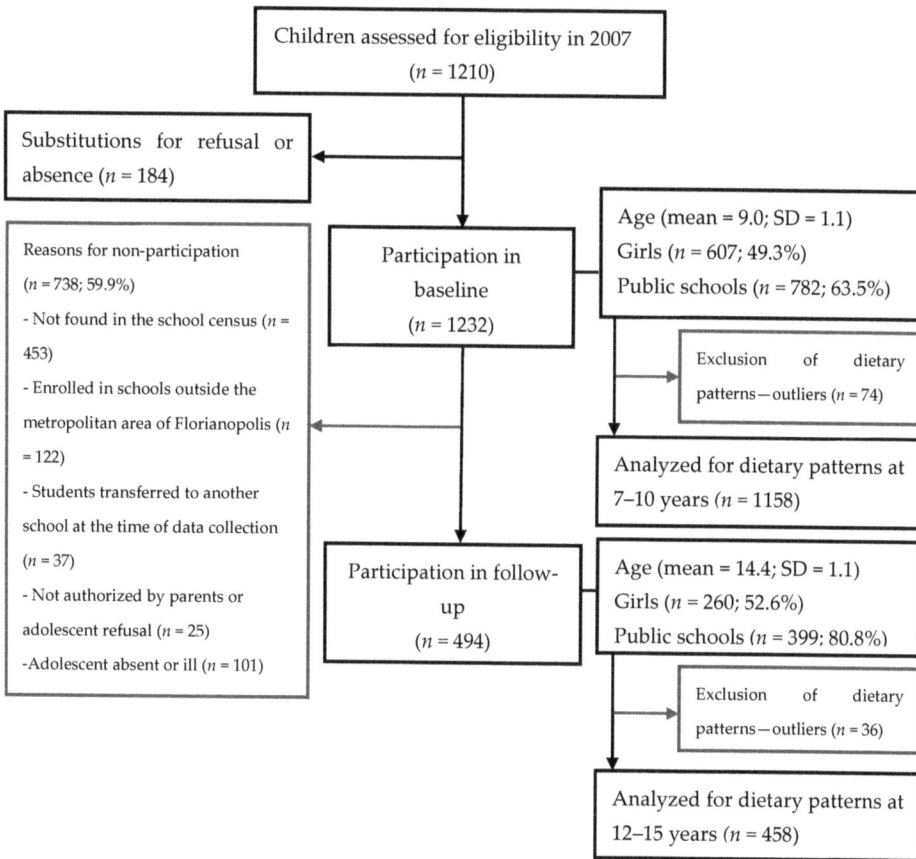

Figure 1. Flowchart of participants in the 2007 survey (7–10-year-olds) and in the 2012 survey (12–15-year-olds).

Both studies were conducted according to the guidelines set out in the Code of Ethics of the World Medical Association (Declaration of Helsinki) and all procedures involving human subjects were approved by the Human Studies Committee of the Federal University of Santa Catarina (07636813.3.0000.0121). Written informed consent was obtained from the parents and oral assent was obtained from the children.

2.2. Dietary Intake

At both time points, dietary data were obtained using the third version of the Previous Day Food Questionnaire (PDFQ-3) [28] based on a single day recall procedure, designed to investigate the consumption frequency of specific foods (not nutrients) as markers of (un)healthy diet and types of physical activities on the previous day. For example, a range of specific foods have been suggested as important dietary determinants of weight status in childhood and adolescence, including fruit and vegetables [29], fat [30], fast-food [31], and sugary drinks [32]. The PDFQ is a paper and pencil questionnaire, designed to be applied in the school setting as a supervised classroom exercise where children are guided by trained researchers following a standardized protocol [28]. The PDFQ-3 was previously validated in a sample of 6–11-year-old schoolchildren, with direct observation of the food eaten at school meals on the previous day as the gold standard, and demonstrated a reasonable average sensitivity (probability of correctly reporting a food intake) of 70.2% and an excellent average specificity (probability of correctly not reporting a food intake) of 96.2% [28]. The food section of the questionnaire covers six daily eating occasions (three main meals and three snacks) ordered chronologically (breakfast and mid-morning snack, lunch and afternoon snack, dinner and evening snack). Each meal and snack is illustrated with 21 pictures of foods/beverages or food groups (bread and biscuits, chocolate milk, coffee with milk, milk, yoghurt, cheese, rice, beans, pasta, beef and poultry, fish and seafood, leafy vegetables, cooked vegetables, vegetable soup, fruits, fruit juices, French fries, pizza and hamburgers, sweets, salty snacks, and soft drinks). The tool does not assess foods or food groups like water, cooking fats, fat, or sugary spreads on bread (e.g., butter or margarine, honey, jam, chocolate or nut-based products), fat content (e.g., low-fat milk or high-fat milk), types of soft drinks and fruit juices (e.g., regular or diet), or types of cooking methods (e.g., frying, baking, roasting).

The foods and food groups illustrated in PDFQ-3 were selected in order to represent the food patterns of children in this age group, foods presented in school menus, and foods recommended in the guidelines for the Brazilian population [33]. Supplementary Figure S1 shows one page of the questionnaire.

The PDFQ-3 was assessed once at each time point for every child, and the day at which the PDFQ-3 was assessed differed between children. This strategy was used in order to describe the daily variability of dietary intake on schooldays (Monday to Thursday) and non-school days (Sunday and holidays) allowing for the analysis of food consumption at the group level. In the 2007 survey, 71.3% (n = 826) of the participants reported food intake on weekdays/schooldays (16.8% on Monday; 22.1% on Tuesday; 17.2% on Wednesday; 15.2% on Thursday), and 28.7% (n = 332) on Sunday/holidays (non-schooldays). As the PDFQ-3 was applied in the school setting and there was no school on Saturdays and Sundays, it was not possible to obtain data representing food consumption for Fridays and Saturdays. Portion sizes were not assessed; therefore, the food intake could not be quantified by weight or energy and instead the (relative) frequency of intake was used as an indicator for the factors. However, number of servings per day (frequency) is routinely used to determine empirical dietary patterns [34–36]. The frequency of food intake was estimated as number of times per day, ranging from 0 to 6 for each food/beverage consumed, assuming that only one serving was consumed on each occasion.

2.3. Physical Activity

In the physical activity section of the PDFQ-3, schoolchildren were asked to report their physical activities (walking/running, playing with a dog, cycling, swimming, playing ball games, jumping rope, athletics, climbing stairs, roller skating/blading, dancing, and helping with household chores). The validation of the physical activity section of the questionnaire using comparisons between the scores generated by the instrument and the number of step counts obtained by pedometers showed mean values for sensitivity and specificity of 78% and 56%, respectively [37]. In the present study, metabolic equivalents (METs) were assigned to each activity reported using the Compendium of Energy Expenditures for Youth [38] and summed for all physical activities (PA) reported by each child. PA in terms of metabolic equivalents (PA MET) were categorized into tertiles (the first tertile was defined as lowest, second tertile as intermediary, and third tertile as highest METs). This scoring method was validated in Brazilian children in a previous study [39].

2.4. Anthropometric and Sociodemographic Measurements

The administrative department of each school provided information on the child's date of birth, sex, and type of school (an important marker of socioeconomic condition in Brazil). Trained research staff measured weight and height of participants following standard techniques [40] in both surveys. Theoretical and practical workshops on measurement techniques were held to standardize the anthropometric measurements in both surveys [41]. Anthropometric measurements were taken with the children wearing light clothes and without shoes. Weight was measured with a digital 180 kg scale (Marte®, model PP, 50 g precision). Height was measured with a portable stadiometer (Alturexata®, 1 mm precision). Body mass index (BMI) was computed as weight (in kg) divided by the square of height (in m). Parents completed a self-administered questionnaire reporting their weight, height, and monthly family income. Monthly family income was defined as a categorical variable taking into account the minimum wage at both time points (<3; $\geq$3 and <5; $\geq$5 and <10; $\geq$10). Maternal weight status was assessed by BMI based on self-reported weight (kg) and height (m). Type of school was constructed as a dichotomous variable (public or private). Children's age was computed as the difference between the date of birth and the date of measurements.

At both time points, children's BMI data was converted into z-scores (according to age and sex) based on the World Health Organization Growth References (WHO-2007) [42]. Weight status of children (baseline) and adolescents (follow-up) were then categorized as non-overweight (N-OW) (BMI-for-age < +1.0 SD) or overweight including obesity (OW) (BMI-for-age $\geq$ +1.0 SD). Underweight (0.8%) and normal weight children were grouped together into the N-OW category, while overweight (non-obese) and obese (6.7%) children were grouped into the OW category. Weight status change was based on individual changes from childhood to early adolescence. In the regression analysis, the change in BMI z-score (BMI z-score at follow-up − BMI z-score at baseline) was modeled as a continuous variable in order to consider the entire distribution of weight status among the whole study population.

2.5. Statistical Analysis

In order to identify DPs in a representative sample of 7–10-year-old schoolchildren, exploratory FA with principal component estimation was applied to the total sample at baseline (n = 1158). A polychoric correlation model for categorical ordered data was used. The number of factors to retain was first examined by the chi-squared test, which showed that the five-factor solution provided the best fit of the a priori model (baseline FA) ($\chi^2(12)$ = 31.51, p < 0.01). However, the four-factor solution produced better interpretability, which was confirmed by the common practice to choose components with Eigenvalues >1.5 to limit the factors [43], and by the examination of the Scree plot (Figure S2). After the choice of the number of factors, the factor loadings of foods items were calculated. Those foods/beverages that showed low loadings for all factors were excluded from the analysis (yoghurt, sweets, fish and vegetable soup), as they did not explain any factor. After the exclusion of those foods, FA was performed again, and four major dietary patterns were considered as best representing the data. The varimax orthogonal rotation was carried out in order to simplify the interpretation of the data, maximizing the higher factor loadings and minimizing the lower ones. Variables with factor loadings $\geq$0.30 or $\leq$−0.30 were considered important for the interpretability of the factors. For the total sample in 2007, the factor scores for each DP were calculated at the individual level by summing the observed standardized frequencies of consumption per food/beverage, weighted according to the absolute factor loadings. The factor scores were standardized and the group mean factor scores were set to zero.

A confirmatory analysis for the complete cases (n = 458) in 2012 was used, in which all factor loadings were the ones evaluated at baseline. This allowed the comparisons in mean factor scores between the same children at follow-up. Using this approach, the changes in factor scores reflected actual differences in the intake frequency of foods/beverages identifying the factor (pattern) rather than a change in the individuals' relative rank position compared to the group mean intake frequency [44].

A high factor score for a given pattern indicated high frequency intake of the foods constituting that food pattern, and a low score indicated low frequency intake of those foods. Factors were labeled by numbers (I, II, III, IV) according to the variance explained and were interpreted according to the food groups that loaded highly on each pattern.

Tracking was defined as how stable the factor scores identified at baseline in the complete-cases sample remained at follow-up. Paired *t* test was used to determine whether the mean factor scores difference between the completers was zero. Spearman's correlation was calculated between the factor scores obtained at each time point. The power analysis of these effects was analyzed considering the effect size measured with Cohen's *d* parameters: <0.2 = small effect, 0.2 to 0.8 = medium, and >0.8 = large [45].

Multivariate linear regression was used to examine the changes in BMI z-scores (defined as the difference between BMI z-score at follow-up and at baseline) associated to changes in each dietary pattern scores (the difference between dietary patterns scores at follow-up and at baseline), simultaneously. The potential confounding variables in the multiple regression models were: child's age (continuous), sex, BMI z-scores (continuous), maternal BMI (continuous), type of school (private or public), monthly family income (categorical), day of the week (school days or Sunday/holidays), and tertiles of PA MET at baseline. The maternal BMI was included in the model, as there is a solid body of evidence on both genetic and environmental parental influence on children's dietary patterns [9,23]. All the covariates were chosen among a range of possible confounders because they were both associated with BMI and with food intake. Interaction terms were not used, as preliminary analyses did not find important examples of interaction, as well as to avoid over-adjustment and chance findings (data not shown).

To investigate if the DPs differed on school days compared with non-school days (Sunday and holidays), exploratory FA with principal component estimation was applied to baseline data for children who reported their food intake on school days using the same analytical approach described above for the complete baseline data. The factor scores obtained on school days were standardized and the group mean factor scores were set to zero and used as a reference. Then, the factor scores for non-school days were computed in a simple confirmatory FA model, in which the loadings on the four factors were those evaluated at school days. One-sample *t* test was used to test the differences between the mean factor scores for non-school days versus school days.

Considering that the sample size available for analyses was restricted to complete cases (*n* = 458), with 80% test power and alpha error of 5%, the study was able to detect an effect size of at least 0.131 for the two-tail paired *t*-test; at least 0.165 for the one-tail Spearman's rho; and at least 0.027 in the multivariate linear regression.

Statistical significance level was set at 5%. Statistical software R [46] was used for factor analysis and Stata 13.0 (Stata Corp., College Station, TX, USA) was used for descriptive and analytical statistics.

3. Results

The total baseline characteristics of participants at age 7 to 10 years (*n* = 1158), including children participating in the follow-up survey (*n* = 458) or lost to follow-up (*n* = 700), are shown in Table 1. There were no differences for age, sex, BMI, prevalence of overweight, mother's weight status, monthly family income, day of the week, and tertiles of PA MET. Nevertheless, a greater proportion of children enrolled in private schools were lost in the follow-up.

Table 1. Characteristics of the study participants by follow-up status.

	Not Followed-Up (*n* = 700)	Followed-Up (*n* = 458)	Total Baseline (*n* = 1158)
		Mean ± SD (95% CI)	
Age (years)	9.1 ± 1.2 (8.9–9.1)	9.0 ± 1.1 (8.9–9.2)	9.0 ± 1.1 (8.9–9.1)
BMI	17.8 ± 2.8 (17.5–18.0)	17.6 ± 2.9 (17.2–17.8)	17.7 ± 2.9 (17.5–17.7)
		% (95% CI)	
Sex			
Boys	49.4 (45.7–53.1)	46.5 (42.0–51.1)	48.3 (45.4–51.2)
Girls	50.6 (46.9–54.3)	53.5 (48.9–58.0)	51.7 (48.8–54.6)
Overweight [a]			
Yes	34.3 (30.9–37.9)	34.3 (30.1–38.8)	34.3 (31.6–37.1)
No	65.7 (62.1–69.1)	65.7 (61.2–69.9)	65.7 (62.9–68.4)
Type of school			
Public	70.4 (66.9–73.7)	86.2 (82.8–89.1)	76.7 (74.2–79.0)
Private	29.6 (26.3–33.1)	13.3 (10.9–17.2)	23.3 (21.0–25.8)
Mother's weight status [b]			
Thin	3.5 (2.3–5.2)	5.5 (3.7–8.1)	4.3 (3.2–5.7)
Normal weight	65.9 (62.2–69.4)	63.0 (58.4–67.5)	64.8 (61.9–67.6)
Overweight	22.6 (19.5–25.9)	20.8 (17.2–24.9)	21.9 (19.5–24.4)
Obese	8.0 (6.2–10.4)	10.6 (8.0–13.9)	9.1 (7.5–10.9)
Monthly family income (minimum wage) [c]			
<3	45.4 (41.4–49.5)	47.3 (42.4–52.3)	46.2 (43.1–49.3)
3–5	20.0 (16.9–23.4)	26.8 (22.7–31.4)	22.7 (20.2–25.5)
5–10	19.9 (16.9–23.4)	15.2 (12.0–19.1)	18.0 (15.8–20.6)
>10	14.7 (12.0–17.8)	10.7 (7.9–14.1)	13.1 (11.1–15.3)
Day of the week [d]			
Non-school days	32.9 (29.5–36.4)	22.3 (18.7–26.3)	28.7 (26.1–31.4)
School days	67.1 (63.6–70.5)	77.7 (73.7–81.3)	71.3 (68.7–73.9)
Tertiles of PA MET			
Lowest	35.0 (31.5–38.6)	32.5 (28.4–37.0)	34.0 (31.3–36.8)
Medium	32.4 (29.1–36.0)	33.0 (28.8–37.4)	32.6 (30.0–35.4)
Highest	32.6 (29.2–36.1)	34.5 (30.3–39.0)	33.3 (30.7–36.1)

PA MET: Physical activities in terms of metabolic equivalents; BMI: Body mass index; WHO: World Health Organization; [a] Overweight (including obesity BMI ≥ +1.0 z-scores—WHO-2007); [b] BMI based on self-reported data on weight and height and classified according to WHO recommendations (Thin—BMI <18.5 kg/m^2, Normal weight—BMI 18.5–24.9 kg/m^2, Overweight non-obese BMI 25–29.9 kg/m^2, Obese—BMI ≥30 kg/m^2); [c] 1 minimum wage = $US 204.30 ($BR 380): September 2007 exchange rate; [d] Day of the week. Missing mother's weight status data (4.0%); Missing income data (15.3%); Missing child's BMI (1.7%).

After computing the FA on the 17 foods/beverages at baseline, four DPs were identified with the highest Eigenvalues that accounted for 47.9% of the total variance of food intake and could be interpreted meaningfully in terms of nutritional characteristics. The detailed structures of the four DPs with their explained variance and loading coefficients are shown in Table 2. The "DP I" had positive high loadings on rice, cooked beans, leafy vegetables, and beef/poultry, while having negative loadings on pasta and fast-food, suggesting that the intake of these foods showed a deviation from this DP. The high loading foods on "DP II" included French fries, salty snacks, soft drinks, and fast-food. The "DP III" loaded highly on fruit juices, cooked vegetables, fruits, pasta, leafy vegetables, cheese and milk, with a negative loading on soft drinks. Finally, the "DP IV" loaded highly on coffee with milk, breads/biscuits, cheese and milk, with negative loadings on chocolate milk and fast-food (Table 2).

Table 2. Structures of four dietary patterns identified by factor analysis with principal component method in a representative sample of 7–10-year-old schoolchildren in 2007.

	Dietary Patterns 2007 (*n* = 1158)			
	DP I	DP II	DP III	DP IV
Variance explained (%)	17.5	10.7	10.0	9.7
Foods and food groups	Factor loadings [a]			
Beans (cooked)	**0.66**	−0.22	0.16	0.08
Beef/poultry	**0.30**	0.08	0.08	0.07
Bread/biscuits	0.04	−0.07	0.19	**0.54**
Cheese	**−0.34**	−0.28	**0.40**	**0.41**
Chocolate milk	−0.17	−0.09	0.21	**−0.58**
Coffee with milk	0.01	0.05	−0.08	**0.90**
Fast-food	**−0.41**	**0.31**	0.04	**−0.31**
French fries	−0.07	**0.85**	0.04	−0.10
Fruit juices	0.07	−0.07	**0.71**	−0.07
Fruits	0.16	0.03	**0.50**	0.00
Leafy vegetables	**0.57**	0.11	**0.40**	0.00
Milk	0.08	−0.08	**0.34**	**0.36**
Pasta	**−0.46**	0.22	**0.49**	0.15
Rice	**0.84**	−0.09	0.08	0.04
Salty snacks	0.08	**0.84**	−0.05	0.09
Soft drinks	−0.27	**0.49**	**−0.32**	−0.02
Vegetables (cooked)	0.21	−0.15	**0.54**	0.04

[a] Factor loading values in bold: ≥ 0.30 or ≤ -0.30.

Table 3 shows mean factor scores of the four dietary patterns at the two time points in the complete cases (*n* = 458), spearman correlations coefficients between factor scores at the two time points, and the effect size for each analysis. Considering the difference between the mean factors scores at the two time points, our sample allows us to conclude that only the scores for DP II differed between the two time points, with a medium effect size. The sample size of the follow-up has sufficient power to show correlations between factor scores of DPs I, III, and IV at the two time points, with a medium effect size. These findings together imply that children presenting higher scores for DP I, DP III, and DP IV at baseline also showed higher scores for the respective DPs at follow-up, and the mean frequencies of consumption of foods constituting these patterns did not increase. On the other hand, no correlation was found for DP II scores between baseline and follow-up and the mean frequency of consumption of the foods constituting the pattern decreased (Table 3).

Table 3. Mean (standard deviation), spearman correlation coefficients, and effect size for corresponding factor scores at each time point in the complete cases (*n* = 458).

	DP I	DP II	DP III	DP IV
	Mean (SD)			
Baseline	−0.04 (1.2)	−0.02 (1.1)	0.07 (1.1)	0.03 (1.3)
Follow-up	0.06 (1.2)	−0.39 (1.0)	−0.07 (1.1)	−0.08 (1.1)
p	0.13	<0.01	0.03	0.15
Effect size	0.07	0.25	0.10	0.07
	Spearman Correlation			
Baseline vs. Follow-up	0.20	0.07	0.22	0.10
p	<0.01	0.12	<0.01	0.03
Effect size	0.41	0.14	0.45	0.20

After controlling for baseline BMI z-scores, maternal BMI, sex, age, type of school, family income, day of the week, and tertiles of PA MET, there was no significant linear association between changes in BMI z-scores and changes in DP scores from childhood to adolescence. The analysis of the change in DP scores showed a small effect size on the change of BMI z-scores (Table 4). Based on the weight status categories defined by WHO-2007, out of the 153 children classified as overweight or obese at baseline, 65.4% (*n* = 100) remained overweight/obese in adolescence (boys: 69.8%; girls: 59.7%). Out of the 297 children classified as non-overweight at baseline, 9.4% (*n* = 28) were found to be overweight/obese (boys: 4.8%; girls: 9.8%) at follow-up.

Table 4. Relation between changes in BMI z-scores and changes in factor scores from ages 7–10 years to 12–15 years in the complete cases.

Change in Dietary Pattern	Change in BMI z-Scores [a]		
	Coefficient	*p*	Effect Size
DP I	0.01	0.92	0.00
DP II	0.02	0.45	0.00
DP III	−0.04	0.19	0.00
DP IV	0.05	0.07	0.01

[a] Outcome change in BMI z-scores (*n* = 450) over the five years since baseline; Adjusted by age (continuous), sex, BMI z-score, maternal BMI, type of school, family income, day of the week (school days or non-school days), and tertiles of PA MET (all baseline).

The FA on the same 17 foods/beverages applied at baseline in the sample who reported food intake on school days also identified four DPs with higher Eigenvalues that explained 49.0% of the food intake variance (Table S1). One-sample *t* test showed that the two DP scores (DP I and DP II) for non-school days were statistically different from zero, i.e., food intake on non-school days differed from school days for these patterns (Table S2).

4. Discussion

The longitudinal analysis of the present study conducted with the complete cases of children and adolescents five years apart showed that, on average, the factor scores for "DP II" (French fries, salty snacks, soft drinks and fast-food) identified at baseline (in 7–10-year-old children) decreased in the follow-up sample (in 12–15-year-olds), whereas no changes were observed for "DP I" (rice, cooked beans, leafy vegetables, beef/poultry), "DP III" (fruit juices, cooked vegetables, fruits, pasta, leafy vegetables, cheese and milk), and "DP IV" (coffee with milk, breads/biscuits, cheese and milk).

Cross-sectional analysis of data obtained at baseline identified four DPs that satisfactorily captured eating behavior (47.9% of food intake variance explained) in this population-based sample of Brazilian schoolchildren. These DPs were also identified in our previous study that extracted DPs by Latent class analysis (LCA) based on the time-of-day of eating events [25] and resembled other patterns identified in Brazilian and international studies conducted in children and adolescents. "DP I" in the present study (including rice and beans) was also identified in studies based on the Brazilian Household Budget Surveys (2002–2003) [47] and (2008–2009) [23]. The latter, conducted in individuals over 10 years of age, confirmed the aggregation of DPs among members of the same family and extracted three major DPs by factor analysis: "Traditional snack" (coffee, rolls, oils and fats, cheese), "Traditional main meal" (rice, beans and other legumes, and meat) and "Fast-food snack" (sandwiches, processed meats, soft drinks, snacks, pizza) [23] in line with "DP I" and "DP II" (salty snacks, French fries, fast-food and sugary beverages) of the present study. The "DP II" in the present study shared various dietary items of high fat and high energy-density items with other studies of children and adolescents in Brazil [21,22], Colombia [48], Canada [49], and European countries [1,35,50,51]. Our "DP III" (fruit juices, cooked vegetables, fruits, pasta, leafy vegetables, cheese and milk) was similar to the "health aware/conscious" pattern associated with lower fat gain in girls between 9 and 11 years of age in the Avon Study in England [52,53].

On average, the factor scores for "DP II" (French fries, salty snacks, soft drinks, and fast-food) identified at baseline (in 7–10-year-old children) decreased in the follow-up sample (12–15-year-olds), whereas no changes were observed for "DP I" (rice, cooked beans, leafy vegetables, and beef/poultry), "DP III" (fruit juices, cooked vegetables, fruits, pasta, leafy vegetables, cheese and milk), and "DP IV" (coffee with milk, breads/biscuits, cheese and milk). Although food consumption was only assessed for one day in the present study and considerable within-subject variation in daily food consumption may occur, our results provide evidence of slight stability of three DP scores (DP I, III, IV) as well as change in "DP II" scores over the five-year follow-up period.

Direct comparisons of the present results with previous DP studies in children and adolescents should consider differences in study design, sample sizes, dietary assessment methods, and statistical methods to derive DPs and to estimate the tracking of DPs. Furthermore, the extent of changes of DP from childhood to adolescence may vary in different populations due to cultural, social, and economic factors. A review of the literature found that the tracking of DPs ranged from weak to moderate between childhood and adolescence [54].

The stability of the mean factor scores for "DP I" (rice, cooked beans, beef/poultry, leafy vegetables) and "DP IV" (milk, coffee with milk, cheese, and breads/biscuits) from childhood to adolescence may be explained by cultural factors. The components of these patterns are traditional foods eaten in Brazilian meals ("DP I" in lunch and/or dinner; "DP IV" in breakfast and/or snacks between meals). These patterns were also identified in cross-sectional studies conducted with children [22,24,25], adolescents [21,22,26], and adults [55] from different regions in Brazil.

We expected to observe an increase in scores for "DP II" (salty snacks, French fries, fast-food, and sugary beverages) at follow-up. However, this was not the case in our study, and the decrease in its factor scores at follow-up might result from a social desirability bias (underreporting). It is also possible that adolescents at follow-up consumed larger portions of the unhealthy foods constituting "DP II", but less frequently. We cannot investigate this hypothesis because the PDFQ-3 did not measure portion sizes. Therefore, energy intake could not be estimated and input variables for DP analysis could not be adjusted for energy intake. The issue of adjusting for energy intake is still controversial in studies of changes in DPs [34].

The present study did not find a significant linear association between changes in DP scores and changes in BMI z-scores. The longitudinal association of a high adherence to unhealthy DPs with increased risk of overweight and obesity was not verified in some earlier studies [12,56]. In the European DONALD study [57], a positive though small association between baseline consumption of high-energy convenience foods and the change in the percentage of body fat over a five-year follow-up was found among boys. A cohort of 5–12-year-old children from low- and middle-income families in Bogota showed that those in the highest quartile of adherence to a snacking pattern had a 0.09 kg/m^2 higher BMI gain and 0.012 mm higher gain in trunk adiposity per year compared to children in the lowest quartile [48].

The strengths of the present study were the longitudinal follow-up design based on a relatively large sample size at baseline, the use of the same validated questionnaire to assess food intake at the two time points, the use of potential confounding variables in the regression analysis, and the application of confirmatory FA to compute factor scores over time. An important feature of our analysis, which was rarely present in previous longitudinal studies on the tracking of DPs [19,44], is that we applied confirmatory FA to calculate factor scores at follow-up by using the factor loadings obtained at baseline. By using this approach to compute the factor scores, the problem of the data dependency and lower reproducibility of factors in different datasets is eliminated [44]. When exploratory FA is used to identify DPs and to investigate their stability over time, the correlation between foods is commonly used to create multiple continuous scores at each time point. A difficulty inherent in this approach is that the DPs obtained are not generally reproducible. The performance of separate exploratory FA at each time point to evaluate tracking may result in high correlations between pattern scores at baseline and at follow-up, despite large changes in the correlations between the specific food items that define a pattern [11].

We acknowledge some limitations in the present study. First, the retention rate in the follow-up study (40.1%) was low, limiting the generalizability of our results to the general population. It could be argued that changes in DP scores from childhood to adolescence were a result of attrition biases. However, children lost to follow-up did not differ significantly from the included participants in DP scores, demographic variables, and weight status at baseline. Therefore, we believe that the low correlations found between the baseline factor scores of DPs I, III, and IV and its scores at follow-up were not affected by such bias. We cannot exclude the possibility that the lack of association found between changes in DPs and changes in BMI z-score could be due to the underrepresentation of adolescents who studied in private schools (wealthier than adolescents from public schools in Brazil) in the follow-up study.

Second, as for all other dietary assessment studies, the self-reported food recall may potentially be subject to misreporting. The PDFQ-3 used in this study proved to be a valid instrument [28] and has been used to assess dietary patterns and behaviors [25,26,58]. The PDFQ-3 was designed to avoid the difficulties associated with children's assessments of portion size, and to simplify the memory task by prompting only the relevant food items eaten on the previous day. The cognitive task required for estimating portion size, frequency, and averaging may not be compatible with the perceptual and conceptual capacities of children who have not reached the stage of abstract reasoning at approximately 10–11 years of age [59,60]. Like some questionnaires validated in other countries [35,61], this approach keeps the questionnaire relatively brief and easy for the child to complete with minimal assistance. Also, the dietary information is derived from the children themselves (without help from parents or guardians). The use of the parent report of a child's diet has also been seen as a limitation [35,62]. In the age range of the present study (7–15 years), children spend a considerable amount of time unsupervised by their parents, who therefore could not validate the children's dietary recall.

The results are based on the frequency of food/beverage and food groups eaten on only one day in each time point in a group of children and conclusions may be applicable to the population rather than to individuals, since a single day of intake may not be representative of usual individual intake. The expected effect of use a food questionnaire that only covers one day of dietary intake is to attenuate the statistical association between changes in adherence to a dietary pattern and changes in BMI z-score [15,63].

The differences in DP between weekdays/schooldays and non-schooldays found in the present study should be highlighted, and in this sense our results are strengthened by a good coverage of the days of the week (school days), including one day of the weekend (Sunday) and holidays to cover the variation in diet at the group level. While the factor scores for "DP I" on weekdays/school days with high loadings for unhealthy foods (fast-foods, French fries, salty snacks, and soft drinks) increased on Sunday/non-school days ($p < 0.01$), the factor scores for "DP II" with high loadings for foods included in Brazilian traditional lunch and/or dinner (rice, beans, beef/poultry) decreased on Sunday/non-school days ($p < 0.01$), thus indicating that specific foods eaten on non-schooldays were less healthy. Changes in daily patterns such as not attending school on the weekend contribute significantly to changes in dietary patterns of food consumption, patterns of physical activity, and ultimately energy balance [64]. Previous research in children indicates that dietary quality is poorer on the weekends compared with weekdays, with significantly higher intakes of total sugars [62], sugar sweetened beverages, confectionery, and lower consumption of fruit and vegetables [62,65]. The potential influence of day-to-day variation of food consumption in the FA merits more attention in future research.

In future studies, information on children's diet from the PDFQ-3 should be integrated with a food frequency questionnaire filled in by parents to complement the measure of food items not covered by the child's questionnaire. In addition, the PDFQ-3 should be applied on various days of the week, including one day of the weekend at each time point, assuring that the child completes the PDFQ-3 on the same day of the week at each time point.

Additionally, although we adjusted for a variety of potential confounding variables, residual confounding cannot be ruled out. In particular, adjustments for social mobility, which expresses life-long changes in family income [5], and which might affect dietary habits and changes in weight status, were not possible due to the lack of information.

5. Conclusions

Four dietary patterns were identified at baseline in schoolchildren aged 7–10 years old: "DP I" (rice, cooked beans, beef/poultry, leafy vegetables), "DP II" (salty snacks, French fries, fast-food, sugary beverages), "DP III" (fruits, cooked and leafy vegetables, fruit juices, pasta, milk, cheese) and "DP IV" (milk, coffee with milk, cheese, breads/biscuits). Slight tracking was observed between factor scores for "DP I", "DP III", and "DP IV" from childhood to adolescence using the complete cases, while the factor scores for "DP II" decreased in follow-up. No significant linear association was shown between changes in BMI z-scores and changes in DP scores over a five-year period.

We cannot be certain that the level of tracking of dietary patterns found in the present study reflected a real finding or resulted from an artifact due to change in intake from a single day in childhood to a single day in adolescence. We intend to address this in the next follow-up of the study by taking repeated dietary assessments during childhood and adolescence.

Supplementary Materials: The following are available online at http://www.mdpi.com/2072-6643/9/10/1098/s1, Figure S1: The Previous Day Food Questionnaire (PDFQ-3), page 2., Figure S2: Scree plot for identification of dietary patterns (components) by factor analysis (FA) with principal component estimation, Table S1: Structures of four dietary patterns identified by factor analysis with the principal component method on baseline cross-sectional data on school days., Table S2: Factor scores on non-school days versus school days (reference) and significance of difference, as assessed by one-sample *t* test.

Acknowledgments: The survey was funded by the Brazilian National Council for Scientific and Technological Development—CNPq (grants 402322/2005-3 and 483955/2011-6), (M.A.A.d.A. grants no. 305148/2011-7 and 308352/2016-5). D.B.L. and A.S.L. received a fellowship from the Brazilian Federal Agency for the Improvement of Higher Education and the Foundation of Research from Santa Catarina State, respectively. The funding sources had no role in the study design; collection, analysis, and interpretation of data; writing of the report; or the decision to submit the article for publication.

Author Contributions: The authors' responsibilities were as follows: D.B.L. and P.F.H. participated in the concept, data analysis and interpretation, and preparation of the paper. M.A.A.d.A. participated in design, ethics submission, supervised the study implementation, interpretation and preparation of the paper. A.S.L., F.B., P.F.D.P. and F.K.V assisted with interpretation and reviewed the paper. D.F.A., J.S. and P.H.d.M.A. assisted with data analysis, interpretation and reviewed the paper. All authors had final approval of the submitted and published versions.

Conflicts of Interest: The authors declare no conflict of interest.

References

1. Mikkila, V.; Rasanen, L.; Raitakari, O.T.; Pietinen, P.; Viikari, J. Consistent dietary patterns identified from childhood to adulthood: The cardiovascular risk in Young Finns Study. *Br. J. Nutr.* **2005**, *93*, 923–931. [CrossRef] [PubMed]

2. Craigie, A.M.; Lake, A.A.; Kelly, S.A.; Adamson, A.J.; Mathers, J.C. Tracking of obesity-related behaviors from childhood to adulthood: A systematic review. *Maturitas* **2011**, *70*, 266–284. [CrossRef] [PubMed]

3. Due, P.; Krølner, R.; Rasmussen, M.; Andersen, A.; TrabDamsgaard, M.; Graham, H.; Holstein, B.E. Pathways and mechanisms in adolescence contribute to adult health inequalities. *Scand. J. Public Health* **2011**, *39*, 62–78. [CrossRef] [PubMed]

4. Totland, T.H.; Gebremariam, M.K.; Lien, N.; Bjelland, M.; Grydeland, M.; Bergh, I.H.; Klepp, K.I.; Andersen, L.F. Does tracking of dietary behaviors differ by parental education in children during the transition into adolescence? *Public Health Nutr.* **2013**, *16*, 673–682. [CrossRef] [PubMed]

5. Arruda, S.P.; da Silva, A.A.; Kac, G.; Goldani, M.Z.; Bettiol, H.; Barbieri, M.A. Socioeconomic and demographic factors are associated with dietary patterns in a cohort of young Brazilian adults. *BMC Public Health* **2014**, *14*, 654. [CrossRef] [PubMed]

6. Popkin, B.M.; Gordon-Larsen, P. The nutrition transition: An overview of world patterns of change. *Nutr. Rev.* **2004**, *62*, S140–S143. [CrossRef] [PubMed]

7. Hawkes, C.; Chopra, M.; Friel, S. Globalization, Trade, and the Nutrition Transition. In *Globalization and Health: Pathways, Evidence and Policy*; Labonté, R., Schrecker, C., Eds.; Routledge: New York, NY, USA, 2009; pp. 235–262.

8. Twisk, J.W.R. *Applied Longitudinal Data Analysis for Epidemiology: A Practical Guide*; Cambridge University Press: Cambridge, UK, 2007.

9. Robinson, S.; Marriott, L.; Poole, J.; Crozier, S.; Borland, S.; Lawrence, W.; Law, C.; Godfrey, K.; Cooper, C.; Inskip, H. Dietary patterns in infancy: The importance of maternal and family influences on feeding practice. *Br. J. Nutr.* **2007**, *98*, 1029–1037. [CrossRef] [PubMed]

10. Northstone, K.; Emmett, P.M. Are dietary patterns stable throughout early and mid-childhood? A birth cohort study. *Br. J. Nutr.* **2008**, *100*, 1069–1076. [CrossRef] [PubMed]

11. Northstone, K.; Emmett, P.M. A comparison of methods to assess changes in dietary patterns from pregnancy to 4 years post-partum obtained using principal components analysis. *Br. J. Nutr.* **2008**, *99*, 1099–1106. [CrossRef] [PubMed]

12. Oellingrath, I.M.; Svendsen, M.V.; Brantsaeter, A.L. Tracking of eating patterns and overweight: A follow-up study of Norwegian schoolchildren from middle childhood to early adolescence. *Nutr. J.* **2011**, *10*, 106. [CrossRef] [PubMed]

13. Bull, C.J.; Northstone, K. Childhood dietary patterns and cardiovascular risk factors in adolescence: Results from the Avon Longitudinal Study of Parents and Children (ALSPAC) cohort. *Public Health Nutr.* **2016**, *19*, 3369–3377. [CrossRef] [PubMed]

14. Lytle, L.A.; Seifert, S.; Greenstein, J.; McGovern, P. How do children's eating patterns and food choices change over time? Results from a cohort study. *Am. J. Health Promot.* **2000**, *14*, 222–228. [CrossRef] [PubMed]

15. Patterson, E.; Warnberg, J.; Kearney, J.; Sjostrom, M. The tracking of dietary intakes of children and adolescents in Sweden over six years: The European Youth Heart Study. *Int. J. Behav. Nutr. Phys. Act.* **2009**, *6*, 91. [CrossRef] [PubMed]

16. Demory-Luce, D.; Morales, M.; Nicklas, T.; Baranowski, T.; Zakeri, I.; Berenson, G. Changes in food group consumption patterns from childhood to young adulthood: The Bogalusa Heart Study. *J. Am. Diet. Assoc.* **2004**, *104*, 1684–1691. [CrossRef] [PubMed]

17. Harris, C.; Flexeder, C.; Thiering, E.; Buyken, A.; Berdel, D.; Koletzko, S.; Bauer, C.P.; Brüske, I.; Koletzko, B.; Standl, M.; et al. Changes in dietary intake during puberty and their determinants: Results from the GINIplus birth cohort study. *BMC Public Health* **2015**, *15*, 841. [CrossRef] [PubMed]

18. Ambrosini, G.L. Childhood dietary patterns and later obesity: A review of the evidence. *Proc. Nutr. Soc.* **2014**, *73*, 137–146. [CrossRef] [PubMed]

19. Ambrosini, G.L.; Emmett, P.M.; Northstone, K.; Jebb, S.A. Tracking a dietary pattern associated with increased adiposity in childhood and adolescence. *Obesity* **2014**, *22*, 458–465. [CrossRef] [PubMed]

20. Wilks, D.C.; Mander, A.P.; Jebb, S.A.; Thompson, S.G.; Sharp, S.J.; Turner, R.M.; Lindroos, A.K. Dietary energy density and adiposity: Employing bias adjustments in a meta-analysis of prospective studies. *BMC Public Health* **2011**, *11*, 48. [CrossRef] [PubMed]

21. Rodrigues, P.R.; Pereira, R.A.; Cunha, D.B.; Sichieri, R.; Ferreira, M.G.; Vilela, A.A.; Gonçalves-Silva, R.M. Factors associated with dietary patterns in adolescents: A school-based study in Cuiabá, Mato Grosso. *Rev. Bras. Epidemiol.* **2012**, *15*, 662–674. [CrossRef] [PubMed]

22. Santos, N.H.; Fiaccone, R.L.; Barreto, M.L.; Silva, L.A.; Silva Rde, C. Association between eating patterns and body mass index in a sample of children and adolescents in Northeastern Brazil. *Cad. Saude Publica* **2014**, *30*, 2235–2245. [CrossRef]

23. Massarani, F.A.; Cunha, D.B.; Muraro, A.P.; Souza Bda, S.; Sichieri, R.; Yokoo, E.M. Familial aggregation and dietary patterns in the Brazilian population. *Cad. Saude Publica* **2015**, *31*, 2535–2545. [CrossRef] [PubMed]

24. Carvalho, C.A.; Fonsêca, P.C.; Nobre, L.N.; Priore, S.E.; FranceschiniSdo, C. Methods of a posteriori identification of food patterns in Brazilian children: A systematic review. *Cien. Saude Colet.* **2016**, *21*, 143–154. [CrossRef] [PubMed]

25. Kupek, E.; Lobo, A.S.; Leal, D.B.; Bellisle, F.; de Assis, M.A. Dietary patterns associated with overweight and obesity among Brazilian schoolchildren: An approach based on the time-of-day of eating events. *Br. J. Nutr.* **2016**, *116*, 1954–1965. [CrossRef] [PubMed]

26. Pinho, M.G.M.; Adami, F.; Benedet, J.; Vasconcelos, F.A.G. Association between screen time and dietary patterns and overweight/obesity among adolescents. *Rev. Nutr.* **2017**, *30*, 377–389. [CrossRef]

27. Leal, D.B.; de Assis, M.A.; González-Chica, D.A.; da Costa, F.F.; de Andrade, D.F.; Lobo, A.S. Changes in total and central adiposity and body fat distribution among 7–10-year-old schoolchildren in Brazil. *Public Health Nutr.* **2015**, *18*, 2105–2114. [CrossRef] [PubMed]

28. Assis, M.A.; Benedet, J.; Kerpel, R.; Vasconcelos, F.A.G.; Di Pietro, P.F.; Kupek, E. Validation of the third version of the Previous Day Food Questionnaire (PDFQ-3) for 6-to-11-years-old schoolchildren. *Cad. Saude Publica* **2009**, *25*, 1816–1826.

29. Ledoux, T.A.; Hingle, M.D.; Baranowski, T. Relationship of fruit and vegetable intake with adiposity: A systematic review. *Obes. Rev.* **2011**, *12*, e143–e150. [CrossRef] [PubMed]

30. Pate, R.R.; O'Neill, J.R.; Liese, A.D.; Janz, K.F.; Granberg, E.M.; Colabianchi, N.; Harsha, D.W.; Condrasky, M.M.; O'Neil, P.M.; Lau, E.Y.; et al. Factors associated with development of excessive fatness in children and adolescents: A review of prospective studies. *Obes. Rev.* **2013**, *14*, 645–658. [CrossRef] [PubMed]

31. Rosenheck, R. Fast-food consumption and increased caloric intake: A systematic review of a trajectory towards weight gain and obesity risk. *Obes. Rev.* **2008**, *9*, 535–547. [CrossRef] [PubMed]

32. Hu, F.B. Resolved: There is sufficient scientific evidence that decreasing sugar-sweetened beverage consumption will reduce the prevalence of obesity and obesity related diseases. *Obes. Rev.* **2013**, *14*, 606–619. [CrossRef] [PubMed]

33. Ministério da Saúde. Guia Alimentar Para a População Brasileira. 2006. Available online: http://bvsms.saude.gov.br/bvs/publicacoes/guia_alimentar_populacao_brasileira_2008.pdf (accessed on 16 July 2015).

34. Newby, P.K.; Tucker, K.L. Empirically derived eating patterns using factor or cluster analysis: A review. *Nutr. Rev.* **2004**, *62*, 177–203. [CrossRef] [PubMed]

35. Pala, V.; Lissner, L.; Hebestreit, A.; Lanfer, A.; Sieri, S.; Siani, A.; Huybrechts, I.; Kambek, L.; Molnar, D.; Tornaritis, M.; et al. Dietary patterns and longitudinal change in body mass in European children: A follow-up study on the IDEFICS multicenter cohort. *Eur. J. Clin. Nutr.* **2013**, *67*, 1042–1049. [CrossRef] [PubMed]

36. Thorpe, M.G.; Milte, C.M.; Crawford, D.; McNaughton, S.A. A comparison of the dietary patterns derived by principal component analysis and cluster analysis in older Australians. *Int. J. Behav. Nutr. Phys. Act.* **2016**, *13*, 30. [CrossRef] [PubMed]

37. Cabral, L.G.A.; Costa, F.F.; Liparotti, J.R. Preliminary validation of the physical activity section of the previous day physical activity and food consumption questionnaire (PDPAFQ). *Rev. Bras. Ativ. Fis. Saude* **2011**, *16*, 100–106.

38. Ridley, K.; Ainsworth, B.E.; Olds, T.S. Development of a Compendium of Energy Expenditures for Youth. *Int. J. Behav. Nutr. Phys. Act.* **2008**, *5*, 1–8. [CrossRef] [PubMed]

39. De Jesus, J.M.; Assis, M.A.A.; Kupek, E. Assessment of physical activity in schoolchildren using a web-based questionnaire. *Rev. Bras. Med. Esporte* **2016**, *22*, 261–266.

40. Lohman, T.G.; Roche, A.F.; Martorell, R. *Anthropometric Standardization Reference Manual*; Human Kinetics: Champaign, IL, USA, 1988.

41. Frainer, D.E.; Adami, F.; Vasconcelos, F.A.; Assis, M.A.; Calvo, M.C.; Kerpel, R. Standardization and reliability of anthropometric measurements for population surveys. *Arch. Latinoam. Nutr.* **2007**, *57*, 335–342. [PubMed]

42. de Onis, M.; Onyango, A.W.; Borghi, E.; Siyam, A.; Nishida, C.; Siekmann, J. Development of a WHO growth reference for school-aged children and adolescents. *Bull. World Health Organ.* **2007**, *85*, 660–667. [CrossRef] [PubMed]

43. Khani, B.R.; Ye, W.; Terry, P.; Wolk, A. Reproducibility and validity of major dietary patterns among Swedish women assessed with a food-frequency questionnaire. *J. Nutr.* **2004**, *134*, 1541–1545. [PubMed]

44. Togo, P.; Osler, M.; Sørensen, T.I.; Heitmann, B.L. A longitudinal study of food intake patterns and obesity in adult Danish men and women. *Int. J. Obes. Relat. Metab. Disord.* **2004**, *28*, 583–593. [CrossRef] [PubMed]

45. Cohen, J. Statistical power analysis. *Curr. Dir. Psychol. Sci.* **1992**, *1*, 98–101. [CrossRef]

46. R Core Team. *R: A Language and Environment for Statistical Computing*; R Foundation for Statistical Computing: Vienna, Austria, 2016.

47. Nascimento, S.; Barbosa, F.S.; Sichieri, R.; Pereira, R.A. Dietary availability patterns of the Brazilian macro-regions. *Nutr. J.* **2011**, *10*, 79. [CrossRef] [PubMed]

48. Shroff, M.R.; Perng, W.; Baylin, A.; Mora-Plazas, M.; Marin, C.; Villamor, E. Adherence to a snacking dietary pattern and soda intake are related to the development of adiposity: A prospective study in school-age children. *Public Health Nutr.* **2014**, *17*, 1507–1513. [CrossRef] [PubMed]

49. Shang, L.; O'Loughlin, J.; Tremblay, A.; Gray-Donald, K. The association between food patterns and adiposity among Canadian children at risk of overweight. *Appl. Physiol. Nutr. Metab.* **2014**, *39*, 195–201. [CrossRef] [PubMed]

50. Craig, L.C.; McNeill, G.; Macdiarmid, J.I.; Masson, L.F.; Holmes, B.A. Dietary patterns of school-age children in Scotland: Association with socio-economic indicators, physical activity and obesity. *Br. J. Nutr.* **2010**, *103*, 319–334. [CrossRef] [PubMed]

51. Moreira, P.; Santos, S.; Padrao, P.; Cordeiro, T.; Bessa, M.; Valente, H.; Barros, R.; Teixeira, V.; Mitchell, V.; Lopes, C.; et al. Food patterns according to sociodemographics, physical activity, sleeping and obesity in Portuguese children. *Int. J. Environ. Res. Public Health* **2010**, *7*, 1121–1138. [CrossRef] [PubMed]

52. Smith, A.D.; Emmett, P.M.; Newby, P.K.; Northstone, K. Dietary patterns and changes in body composition in children between 9 and 11 years. *Food Nutr. Res.* **2014**, *58*. [CrossRef] [PubMed]

53. Emmett, P.M.; Jones, L.R.; Northstone, K. Dietary patterns in the Avon Longitudinal Study of Parents and Children. *Nutr. Rev.* **2015**, *73*, 207–230. [CrossRef] [PubMed]

54. Madruga, S.W.; Araújo, C.L.; Bertoldi, A.D.; Neutzling, M.B. Tracking of dietary patterns from childhood to adolescence. *Rev. Saude Publica* **2012**, *46*, 376–386. [CrossRef] [PubMed]

55. de Oliveira Santos, R.; Fisberg, R.M.; Marchioni, D.M.; Troncoso Baltar, V. Dietary patterns for meals of Brazilian adults. *Br. J. Nutr.* **2015**, *114*, 822–828. [CrossRef] [PubMed]

56. Alexy, U.; Sichert-Hellert, W.; Kersting, M.; Schultze-Pawlitschko, V. Pattern of long-term fat intake and BMI during childhood and adolescence—Results of the DONALD Study. *Int. J. Obes. Relat. Metab. Disord.* **2004**, *28*, 1203–1209. [CrossRef] [PubMed]

57. Alexy, U.; Libuda, L.; Mersmann, S.; Kersting, M. Convenience foods in children's diet and association with dietary quality and body weight status. *Eur. J. Clin. Nutr.* **2011**, *65*, 160–166. [CrossRef] [PubMed]

58. Assis, M.A.; Calvo, M.C.; Kupek, E.; Assis Guedes de Vasconcelos, F.; Campos, V.C.; Machado, M.; Costa, F.F.; de Andrade, D.F. Qualitative analysis of the diet of a probabilistic sample of schoolchildren from Florianópolis, Santa Catarina State, Brazil, using the Previous Day Food Questionnaire. *Cad. Saude Publica* **2010**, *26*, 1355–1365. [CrossRef] [PubMed]

59. Baranowski, T.; Domel, S. A cognitive model of children's reporting of food intake. *Am. J. Clin. Nutr.* **1994**, *59* (Suppl. 1), 212S–217S. [PubMed]

60. Livingstone, M.B.; Robson, P.J.; Wallace, J.M. Issues in dietary intake assessment of children and adolescents. *Br. J. Nutr.* **2004**, *92* (Suppl. 2), S213–S222. [CrossRef] [PubMed]

61. Magarey, A.; Golley, R.; Spurrier, N.; Goodwin, E.; Ong, F. Reliability and validity of the Children's Dietary Questionnaire: A new tool to measure children's dietary patterns. *Int. J. Pediatr. Obes.* **2009**, *4*, 257–265. [CrossRef] [PubMed]

62. Rothausen, B.W.; Matthiessen, J.; Andersen, L.F.; Brockhoff, P.B.; Tetens, I. Dietary patterns on weekdays and weekend days in 4–14-year-old Danish children. *Br. J. Nutr.* **2013**, *109*, 1704–1713. [CrossRef] [PubMed]

63. Junior, E.V.; Fisberg, R.M.; Cesar, C.L.G.; Marchioni, D.M.L. Sources of variation of energy and nutrient intake among adolescents in São Paulo, Brazil. *Cad. Saude Publica* **2010**, *26*, 2129–2137. [CrossRef]

64. McCarthy, S. Weekly patterns, diet quality and energy balance. *Physiol. Behav.* **2014**, *134*, 55–59. [CrossRef] [PubMed]

65. Svensson, A.; Larsson, C.; Eiben, G.; Lanfer, A.; Pala, V.; Hebestreit, A.; Huybrechts, I.; Fernández-Alvira, J.M.; Russo, P.; Koni, A.C.; et al. European children's sugar intake on weekdays versus weekends: The IDEFICS study. *Eur. J. Clin. Nutr.* **2014**, *68*, 822–828. [CrossRef] [PubMed]

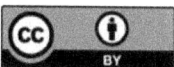

MDPI

St. Alban-Anlage 66

4052 Basel, Switzerland

Tel. +41 61 683 77 34

Fax +41 61 302 89 18

http://www.mdpi.com

Nutrients Editorial Office

E-mail: nutrients@mdpi.com

http://www.mdpi.com/journal/nutrients